Colorectal Cancer

Colorectal Cancer

Diagnosis and Clinical Management

EDITED BY

John H. Scholefield FRCS, ChM

Head, Division of GI Surgery
Professor of Surgery
University Hospital
Nottingham, UK

Cathy Eng MD, FACP

Associate Professor
Associate Medical Director, Colorectal Center
The University of Texas M.D. Anderson Cancer Center
Houston, TX, USA

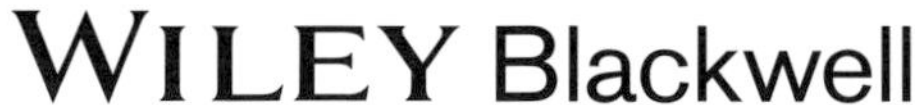

Registered office: John Wiley & Sons, Ltd, The Atrium, Southern Gate, Chichester, West Sussex, PO19 8SQ, UK

Editorial offices: 9600 Garsington Road, Oxford, OX4 2DQ, UK
The Atrium, Southern Gate, Chichester, West Sussex, PO19 8SQ, UK
111 River Street, Hoboken, NJ 07030-5774, USA

For details of our global editorial offices, for customer services and for information about how to apply for permission to reuse the copyright material in this book please see our website at www.wiley.com/wiley-blackwell

Library of Congress Cataloging-in-Publication Data

Colorectal cancer (Scholefield)
Colorectal cancer : diagnosis and clinical management / edited by John H. Scholefield, Cathy Eng.
p. ; cm.
Includes bibliographical references and index.
ISBN 978-0-470-67480-2 (cloth) – ISBN 978-1-118-33791-2 – ISBN 978-1-118-33789-9 (ePub) – ISBN 978-1-118-33790-5
I. Scholefield, John H., editor of compilation. II. Eng, Cathy, editor of compilation. III. Title.
[DNLM: 1. Colorectal Neoplasms–therapy. 2. Colorectal Neoplasms–diagnosis. 3. Colorectal Neoplasms–prevention & control. WI 529]
RC280.C6
616.99′4347–dc23 2013042716

A catalogue record for this book is available from the British Library.

Wiley also publishes its books in a variety of electronic formats. Some content that appears in print may not be available in electronic books.

Cover image: Coloured X-ray of cancer of the colon © SCIENCE PHOTO LIBRARY
Cover design by Meaden Creative

Set in 9.5/13pt Meridien by Aptara Inc., New Delhi, India
Printed and bound in Singapore by Markono Print Media Pte Ltd

1 2014

Contents

Contributors

Carmen Allegra MD
Professor
Department of MedicineChief
Division of Hematology/Oncology
University of Florida
Gainesville, FL, USA

Thomas A. Aloia, MD, FACS
Associate Professor
Department of Surgical Oncology
The University of Texas MD Anderson Cancer Center
Houston, TX, USA

Simon P. Bach MBBS, MD, FRCS
Senior Lecturer
Academic Department of Surgery
University Hospital Birmingham NHS Trust
Birmingham, UK

Sarah Bannon, MS, CGC
Genetic Counselor
Department of Surgical Oncology
The University of Texas MD Anderson Cancer Center
Houston, Texas, USA

Tanios Bekaii-Saab MD
Section Chief, Gastrointestinal Oncology
Chair, CCC Gastrointestinal Disease Research Group
Associate Professor of Medicine and Pharmacology
The Ohio State University Comprehensive Cancer Center
Columbus, OH, USA

Amanda B. Cooper, MD
Clinical Fellow in Hepato-pancreato-biliary Surgery
Department of Surgical Oncology
The University of Texas MD Anderson Cancer Center
Houston, TX, USA

Steven A. Curley MD, FACS
Professor
Department of Surgical Oncology
The University of Texas MD Anderson Cancer Center
Houston, TX, USA

Brian G. Czito MD
Gary Hock and Lynn Proctor Associate Professor
Department of Radiation Oncology
Duke University Medical Center
Durham, NC, USA

Karen C. Daily DO
Assistant Professor
Department of Medicine
Division of Hematology/Oncology
University of Florida
Gainesville, FL, USA

Egidio Del Fabbro MD
Director, Palliative Care
Division of Hematology/Oncology and Palliative Care;
Associate Professor
Virginia Commonwealth University
Richmond, VA, USA

Sunil Dolwani MBBS MD
Consultant Gastroenterologist & Hon Senior Lecturer
Institute of Cancer and Genetics
Cardiff University School of Medicine
Cardiff, Wales

Marsha L. Frazier PhD
Professor
Department of Epidemiology
The University of Texas MD Anderson Cancer Center
Houston, TX, USA

David Jayne
Professor of Surgery
Translational Anaesthesia & Surgery
St. James's University Hospital
Leeds, UK

Daedong Kim MD, PhD
Assistant Professor of Surgery
Department of GI Medical Oncology
The University of Texas MD Anderson Cancer Center
Houston, TX, USA;
Department of Surgery
Catholic University of Daegu
Daegu, Korea

Yusuke Kinugasa MD
Chief
Division of Colon and Rectal Surgery
Shizuoka Cancer Center Hospital
Shizuoka, Japan

Paula McDonald
Screening Laboratory Team Leader
Scottish Bowel Screening Centre
King's Cross Hospital
Dundee, UK

Ludmila Katherine Martin MD
Fellow, Oncology/Hematology
The Ohio State University Comprehensive
Cancer Center
Columbus, OH, USA

Dipen Maru, MD
Associate Professor
Department of Pathology and Translational Molecular Pathology
The University of Texas MD Anderson Cancer Center
Houston, TX, USA

Timothy J. Moore, BM, FRCS
Consultant Colorectal Surgeon
Hampshire Hospitals NHS Foundation Trust
Royal Hampshire County Hospital
Winchester, UK

Brendan J. Moran MB, Bchir, FRCSI
Senior Lecturer, Cancer Sciences Division
Southampton University;
Consultant Colorectal Surgeon
Hampshire Hospitals NHS Foundation Trust
Basingstoke and North Hampshire Hospital
Basingstoke, UK

Maureen E. Mork, MS, CGC
Genetic Counselor
Department of Gastroenterology, Hepatology & Nutrition
The University of Texas MD Anderson Cancer Center
Houston, Texas, USA

Manisha Palta, MD
Assistant Professor
Department of Radiation Oncology
Duke University Medical Center
Durham, NC, USA

Mala Pande PhD, MPH, MBBS
Assistant Professor
Department of Gastroenterology, Hepatology and Nutrition
The University of Texas MD Anderson Cancer Center
Houston, TX, USA

Thomas D. Pinkney, MBChB, MMedEd, FRCS
Senior Lecturer and Honorary Consultant Colorectal Surgeon
Academic Department of Surgery
University Hospital Birmingham NHS Trust
Birmingham, UK

Maura Polansky MS, MHPE, PA-C
Program Director, Physician Assistant
Educational Programs
The University of Texas MD Anderson Cancer Center
Houston, TX, USA

Krish Ragunath MD DNB MPhil FRCP(Edin) FRCP(Lond)
Head of Endoscopy & Consultant Gastroenterologist
Nottingham Digestive Diseases Centre, NIHR Biomedical Research Unit
Queens Medical Centre Campus, Nottingham University Hospitals NHS Trust
Nottingham, UK

Miguel A. Rodriguez-Bigas, MD
Professor of Surgery
Department of Surgical Oncology
The University of Texas MD Anderson Cancer Center
Houston, TX, USA

John H. Scholefield FRCS, ChM
Head, Division of GI Surgery
Professor of Surgery
University Hospital
Nottingham
UK

Rajvinder Singh MBBS MPhil FRACP AM FRCP
Clinical Associate Professor & Consultant Gastroenterologist
Lyell McEwin Hospital
University of Adelaide
Adelaide
Australia

Stephen Staal MD
Professor, Department of Medicine
Division of Hematology / Oncology
University of Florida
Gainesville, FL, USA

Robert JC Steele MD, FRCS
Professor of Surgery
Head of Academic Surgery
Centre for Academic Clinical Practice
Centre for Research into Cancer Prevention and Screening
Ninewells Hospital & Medical School
Dundee, UK

Kenichi Sugihara MD, DMSc
Professor,
Department of Surgical Oncology, Graduate School
Tokyo Medical and Dental University
Tokyo, Japan

Gregory Taylor
Clinical Lecturer in Surgery
Translational Anaesthesia and Surgery
St James's University Hospital
Leeds, UK

Shunsuke Tsukamoto
Chief
Division of Colon and Rectal Surgery
National Cancer Center Hospital
Shizuoka, Japan

Noriya Uedo MD
Vice-director
Department of Gastrointestinal Oncology
Osaka Medical Center for Cancer and Cardiovascular Diseases
Osaka, Japan

Jean-Nicolas Vauthey, MD, FACS
Professor
Department of Surgical Oncology
The University of Texas MD Anderson Cancer Center
Houston, TX, USA

Jenny Wei MD
Fellow, Department of Palliative Care and Rehabilitation Medicine
University of Texas, MD Anderson Cancer Center
Houston, TX, USA

Christopher G. Willett, MD
Professor and Chair
Department of Radiation Oncology
Duke University Medical Center
Durham, NC, USA

PART 1
Diagnosis

CHAPTER 1

Epidemiology

Mala Pande & Marsha L. Frazier
The University of Texas MD Anderson Cancer Center, Houston, TX, USA

KEY POINTS

Descriptive epidemiology: assessment of the distribution of colorectal cancer

- Ecological studies of populations are used to determine variation in rates. Incidence, mortality rate, time trends, and prevalence are some key measures.
- The burden of colorectal cancer varies globally: the incidence rate is 10 times higher and the mortality rate 5 times higher in countries with the highest rates than in countries with the lowest rates.
- Worldwide, colorectal cancer is the third most common cancer in men, the second most common cancer in women, and the fourth leading cause of cancer deaths.
- In the United States, colorectal cancer is the third most common cancer in both men and women (9% of the estimated incident cancer cases in both men and women in 2012) and the third leading cause of cancer deaths (9% of estimated cancer deaths in both men and women in 2012).
- There are geographic variations in incidence and mortality, with higher incidence but lower mortality rates in developed countries than in developing countries.
- Colorectal cancer incidence rates have been declining in the United States, and have been stable or declining in most developed countries but are rising in developing countries.
- The increasing risk of colorectal cancer in developing countries may be attributable to increased longevity, and adverse lifestyle changes including smoking, lack of physical activity, and adoption of a westernized diet.
- Colorectal cancer incidence and mortality rate vary by geographic location, age, sex, race/ethnicity, and over time.
- The prevalence of colorectal cancer is high because it has a relatively good prognosis. As a result, there are over 1 million colorectal cancer survivors in the United States.

Analytic epidemiology: assessment of determinants of colorectal cancer:

- Cross-sectional, case-control, and cohort study designs can be used to determine the association of suspected environmental, lifestyle, and other exposures with colorectal cancer risk. Randomized controlled trials are the gold standard for determining cause and effect.

Colorectal Cancer: Diagnosis and Clinical Management, First Edition. Edited by John H. Scholefield and Cathy Eng.

- Factors that increase the risk of colorectal cancer include older age, African-American race/ethnicity, inherited predisposition syndromes, family history of colorectal cancer or colorectal polyps, inflammatory bowel disease, personal history of colorectal cancer or polyps, diabetes, obesity, physical inactivity, smoking, and alcohol.
- Many other probable risk factors are under investigation.

Introduction

In the last decade, cancer has become the leading cause of death in economically developed countries and the second leading cause of death in developing countries. Globally, colorectal cancer (CRC) is the third most common cancer in men, the second most common cancer in women, and the fourth leading cause of cancer deaths. In 2008, an estimated 665,000 men and 570,000 women were diagnosed with CRC, and 668,000 deaths were attributable to CRC, accounting for 8% of all cancer deaths [1].

Colorectal cancer incidence worldwide

There is almost a 10-fold variation in CRC incidence rates (proportion of newly diagnosed cases per year) worldwide for both sexes. CRC incidence rates are highest in Australia/New Zealand and Western Europe and lowest in Middle Africa and South-Central Asia [1] (Figure 1.1).

Although developed countries account for almost two-thirds of CRC cases (with the exception of a few countries in Eastern Europe, Eastern Asia, and Spain), the rates in developed countries have mostly remained stable or declined over time, whereas rates in developing countries are rising [1;2]. These differences may be attributable to changes in lifestyle and environmental factors as well as underlying genetic susceptibility. The rapid increase in the cancer burden in developing countries is possibly due to population growth and aging, and adverse lifestyle changes such as increased smoking, physical inactivity, and westernized diets [3]. Worldwide, the age-standardized rate (ASR) for CRC incidence is 17.3 per 100,000 population and the cumulative risk for CRC from birth to age 74 years is 0.9% [1]. The incidence of CRC is higher in men than in women (overall male:female ratio of age-standardized rates is 1.4:1). Country-specific rates for CRC incidence and mortality are available from the GLOBCAN database from the World Health Organization's International Agency for Research on Cancer (*http://globocan.iarc.fr/*).

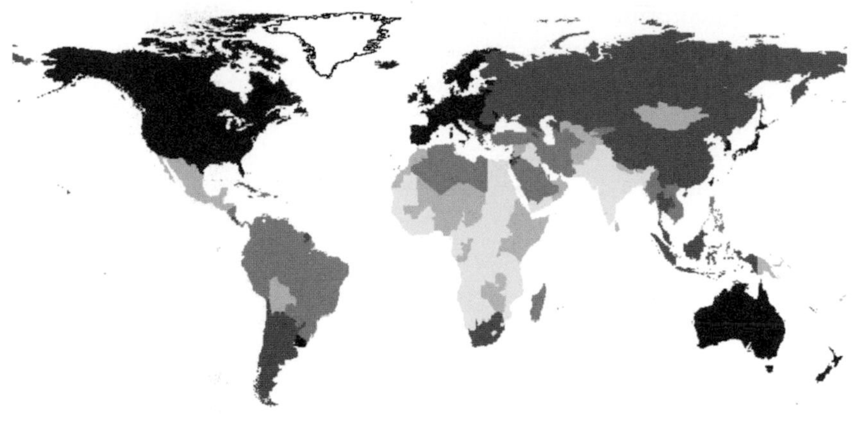

< 4.6 < 7.5 < 12.5 < 24.2 < 42.1

GLOBOCAN 2008 (IARC) - 27.3.2012

Figure 1.1 Estimated age-standardized incidence rate per 100,000 colorectum: both sexes, all ages [1].

Colorectal cancer incidence, time trends, and lifetime risk in the United States (US)

It is estimated that 143,460 men and women (73,420 men and 70,040 women) will be diagnosed with CRC in the US in 2012 [4]. Of all CRCs diagnosed, about 72% affect the colon and the remaining 28% affect the rectum. Incidence rates for CRC in the US have declined roughly by 2–3% every year over the last 15–20 years [5], largely attributable to the advent of CRC screening, which allows for early detection and removal of precancerous polyps [6]. The lifetime incidence of CRC in the US is 5%, or 1 in 20 people are predicted to get CRC over their lifetime. The incidence of CRC is 25% higher in men than in women, and most (>90%) cases occur in men and women older than 50 years. Rates vary significantly by race/ethnicity; the incidence of CRC in African-American men is 20% higher than in white men [3].

Colorectal cancer mortality worldwide

CRC is the fourth most common cause of death from cancer, accounting for 8% of all cancer deaths worldwide. Globally, mortality rates continue to increase for deaths due to CRC (the ASR is 8.2/100,000). Cancer survival tends to be poorer in developing countries, possibly because cancer is diagnosed at later stages and patients have limited access to timely and standard care [3]. There is less variability in mortality rates worldwide (6 times higher in men and 5 times higher in women, in countries with the highest rates than in countries with the lowest rates), with the highest estimated mortality rates in both sexes in Central and Eastern Europe (20.1/100,000 for men and 12.2/100,000 for women), and the lowest in Middle Africa (3.5/100,000 for men and 2.7/100,000 for women) [1].

The mortality rate for CRC is roughly half the incidence rate, so its prognosis is relatively good. Thus, CRC has a high 5-year prevalence (number of cases in the population at a given time), with an estimated 3.26 million people alive with CRC diagnosed within the past 5 years [1;7]. The decrease in mortality may be due to changes in incidence, progress in therapy, improved early detection due to widespread screening, diagnosis at earlier stages (when the cancer is more amenable to treatment), and many other factors [8].

Colorectal cancer mortality in the US

An estimated 51,690 people will die of CRC in 2012 [4]. CRC-related deaths in the US have been declining steadily from 1975 to 2009, with an annual percentage change of 0.5–4% [4]. The US mortality rate for CRC from 2005 to 2009 was 16.7 per 100,000 patients per year. However, mortality rates varied significantly by both sex and race/ethnicity. Mortality rates are highest for African-American men (29.8/100,000) and lowest for Asian-Pacific Islander women (9.6/100,000). The largest proportion (29%) of CRC deaths occurred in patients aged 75–84 years, and the median age at death was 74 years [4]. The mortality rate for CRC is roughly one-third the incidence rate, resulting in a high prevalence of patients diagnosed with CRC. On January 1, 2009, over 1.14 million people with a history of CRC were alive in the US [4]. The 5-year survival rate for CRC is related to the stage at diagnosis; CRC diagnosed at the local stage has a 5-year survival rate of 90%, but the rate drops to only 12% if CRC is diagnosed after it has metastasized [9]. Overall, the US has one of the highest 5-year survival rates for CRC in the world: 61% for patients diagnosed at any stage.

Colorectal cancer risk factors

Epidemiologic studies have identified many factors that may increase or decrease risk of CRC. Some of these factors, such as a personal or family history of CRC or a history of inflammatory bowel disease, are non-modifiable, but many lifestyle risk factors, such as smoking, alcohol use, and lack of physical activity, are modifiable. It was recently reported that following a healthy lifestyle that includes being physically active for at least 30 minutes per day, following a healthy diet, controlling abdominal adiposity, not smoking, and not drinking alcohol in excess could have prevented 23% of the CRC cases in a cohort of more than 50,000 people aged 50–64 years, who were cancer-free at baseline and followed up for an average of 10 years [10]. Genetic susceptibility due to inherited germline mutations is the cause of CRC in about 5% of patients; however, most cases are sporadic, not familial.

Age

Age is a major risk factor influencing CRC incidence and death rate, because both rates increase with age. Over 90% of new CRC cases and deaths occur in people older than 50 years. However, CRC incidence rates in that age group have been steadily declining since the mid-1980s, whereas incidence rates in people younger than 50 years have consistently increased since the early 1990s [11]. Researchers are not sure what is causing the increase in younger adults, but a recent study found that young-onset CRC was more prevalent than later-onset CRC among patients of non-white race/ethnicity, patients who had no insurance or Medicaid insurance, and patients living in the Southern and Western US [11]. Younger patients also had a more advanced stage at diagnosis, location distal to the splenic flexure or in the rectum, a mucinous or signet ring histologic subtype, and poor or no cell differentiation [11].

Sex

Worldwide, and in the US, men are at greater risk for CRC than women, but the reasons for the difference in CRC incidence and mortality rates by sex are not well understood. The sex-specific differences may be related to hormonal risk factors, differences in screening and access to medical care, and sex-specific genetic and molecular interactions with environmental risk factors [12]. Sex also affects the CRC site, men having a higher incidence of rectal cancers (31% of CRCs) than women (24%) [9].

Race/ethnicity

The burden of CRC varies significantly by race/ethnicity (Figure 1.2). African-Americans have the highest incidence and mortality rates in the US, followed by non-Hispanic whites. CRC incidence rates are lowest in Hispanics. CRC-related mortality rates have declined over time for all races/ethnicities, but the

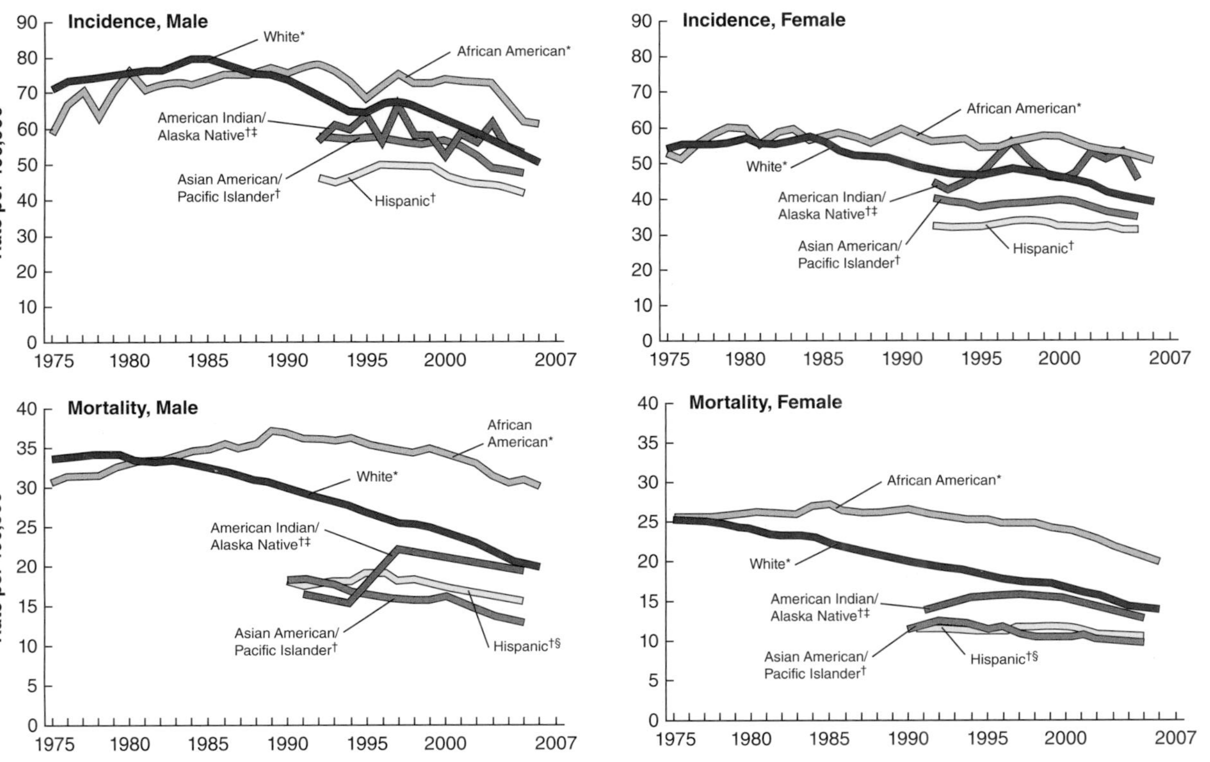

Rates are per 100,000 and age adjusted to the 2000 US standard population. *Rates are two-year moving averages. †Rates are three-year moving averages. ‡Rates are based on Contract Health Service Delivery Areas; mortality rates are for fixed time intervals: 1990–1992, 1993–1995, 1996–1998, 1999–2002, and 2003–2007. §Due to incomplete data, rates exclude deaths from Connecticut, District of Columbia, Louisiana, Maine, Maryland, Minnesota, Mississippi, New Hampshire, New York, North Dakota, Oklahoma, Vermont, and Virginia.

Sources: Incidence – Surveillance, Epidemiology, and End Results (SEER) Program; Mortality – National Center for Health Statistics, Centers for Disease Control and Prevention, as provided by the SEER Program, National Cancer Institute.

Figure 1.2 Trends in CRC incidence and mortality rate by race-ethnicity and sex, 1975–2007 [4].

decline has been significantly larger among US whites than among African-Americans.

Geographic differences

CRC incidence rates vary globally and between US states. Developed nations have higher CRC incidence rates than developing nations; the highest rates are seen in Australia and Canada, and the lowest rates are seen in Middle Africa (Figure 1.1). Incidence rates have rapidly increased in countries that have recently transitioned from relatively low-income to high-income economies, such as Japan, Singapore, and some Eastern European countries (Figure 1.3) [13;14]. Geographic variation in rates is also observed between US states/regions; socioeconomic factors contribute to this variation by influencing access to screening and treatment.

Geographic distribution of CRC in the US also varies by race/ethnicity and sex. CRC incidence rates (per 100,000) among white men range from 44.4 in Utah to 68.7 in North Dakota, and incidence rates among African-American men range from 46.4 in Arizona to 82.4 in Kentucky. Similar variations across states are seen among white women (ranging from 31.8 in Utah to 48.6 in West Virginia) and African-American women (ranging from 34.8 in New Mexico to 61.5 in West Virginia) [9].

Genetic predisposition

Roughly 5% of CRC cases are attributable to a genetic predisposition. That is, inherited mutations in certain key genes result in a greatly increased lifetime risk of CRC. Several genetic susceptibility syndromes predispose people to CRC, the most common of which is Lynch syndrome. People with Lynch syndrome inherit germline mutations in one of the DNA mismatch repair genes, *MLH1, MSH2, MSH6,* or *PMS2,* and this predisposes them to cancers of the colorectum, endometrium, ovary, stomach, small intestine, hepatobiliary tract, urinary tract, brain, and skin. These mutations have an autosomal dominant pattern of inheritance, so offspring have a 50% probability of being affected. Other characteristics of CRC associated with genetic susceptibility include an earlier age at onset (the median age at CRC diagnosis is 45 years in patients with Lynch syndrome), multiple family members may be affected, and patients are susceptible to develop other primary cancers besides CRC. Cancers are largely right-sided in patients with Lynch syndrome as compared to left-sided in sporadic CRC, and tumors in patients with Lynch syndrome display characteristic microsatellite instability. Histologically, tumors in these patients exhibit poor differentiation, tumor-infiltrating lymphocytes, and mucinous, signet ring, or cribriform histology.

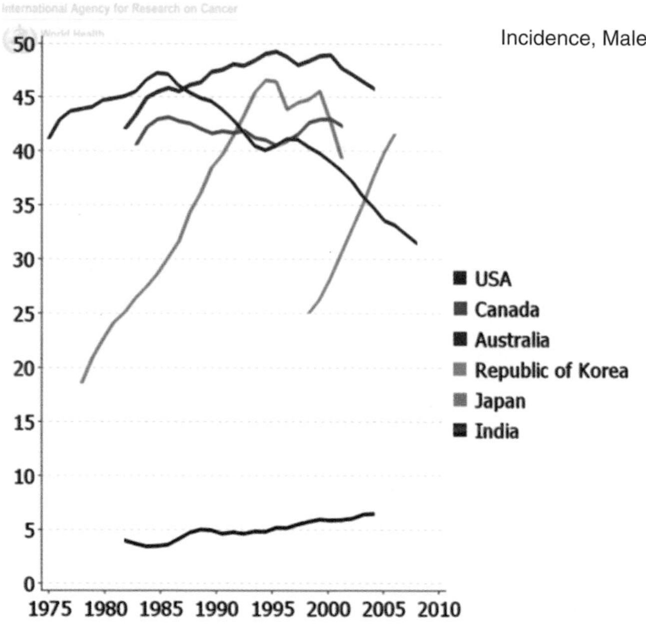

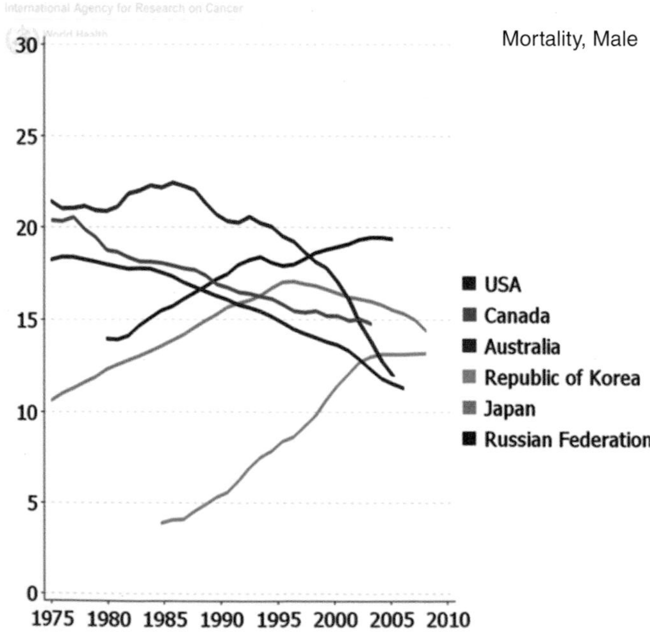

Figure 1.3 Trends in colorectal cancer incidence and mortality rate in selected countries (aged-standardized (world) per 100,000 men) [1].

Immunohistochemical staining of the tumors for loss of DNA mismatch repair protein, microsatellite instability testing, and family history are the hallmarks of screening for suspected Lynch syndrome mutation carriers prior to definitive mismatch repair gene mutation testing.

Other, less common genetic susceptibility syndromes include familial adenomatous polyposis, Peutz-Jeghers syndrome, and mutY homolog (*MUTYH*)-associated polyposis [15].

Familial adenomatous polyposis accounts for less than 1% of CRCs and is caused by mutations in the *APC* gene; its characteristic phenotype is early-onset of multiple (up to thousands) adenomas, which lead to CRC if untreated. An attenuated form of familial adenomatous polyposis with a less severe polyposis phenotype is due to mutations in *APC* at different sites. Peutz-Jeghers syndrome is another rare syndrome, caused by mutations in the *STK11* (also called *LKB1*) gene. Patients with Peutz-Jeghers syndrome develop characteristic hyperpigmentation of the lips, fingers, and toes and are at increased risk of developing hamartomatous polyps in the digestive tract and of breast, colorectal, and other cancers. Patients with *MUTYH*-associated polyposis present with multiple colorectal adenomas or CRC as a result of autosomal recessively inherited biallelic mutations in the base excision repair gene *MUTYH* [15].

Family history

Family history is an important risk factor for CRC, even without the increased familial risk due to genetic predisposition syndromes. Familial risk is likely to be an interaction of genetic and environmental causes [16]. Having a first-degree relative (parent, sibling, or child) with CRC increases CRC risk to almost double that of the general population, and CRC risk is increased further if two first-degree relatives are affected or if a family member is diagnosed with CRC at younger than 60 years [17;18]. A family history of large (>1 cm) adenoma or histologically advanced adenoma is associated with roughly the same risk of CRC as a family history of CRC [18]. Those with a history of one or two small (<1 cm) adenomas are not considered at substantially increased risk [19]. However, a recent review has reported that the risk associated with a family history of adenomas or CRC may be overestimated because of the likelihood of looking for cancer in families who already have a history of CRC (as people with a family history of CRC are more likely to be screened than others) and because the family history for colon polyps may be inaccurate [20].

A possible genetic basis for familial CRC has been investigated by recent genome-wide association studies (GWAS) examining genetic variation across the genome for markers of CRC risk. However, the genetic polymorphisms identified by these studies are largely low-penetrance markers and account for only a small proportion of familial aggregation of CRC [21]. A study estimated that the contribution of 10 GWAS loci to variance in familial CRC risk was only 9% [22]. Larger, more powerful studies, including meta-analyses, are finding additional susceptibility loci [23] that may account for a larger proportion of familial CRC, supporting the idea that familial CRC results from the effects of many low-penetrance genes [24].

Personal medical history

A history of adenomas, prior CRC, and inflammatory bowel disease significantly increases the risk of CRC. Patients with a prior history of large (>1 cm) adenomatous polyps or villous or tubulovillous polyps, particularly a history of multiple polyps, are considered to be at increased risk of CRC [25–27]. Among CRC patients with a history of resection of a single CRC, 1.5–3% are likely to develop metachronous primary CRC during the first 5 years postoperatively [28].

Patients with a history of inflammatory bowel disease are at an increased lifetime risk of CRC, particularly patients with ulcerative colitis. The overall incidence of CRC in patients with inflammatory bowel disease was 95 cases per 100,000 in a population-based study in Sweden [29]. CRC risk may differ by sex; in a large Swedish cohort, the CRC risk for men was 60% higher than for women, and the cumulative incidence of CRC 40 years after the diagnosis of inflammatory bowel disease was 8.3% for men and 3.5% for women [30].

The CRC risk associated with ulcerative colitis depends on the activity and duration of the colitis, extent of colon involvement, and involved site in the colon [31;32] Age and extent of disease at diagnosis are also independent predictors of increased CRC risk [33]. In a population-based Swedish cohort of patients with ulcerative colitis, pancolitis was associated with a 15 times higher incidence of CRC as compared to the general population, and left-sided colitis was associated with a 3 times higher incidence, but the CRC incidence associated with proctitis or proctosigmoiditis was not significantly increased compared with the expected CRC incidence in the general population [33]. The likelihood of developing cancer begins 8–10 years after diagnosis of pancolitis and 15–20 years after diagnosis of more localized colitis [33]. The cumulative incidence of CRC is approximately 5–10% after 20 years and 12–20% after 30 years with colitis [33–36], although some studies have reported lower cumulative incidence rates, possibly due to improved surveillance [37;38].

The risk of CRC is not as well documented in patients with Crohn's disease as in patients with ulcerative colitis. Some studies have reported an increased CRC risk for Crohn's disease of long duration similar to that for ulcerative colitis [39–42], whereas other studies have found no clear increase in CRC risk associated with Crohn's disease [31;43;44].

In a study comparing CRC outcomes in Crohn's disease and ulcerative colitis, the times until CRC development were similar for the two diseases (median 15 and 18 years, respectively), although the median age at CRC diagnosis was higher in Crohn's disease patients than in those with ulcerative colitis (55 and 43 years, respectively) [45]. It is well documented that CRC in inflammatory bowel disease is preceded by dysplasia, necessitating a regimen of increased surveillance for these patients for early detection and possible prophylactic colectomy to prevent CRC.

Prior abdominal radiation may also affect CRC risk. Two recent studies have reported that abdominal radiation for childhood malignancies may increase CRC risk for adult survivors [46;47].

Obesity

Increasing rates of obesity worldwide and particularly in the US are of growing concern, because obesity has been linked to many types of cancer, including CRC [48]. In a large prospective cohort of male health professionals, increasing body mass index (BMI) was associated with an increasing trend in risk for CRC [49]. Furthermore, abdominal adiposity was also associated with risk of CRC, even after adjusting for BMI [49]. Similarly, in an analysis of obesity and CRC risk among women in the Nurses' Health Study prospective cohort, compared with women of normal weight, obese women were 1.5 times more likely to develop CRC [50]. In a meta-analysis of 29 studies, each 5 kg/m^2 increase in BMI was associated with a 24% increase in risk of colon cancer and a 9% increase in risk of rectal cancer in men and with a 9% increase in risk of colon cancer in women [48]. Obesity also increases the risk of dying from CRC [51]. The epidemiologic evidence for the impact of dietary and lifestyle factors on risk of colon and rectal cancer is shown in Figure 1.4.

Diabetes mellitus

The association between diabetes mellitus and increased risk for CRC is becoming increasingly strong [52–55]. A recent meta-analysis concluded that there was a 38% increase in risk for colon cancer and a 20% increase in risk for rectal cancer in patients with diabetes compared with those without diabetes, and the association was evident even after controlling for other risk factors including smoking, obesity, and physical activity. It has been postulated that hyperinsulinemia links diabetes to CRC. Studies have shown that insulin is an important growth factor for colonic mucosal cells and stimulates colonic tumor cells [56;57]. This is further supported by evidence of

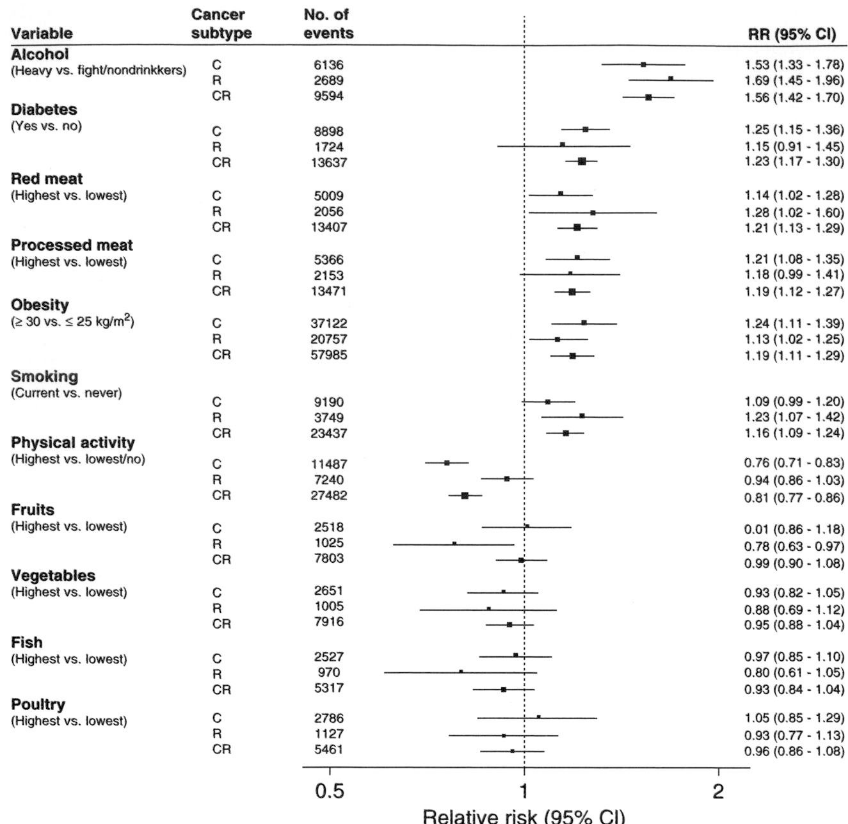

Variable
Cancer subtype
No. of events
RR (95% CI)
Alcohol
(Heavy vs. fight/nondrinkkers)
C 6136 1.53 (1.33 - 1.78)
R 2689 1.69 (1.45 - 1.96)
CR 9594 1.56 (1.42 - 1.70)
Diabetes
(Yes vs. no)
C 8898 1.25 (1.15 - 1.36)
R 1724 1.15 (0.91 - 1.45)
CR 13637 1.23 (1.17 - 1.30)
Red meat
(Highest vs. lowest)
C 5009 1.14 (1.02 - 1.28)
R 2056 1.28 (1.02 - 1.60)
CR 13407 1.21 (1.13 - 1.29)
Processed meat
(Highest vs. lowest)
C 5366 1.21 (1.08 - 1.35)
R 2153 1.18 (0.99 - 1.41)
CR 13471 1.19 (1.12 - 1.27)
Obesity
(≥ 30 vs. ≤ 25 kg/m2)
C 37122 1.24 (1.11 - 1.39)
R 20757 1.13 (1.02 - 1.25)
CR 57985 1.19 (1.11 - 1.29)
Smoking
(Current vs. never)
C 9190 1.09 (0.99 - 1.20)
R 3749 1.23 (1.07 - 1.42)
CR 23437 1.16 (1.09 - 1.24)
Physical activity
(Highest vs. lowest/no)
C 11487 0.76 (0.71 - 0.83)
R 7240 0.94 (0.86 - 1.03)
CR 27482 0.81 (0.77 - 0.86)
Fruits
(Highest vs. lowest)
C 2518 0.01 (0.86 - 1.18)
R 1025 0.78 (0.63 - 0.97)
CR 7803 0.99 (0.90 - 1.08)
Vegetables
(Highest vs. lowest)
C 2651 0.93 (0.82 - 1.05)
R 1005 0.88 (0.69 - 1.12)
CR 7916 0.95 (0.88 - 1.04)
Fish
(Highest vs. lowest)
C 2527 0.97 (0.85 - 1.10)
R 970 0.80 (0.61 - 1.05)
CR 5317 0.93 (0.84 - 1.04)
Poultry
(Highest vs. lowest)
C 2786 1.05 (0.85 - 1.29)
R 1127 0.93 (0.77 - 1.13)
CR 5461 0.96 (0.86 - 1.08)
0.5
1
2
Relative risk (95% CI)
C, colon; R, rectal; CR, colorectal

Figure 1.4 The impact of dietary and lifestyle risk factors on risk of colorectal cancer: A quantitative overview of the epidemiologic evidence citation [84]. Reproduced with permission of John Wiley & Sons Ltd.

associations between CRC risk and insulin biomarkers such as serum levels of insulin-like growth factor (IGF1), IGF binding protein-3 (IGFBP-3), and C-peptide [58;59]. Type 2 diabetes mellitus has also been linked to an increased mortality rate in patients with CRC; patients with CRC and type 2 diabetes were found to be at a higher risk of dying than CRC patients without diabetes [60].

Physical activity

There is strong evidence linking physical activity with decreased risk of CRC. In a meta-analysis of 52 cohort and case-control studies, an inverse association between physical activity and colon cancer was found in both men (relative risk [RR] 0.76; 95% confidence interval [CI] 0.71–0.82) and women (RR 0.79; 95% CI 0.71–0.88) [61]. Regular leisure time and occupational physical activity are also associated with protection from CRC.

Diet

Fruits and vegetables

The relationship between consumption of fruits and vegetables and CRC risk has been inconclusive. Some studies have found an inverse association between fruit and vegetable intake and CRC risk, comparing highest with lowest intakes of fruits and vegetables (RR 0.92; 95% CI 0.86–0.99) [62], whereas other large cohort and pooled studies have shown a weak or no protective effect [63;64]. The weak protective effect appears to be limited to distal colon cancers. Measurement of dietary exposures that depends on dietary recall can be challenging, and the imprecision of this measure may explain the heterogeneity in results.

Red meat consumption

Consumption of red meat or processed meat has been found to be associated with increased risk of CRC in many studies. A meta-analysis of prospective studies found a 22% (RR 1.22; 95% CI 1.11–1.34) increase in risk of CRC in the highest compared with the lowest intake of red and processed meats [65]. In addition, there was a dose-response relationship: for every 100 g/day increase in consumption, the CRC risk increased by 14%, and the associations with CRC risk were similar for colon and rectal cancer [65]. It has been hypothesized that the association between red meat and CRC is related to the cooking process. High-temperature cooking of meats, including barbecuing, has been found to increase the risk of both adenomas and CRC, likely through the production of polycyclic aromatic hydrocarbons and other cooking-related mutagens generated when meat is charred [66]. Other potential factors implicated in mediating CRC risk associated with red meat consumption include high iron and fat content in meat, and genetic variation in carcinogen-metabolizing enzymes that may influence the mutagenicity of the carcinogenic compounds in red meat [66–68].

Fiber

Results from studies of dietary fiber and CRC risk have been inconsistent. In many studies, fiber was found to be associated with a decreased risk of adenomas and CRC, but others found no association or only a modest association. The World Cancer Research Fund/American Institute for Cancer Research reported a meta-analysis showing strong evidence that consumption of foods containing dietary fiber, in particular fiber from cereals and whole grains, protects against CRC [13;69]. There is a biological rationale for fiber's possible protective role against CRC, because fiber dilutes fecal content, decreases its transit time, and increases its bulk, but the exact mechanism is not well understood [13].

Calcium and dairy

Dietary or supplemental calcium has been associated with a protective effect in CRC risk in several large cohort studies and pooled analyses, showing a 24–35% reduction in risk in the highest compared with the lowest levels of calcium intake [70–72]. However, in a large randomized controlled trial of 36,282 post-menopausal women who were given either a combination of calcium and vitamin D or a placebo, no significant difference in CRC rates between groups was observed during a mean follow-up time of 7 years [73]. Results of a longer follow-up from this study are pending. Overall, the evidence indicates a probable protective role of calcium on CRC risk as well as a plausible mechanism for this effect: calcium reduces cellular proliferation and promotes differentiation and apoptosis in normal and tumor colorectal cells [74].

In a meta-analysis of 19 cohort studies, higher levels of intake of milk and other dairy products were associated with a modest reduction in risk for colon but not rectal cancer [75].

Fish

A meta-analysis found evidence that fish consumption has a modest protective effect on CRC risk; the highest fish intake was associated with a lower incidence of CRC than the lowest fish intake (summary odds ratio 0.88; 95% CI 0.80–0.95) [76]. However, although suggestive, the evidence is still considered too limited to draw a conclusion [13].

Garlic

Studies investigating garlic consumption have suggested an inverse association between higher garlic intake and risk of CRC.

Smoking

Cigarette smoking is a preventable risk factor that is linked to many types of cancer, including CRC [77]. A large meta-analysis of more than 100 studies found an 18% increase in risk of developing CRC among smokers compared with non-smokers (RR 1.18; 95% CI 1.11–1.25) [78]. Smoking was also associated with an increased risk of dying from CRC (RR 1.25; 95% CI 1.14–1.37) [78]. The associations between smoking and both CRC incidence and mortality were stronger for rectal cancer than colon cancer. Colon polyps, which are precursors of CRC, have also been linked to smoking. The influence of smoking on the risk of more advanced adenomatous polyps is particularly strong; smoking has been linked to both the formation and aggressiveness of adenomas [79]. Smoking may also modify CRC risk in patients with Lynch syndrome [80].

Alcohol

Alcohol consumption has been associated with an increased risk of CRC. In a meta-analysis of alcohol drinking and CRC risk across 27 cohort and 34 case-control studies, risk was increased by 21% for moderate drinkers (2–3 drinks/day) and by 52% for heavy drinkers (≥4 drinks/day) compared with non-drinkers and occasional drinkers [81]. Furthermore, in a dose-response analysis, RR increased with the amount of alcohol consumed, ranging from 7% in light drinkers (10 g/day) to 82% in those consuming 100 g/day [81]. It has been proposed that the risk may be mediated through the folate-related DNA methylation pathway, since alcohol may interfere with folate absorption and act as a methyl group antagonist [82;83].

Drugs and supplements

Many compounds such as aspirin and other non-steroidal anti-inflammatory drugs (NSAIDs), COX-2 selective inhibitors, resistant starch, sulindac, hormones, bisphosphonates, statins, and supplements such as calcium, vitamin D, selenium, and folates may have a chemopreventive effect on colorectal adenomas and CRC. Promising preliminary evidence from observational and animal studies followed by confirmation in well-designed randomized clinical trials is required to assess any cancer prevention benefits at the population level. To date, none of the above agents is recommended for chemoprevention of CRC in the general population.

There is strong evidence that aspirin [85] and COX-2 selective inhibitors such as celecoxib and rofecoxib [86–88] reduce the risk of CRC. However, the harms, such as risk of bleeding and cardiovascular toxicity, outweigh the benefits. Therefore, the consensus statement from the US Preventive Services Task Force advises that these agents should not be used for the prevention of CRC in asymptomatic adults at average risk for CRC [89]. A randomized controlled trial of difluoromethylornithine and sulindac (an NSAID) in patients with a previously resected adenoma found a significant reduction in adenoma recurrence, but the therapy was associated with drug-related ototoxicity [90].

A recent retrospective study found that regular use of aspirin after diagnosis of locally advanced CRC was associated with longer survival in patients with mutated-PIK3CA (phosphatidylinositol-4,5-bisphosphonate 3-kinase, catalytic subunit alpha polypeptide gene) but not among patients with wild-type PIK3CA cancer. Experimental evidence suggests that aspirin downregulates PI3K signaling through inhibition of cyclooxygenase-2 [91]. Yet the presence of the PIK3CA mutation is infrequent and is present only in 10–20% of all CRC patients. Therefore, adjuvant aspirin therapy may be indicated for specific subgroups of patients such as those with PIK3CA-mutated CRC. A prospective clinical trial to validate the beneficial role of aspirin in this specific patient population may be worth pursuing.

A meta-analysis has shown that post-menopausal hormone therapy has a protective effect against CRC [92]. However, use of hormone therapy for CRC chemoprevention is not recommended because of the associated risks of side effects with long-term use.

Certain drugs that are commonly used to treat other diseases, such as statins for cardiovascular disease and bisphosphonates for osteoporosis, also may protect against CRC [93–95].

Low vitamin D levels have been linked to increased CRC risk [95]. Vitamin D and calcium are interlinked, but as noted earlier, no significant difference in CRC rates was observed in a randomized controlled trial of vitamin D and calcium versus placebo [73].

The exact role of folic acid and folates in CRC chemoprevention is still unclear. A protective effect of folic acid supplementation was found for adenomas and CRC, particularly with prior longer-term use [97]. In contrast, two randomized controlled trials found that folic acid resulted in no reduction in risk for recurrent adenomas [98;99], and one randomized controlled trial suggested that folic acid increased adenoma risk [98]. However, an increased risk of CRC due to folic acid supplementation was not supported in another large cancer prevention cohort [100].

Conclusion

CRC is one of the common cancers with a significant global public health burden. Epidemiologic studies have identified demographic, lifestyle, clinical and genetic factors that influence CRC risk. Knowledge of these risk factors can be applied to promote CRC prevention with the ultimate objective to reduce the morbidity and mortality from CRC.

TIPS AND TRICKS / KEY PITFALLS

- Variations in global, national, and regional rates provide clues for epidemiologic investigation into key genetic, environmental, and lifestyle risk factors.
- Population-based studies provide evidence for colorectal cancer prevention strategies, for example, lifestyle modifications such as avoiding smoking and excessive alcohol intake, engaging in regular physical activity, and maintaining optimal weight.
- Other probable risk and protective factors that may influence the development of colorectal cancer, such as dietary factors including consumption of fruits, vegetables, and fish, have inconsistent or insufficient evidence and therefore cannot yet be translated to the clinic.

CASE STUDY AND MULTIPLE-CHOICE QUESTIONS

Case 1

Colorectal cancer incidence rates in developed countries have remained stable or decreased over the last 10 years, whereas rates in developing countries have been rising.

1 Which of the following could contribute to a decrease in rates (there may be more than one correct answer)?

A. Availability of colorectal cancer screening.

B. Consumption of red meat.

C. Aging population.

D. Sedentary lifestyle.

2 Which of the following could contribute to an increase in colorectal cancer incidence rates (there may be more than one correct answer)?

A. Availability of colorectal cancer screening.

B. Consumption of red meat.

C. Aging population.

D. Sedentary lifestyle.

Case 2

An obese, diabetic patient who smokes and has a history of rectal polyps has a brother who was recently diagnosed with colon cancer. The patient is concerned about his risk for developing colorectal cancer.

1 What is his risk profile?

A. Low risk

B. Average risk

C. More than average risk

2 What can he do to reduce his risk (more than 1 answer may be correct)?

A. Quit smoking

B. Exercise regularly

C. Get regular screening

D. Take folic acid supplements

References

1 Ferlay J, Shin HR, Bray F, Forman D, Mathers C, Parkin DM. Cancer incidence and mortality worldwide. GLOBOCAN 2008. *Int J Cancer* 2010 Dec 15; 127(12): 2893–917. IARC CancerBase No. 10 [Internet]. Lyon, France: International Agency for Research on Cancer; 2010. Available at *http://globocan.iarc.fr*. Accessed on March 27, 2012.

2 Center MM, Jemal A, Ward E. International trends in colorectal cancer incidence rates. *Cancer Epidemiol Biomark Prev* 2009 Jun; 18(6): 1688–94.

3 Jemal A, Bray F, Center MM, Ferlay J, Ward E, Forman D. Global cancer statistics. *CA Cancer J Clin* 2011 Mar; 61(2): 69–90.

4 Howlader N, Noone AM, Krapcho M, Neyman N, Amonou R, Altekruse SF, et al. (eds). *SEER Cancer Statistics Review, 1975–2009 (Vintage 2009 Populations)*. Bethesda, MD: National Cancer Institute; 2012 Apr. Available at *http://seer.cancer.gov/csr/1975_2009_pops09/*. Based on November 2011 SEER data submission.

5 Kohler BA, Ward E, McCarthy BJ, Schymura MJ, Ries LA, Eheman C, et al. Annual report to the nation on the status of cancer, 1975–2007, featuring tumors of the brain and other nervous system. *J Natl Cancer Inst* 2011 May 4; 103(9): 714–36.

6 Edwards BK, Ward E, Kohler BA, Eheman C, Zauber AG, Anderson RN, et al. Annual report to the nation on the status of cancer, 1975–2006, featuring colorectal cancer trends and impact of interventions (risk factors, screening, and treatment) to reduce future rates. *Cancer* 2010 Feb 1; 116(3): 544–73.

7 Bray F, Ren JS, Masuyer E, Ferlay J. Global estimates of cancer prevalence for 27 sites in the adult population in 2008. *Int J Cancer* 2013 Mar 1; 132(5): 1133–45.

8 Troisi RJ, Freedman AN, Devesa SS. Incidence of colorectal carcinoma in the US: an update of trends by gender, race, age, subsite, and stage, 1975–1994. *Cancer* 1999 Apr 15; 85(8): 1670–6.

9 American Cancer Society. *Colorectal Cancer Facts and Figures* 2011–2013. Atlanta, GA: 2011.

10 Kirkegaard H, Johnsen NF, Christensen J, Frederiksen K, Overvad K, Tjonneland A. Association of adherence to lifestyle recommendations and risk of colorectal cancer: a prospective Danish cohort study. *BMJ* 2010; 341: c5504.

11 You YN, Xing Y, Feig BW, Chang GJ, Cormier JN. Young-onset colorectal cancer: is it time to pay attention? *Arch Intern Med* 2012 Feb 13; 172(3): 287–9.

12 Murphy G, Devesa SS, Cross AJ, Inskip PD, McGlynn KA, Cook MB. Sex disparities in colorectal cancer incidence by anatomic subsite, race and age. *Int J Cancer* 2011 Apr 1; 128(7): 1668–75.

13 World Cancer Research Fund and American Institute for Cancer Research. Colorectal cancer report 2010: *Food, Nutrition, Physical Activity, and the Prevention of Colorectal Cancer.* 2011.

14 Curado MP, Edwards B, Shin HR, Storm H, Ferlay J, Heanue M, et al. *Cancer Incidence in Five Continents. [IX]*. 2007. Lyon, IARC Scientific Publications No. 160. IARC.

15 Aretz S, Genuardi M, Hes FJ. Clinical utility gene card for: MUTYH-associated polyposis (MAP): Autosomal recessive colorectal adenomatous polyposis, Multiple colorectal adenomas, Multiple adenomatous polyps (MAP) – update 2013 Jan; 21(1). *Eur J Hum Genet* 2013 Jan; 21(1).

16 Mucci LA, Wedren S, Tamimi RM, Trichopoulos D, Adami HO. The role of gene-environment interaction in the aetiology of human cancer: examples from cancers of the large bowel, lung and breast. *J Intern Med* 2001 Jun; 249(6): 477–93.

17 Fuchs CS, Giovannucci EL, Colditz GA, Hunter DJ, Stampfer MJ, Rosner B, et al. Dietary fiber and the risk of colorectal cancer and adenoma in women. *N Engl J Med* 1999 Jan 21; 340(3): 169–76.

18 Winawer SJ, Zauber AG, Gerdes H, O'Brien MJ, Gottlieb LS, Sternberg SS, et al. Risk of colorectal cancer in the families of patients with adenomatous polyps. National Polyp Study Workgroup. *N Engl J Med* 1996 Jan 11; 334(2): 82–7.

19 Atkin WS, Morson BC, Cuzick J. Long-term risk of colorectal cancer after excision of rectosigmoid adenomas. *N Engl J Med* 1992 Mar 5; 326(10): 658–62.

20 Imperiale TF, Ransohoff DF. Risk for colorectal cancer in persons with a family history of adenomatous polyps: a systematic review. *Ann Intern Med* 2012 May 15; 156(10): 703–9.

21 von HS, Picelli S, Edler D, Lenander C, Dalen J, Hjern F, et al. Association studies on 11 published colorectal cancer risk loci. *Br J Cancer* 2010 Aug 10; 103(4): 575–80.

22 Niittymaki I, Kaasinen E, Tuupanen S, Karhu A, Jarvinen H, Mecklin JP, et al. Low-penetrance susceptibility variants in familial colorectal cancer. *Cancer Epidemiol Biomark Prev* 2010 Jun; 19(6): 1478–83.

23 Dunlop MG, Dobbins SE, Farrington SM, Jones AM, Palles C, Whiffin N, et al. Common variation near CDKN1A, POLD3 and SHROOM2 influences colorectal cancer risk. *Nat Genet* 2012 Jul; 44(7): 770–6.

24 Jasperson KW, Tuohy TM, Neklason DW, Burt RW. Hereditary and familial colon cancer. *Gastroenterology* 2010 Jun; 138(6): 2044–58.

25 Ahsan H, Neugut AI, Garbowski GC, Jacobson JS, Forde KA, Treat MR, et al. Family history of colorectal adenomatous polyps and increased risk for colorectal cancer. *Ann Intern Med* 1998 Jun 1; 128(11): 900–5.

26 Cottet V, Pariente A, Nalet B, Lafon J, Milan C, Olschwang S, et al. Colonoscopic screening of first-degree relatives of patients with large adenomas: increased risk of colorectal tumors. *Gastroenterology* 2007 Oct; 133(4): 1086–92.

27 Nakama H, Zhang B, Fukazawa K, Abdul Fattah AS. Family history of colorectal adenomatous polyps as a risk factor for colorectal cancer. *Eur J Cancer* 2000 Oct; 36(16): 2111–4.

28 Mulder SA, Kranse R, Damhuis RA, Ouwendijk RJ, Kuipers EJ, van Leerdam ME. The incidence and risk factors of metachronous colorectal cancer: an indication for follow-up. *Dis Colon Rectum* 2012 May; 55(5): 522–31.

29 Soderlund S, Brandt L, Lapidus A, Karlen P, Brostrom O, Lofberg R, et al. Decreasing time-trends of colorectal cancer in a large cohort of patients with inflammatory bowel disease. *Gastroenterology* 2009 May; 136(5): 1561–7.
30 Soderlund S, Granath F, Brostrom O, Karlen P, Lofberg R, Ekbom A, et al. Inflammatory bowel disease confers a lower risk of colorectal cancer to females than to males. *Gastroenterology* 2010 May; 138(5): 1697–703.
31 Jess T, Loftus EV, Jr., Velayos FS, Harmsen WS, Zinsmeister AR, Smyrk TC, et al. Risk of intestinal cancer in inflammatory bowel disease: a population-based study from olmsted county, Minnesota. *Gastroenterology* 2006 Apr; 130(4): 1039–46.
32 Rutter MD, Saunders BP, Wilkinson KH, Rumbles S, Schofield G, Kamm MA, et al. Thirty-year analysis of a colonoscopic surveillance program for neoplasia in ulcerative colitis. *Gastroenterology* 2006 Apr; 130(4): 1030–8.
33 Ekbom A, Helmick C, Zack M, Adami HO. Ulcerative colitis and colorectal cancer. A population-based study. *N Engl J Med* 1990 Nov 1; 323(18): 1228–33.
34 Katzka I, Brody RS, Morris E, Katz S. Assessment of colorectal cancer risk in patients with ulcerative colitis: experience from a private practice. *Gastroenterology* 1983 Jul; 85(1): 22–9.
35 Lennard-Jones JE, Melville DM, Morson BC, Ritchie JK, Williams CB. Precancer and cancer in extensive ulcerative colitis: findings among 401 patients over 22 years. *Gut* 1990 Jul; 31(7): 800–6.
36 Mir-Madjlessi SH, Farmer RG, Easley KA, Beck GJ. Colorectal and extracolonic malignancy in ulcerative colitis. *Cancer* 1986 Oct 1; 58(7): 1569–74.
37 Langholz E, Munkholm P, Davidsen M, Binder V. Colorectal cancer risk and mortality in patients with ulcerative colitis. *Gastroenterology* 1992 Nov; 103(5): 1444–51.
38 Winther KV, Jess T, Langholz E, Munkholm P, Binder V. Long-term risk of cancer in ulcerative colitis: a population-based cohort study from Copenhagen County. *Clin Gastroenterol Hepatol* 2004 Dec; 2(12): 1088–95.
39 Ekbom A, Helmick C, Zack M, Adami HO. Increased risk of large-bowel cancer in Crohn's disease with colonic involvement. *Lancet* 1990 Aug 11; 336(8711): 357–9.
40 Friedman S, Rubin PH, Bodian C, Goldstein E, Harpaz N, Present DH. Screening and surveillance colonoscopy in chronic Crohn's colitis. *Gastroenterology* 2001 Mar; 120(4): 820–6.
41 Maykel JA, Hagerman G, Mellgren AF, Li SY, Alavi K, Baxter NN, et al. Crohn's colitis: the incidence of dysplasia and adenocarcinoma in surgical patients. *Dis Colon Rectum* 2006 Jul; 49(7): 950–7.
42 Rubio CA, Befrits R. Colorectal adenocarcinoma in Crohn's disease: a retrospective histologic study. *Dis Colon Rectum* 1997 Sep; 40(9): 1072–8.
43 Fireman Z, Grossman A, Lilos P, Hacohen D, Bar MS, Rozen P, et al. Intestinal cancer in patients with Crohn's disease. A population study in central Israel. *Scand J Gastroenterol* 1989 Apr; 24(3): 346–50.
44 Gollop JH, Phillips SF, Melton LJ, III, Zinsmeister AR. Epidemiologic aspects of Crohn's disease: a population based study in Olmsted County, Minnesota, 1943–1982. *Gut* 1988 Jan; 29(1): 49–56.
45 Choi PM, Zelig MP. Similarity of colorectal cancer in Crohn's disease and ulcerative colitis: implications for carcinogenesis and prevention. *Gut* 1994 Jul; 35(7): 950–4.

46 Henderson TO, Oeffinger KC, Whitton J, Leisenring W, Neglia J, Meadows A, et al. Secondary gastrointestinal cancer in childhood cancer survivors: a cohort study. *Ann Intern Med* 2012 Jun 5; 156(11): 757–66.

47 Nottage K, McFarlane J, Krasin MJ, Li C, Srivastava D, Robison LL, et al. Secondary colorectal carcinoma after childhood cancer. *J Clin Oncol* 2012 Jul 10; 30(20): 2552–8.

48 Renehan AG, Tyson M, Egger M, Heller RF, Zwahlen M. Body-mass index and incidence of cancer: a systematic review and meta-analysis of prospective observational studies. *Lancet* 2008 Feb 16;371(9612): 569–78.

49 Giovannucci E, Ascherio A, Rimm EB, Colditz GA, Stampfer MJ, Willett WC. Physical activity, obesity, and risk for colon cancer and adenoma in men. *Ann Intern Med* 1995 Mar 1; 122(5): 327–34.

50 Martinez ME, Giovannucci E, Spiegelman D, Hunter DJ, Willett WC, Colditz GA. Leisure-time physical activity, body size, and colon cancer in women. Nurses' Health Study Research Group. *J Natl Cancer Inst* 1997 Jul 2; 89(13): 948–55.

51 Calle EE, Rodriguez C, Walker-Thurmond K, Thun MJ. Overweight, obesity, and mortality from cancer in a prospectively studied cohort of US adults. *N Engl J Med* 2003 Apr 24; 348(17): 1625–38.

52 He J, Stram DO, Kolonel LN, Henderson BE, Le ML, Haiman CA. The association of diabetes with colorectal cancer risk: the Multiethnic Cohort. *Br J Cancer* 2010 Jun 29; 103(1): 120–6.

53 Larsson SC, Orsini N, Wolk A. Diabetes mellitus and risk of colorectal cancer: a meta-analysis. *J Natl Cancer Inst* 2005 Nov 16; 97(22): 1679–87.

54 Yang YX, Hennessy S, Lewis JD. Type 2 diabetes mellitus and the risk of colorectal cancer. *Clin Gastroenterol Hepatol* 2005 Jun; 3(6): 587–94.

55 Yuhara H, Steinmaus C, Cohen SE, Corley DA, Tei Y, Buffler PA. Is diabetes mellitus an independent risk factor for colon cancer and rectal cancer? *Am J Gastroenterol* 2011 Nov; 106(11): 1911–21.

56 Giovannucci E. Insulin and colon cancer. *Cancer Causes Control* 1995 Mar; 6(2): 164–79.

57 Watkins LF, Lewis LR, Levine AE. Characterization of the synergistic effect of insulin and transferrin and the regulation of their receptors on a human colon carcinoma cell line. *Int J Cancer* 1990 Feb 15; 45(2): 372–5.

58 Ma J, Pollak MN, Giovannucci E, Chan JM, Tao Y, Hennekens CH, et al. Prospective study of colorectal cancer risk in men and plasma levels of insulin-like growth factor (IGF)-I and IGF-binding protein-3. *J Natl Cancer Inst* 1999 Apr 7; 91(7): 620–5.

59 Ma J, Giovannucci E, Pollak M, Leavitt A, Tao Y, Gaziano JM, et al. A prospective study of plasma C-peptide and colorectal cancer risk in men. *J Natl Cancer Inst* 2004 Apr 7; 96(7): 54–53.

60 Dehal AN, Newton CC, Jacobs EJ, Patel AV, Gapstur SM, Campbell PT. Impact of diabetes mellitus and insulin use on survival after colorectal cancer diagnosis: the Cancer Prevention Study-II Nutrition Cohort. *J Clin Oncol* 2012 Jan 1; 30(1): 53–9.

61 Wolin KY, Yan Y, Colditz GA, Lee IM. Physical activity and colon cancer prevention: a meta-analysis. *Br J Cancer* 2009 Feb 24; 100(4): 611–6.

62 Slattery ML, Boucher KM, Caan BJ, Potter JD, Ma KN. Eating patterns and risk of colon cancer. *Am J Epidemiol* 1998 Jul 1; 148(1): 4–16.

63 Koushik A, Hunter DJ, Spiegelman D, Beeson WL, van den Brandt PA, Buring JE, et al. Fruits, vegetables, and colon cancer risk in a pooled analysis of 14 cohort studies. *J Natl Cancer Inst* 2007 Oct 3; 99(19): 1471–83.

64 Lee JE, Chan AT. Fruit, vegetables, and folate: cultivating the evidence for cancer prevention. *Gastroenterology* 2011 Jul; 141(1): 16–20.

65 Chan DS, Lau R, Aune D, Vieira R, Greenwood DC, Kampman E, et al. Red and processed meat and colorectal cancer incidence: meta-analysis of prospective studies. *PLoS One* 2011; 6(6): e20456.

66 Cross AJ, Ferrucci LM, Risch A, Graubard BI, Ward MH, Park Y, et al. A large prospective study of meat consumption and colorectal cancer risk: an investigation of potential mechanisms underlying this association. *Cancer Res* 2010 Mar 15; 70(6): 2406–14.

67 Chan AT, Tranah GJ, Giovannucci EL, Willett WC, Hunter DJ, Fuchs CS. Prospective study of N-acetyltransferase-2 genotypes, meat intake, smoking and risk of colorectal cancer. *Int J Cancer* 2005 Jul 1; 115(4): 648–52.

68 Shin A, Shrubsole MJ, Rice JM, Cai Q, Doll MA, Long J, et al. Meat intake, heterocyclic amine exposure, and metabolizing enzyme polymorphisms in relation to colorectal polyp risk. *Cancer Epidemiol Biomark Prev* 2008 Feb; 17(2): 320–9.

69 Aune D, Chan DS, Lau R, Vieira R, Greenwood DC, Kampman E, et al. Dietary fibre, whole grains, and risk of colorectal cancer: systematic review and dose-response meta-analysis of prospective studies. *BMJ* 2011; 343: d6617.

70 Cho E, Smith-Warner SA, Spiegelman D, Beeson WL, van den Brandt PA, Colditz GA, et al. Dairy foods, calcium, and colorectal cancer: a pooled analysis of 10 cohort studies. *J Natl Cancer Inst* 2004 Jul 7; 96(13): 1015–22.

71 Park Y, Leitzmann MF, Subar AF, Hollenbeck A, Schatzkin A. Dairy food, calcium, and risk of cancer in the NIH-AARP Diet and Health Study. *Arch Intern Med* 2009 Feb 23; 169(4): 391–401.

72 Wu K, Willett WC, Fuchs CS, Colditz GA, Giovannucci EL. Calcium intake and risk of colon cancer in women and men. *J Natl Cancer Inst* 2002 Mar 20; 94(6): 437–46.

73 Wactawski-Wende J, Kotchen JM, Anderson GL, Assaf AR, Brunner RL, O'Sullivan MJ, et al. Calcium plus vitamin D supplementation and the risk of colorectal cancer. *N Engl J Med* 2006 Feb 16; 354(7): 684–96.

74 Lamprecht SA, Lipkin M. Cellular mechanisms of calcium and vitamin D in the inhibition of colorectal carcinogenesis. *Ann N Y Acad Sci* 2001 Dec; 952: 73–87.

75 Aune D, Lau R, Chan DS, Vieira R, Greenwood DC, Kampman E, et al. Dairy products and colorectal cancer risk: a systematic review and meta-analysis of cohort studies. *Ann Oncol* 2012 Jan; 23(1): 37–45.

76 Wu S, Feng B, Li K, Zhu X, Liang S, Liu X, et al. Fish consumption and colorectal cancer risk in humans: a systematic review and meta-analysis. *Am J Med* 2012 Jun; 125(6): 551–9.

77 American Cancer Society. *Cancer Facts and Figures 2012*. Atlanta: American Cancer Society; 2012.

78 Botteri E, Iodice S, Bagnardi V, Raimondi S, Lowenfels AB, Maisonneuve P. Smoking and colorectal cancer: a meta-analysis. *JAMA* 2008 Dec 17; 300(23): 2765–78.

79 Botteri E, Iodice S, Raimondi S, Maisonneuve P, Lowenfels AB. Cigarette smoking and adenomatous polyps: a meta-analysis. *Gastroenterology* 2008 Feb; 134(2): 388–95.

80 Pande M, Lynch PM, Hopper JL, Jenkins MA, Gallinger S, Haile RW, et al. Smoking and colorectal cancer in Lynch syndrome: results from the Colon Cancer Family Registry and the University of Texas MD Anderson Cancer Center. *Clin Cancer Res* 2010 Feb 15; 16(4): 1331–9.

81 Fedirko V, Tramacere I, Bagnardi V, Rota M, Scotti L, Islami F, et al. Alcohol drinking and colorectal cancer risk: an overall and dose-response meta-analysis of published studies. *Ann Oncol* 2011 Sep; 22(9): 1958–72.

82 Giovannucci E, Rimm EB, Ascherio A, Stampfer MJ, Colditz GA, Willett WC. Alcohol, low-methionine–low-folate diets, and risk of colon cancer in men. *J Natl Cancer Inst* 1995 Feb 15; 87(4): 265–73.

83 Harnack L, Jacobs DR, Jr., Nicodemus K, Lazovich D, Anderson K, Folsom AR. Relationship of folate, vitamin B-6, vitamin B-12, and methionine intake to incidence of colorectal cancers. *Nutr Cancer* 2002; 43(2): 152–8.

84 Huxley RR, Ansary-Moghaddam A, Clifton P, Czernichow S, Parr CL, Woodward M. The impact of dietary and lifestyle risk factors on risk of colorectal cancer: a quantitative overview of the epidemiological evidence. *Int J Cancer* 2009; 125: 171–80.

85 Flossmann E, Rothwell PM. Effect of aspirin on long-term risk of colorectal cancer: consistent evidence from randomised and observational studies. *Lancet* 2007 May 12; 369(9573): 1603–13.

86 Arber N, Eagle CJ, Spicak J, Racz I, Dite P, Hajer J, et al. Celecoxib for the prevention of colorectal adenomatous polyps. N *Engl J Med* 2006 Aug 31; 355(9): 885–95.

87 Baron JA, Sandler RS, Bresalier RS, Quan H, Riddell R, Lanas A, et al. A randomized trial of rofecoxib for the chemoprevention of colorectal adenomas. *Gastroenterology* 2006 Dec; 131(6): 1674–82.

88 Bertagnolli MM, Eagle CJ, Zauber AG, Redston M, Solomon SD, Kim K, et al. Celecoxib for the prevention of sporadic colorectal adenomas. *N Engl J Med* 2006 Aug 31; 355(9): 873–84.

89 Chan AT, Giovannucci EL. Primary prevention of colorectal cancer. *Gastroenterology* 2010 Jun; 138(6): 2029–43.

90 Meyskens FL, Jr., McLaren CE, Pelot D, Fujikawa-Brooks S, Carpenter PM, Hawk E, et al. Difluoromethylornithine plus sulindac for the prevention of sporadic colorectal adenomas: a randomized placebo controlled, double-blind trial. *Cancer Prev Res (Phila)* 2008 Jun; 1(1): 32–8.

91 Liao X, Lochhead P, Nishihara R, Morikawa T, Kuchiba A, Yamauchi M, et al. Aspirin use, tumor PIK3CA mutation, and colorectal-cancer survival. *N Engl J Med* 2012 Oct 25; 367(17): 1596–606.

92 Green J, Czanner G, Reeves G, Watson J, Wise L, Roddam A, et al. Menopausal hormone therapy and risk of gastrointestinal cancer: nested case-control study within a prospective cohort, and meta-analysis. *Int J Cancer* 2012 May 15; 130(10): 2387–96.

93 Poynter JN, Gruber SB, Higgins PD, Almog R, Bonner JD, Rennert HS, et al. Statins and the risk of colorectal cancer. *N Engl J Med* 2005 May 26; 352(21): 2184–92.

94 Rennert G, Pinchev M, Rennert HS, Gruber SB. Use of bisphosphonates and reduced risk of colorectal cancer. *J Clin Oncol* 2011 Mar 20; 29(9): 1146–50.

95 Singh H, Nugent Z, Demers A, Mahmud S, Bernstein C. Exposure to bisphosphonates and risk of colorectal cancer: a population-based nested case-control study. *Cancer* 2012 Mar 1; 118(5): 1236–43.

96 Chung M, Lee J, Terasawa T, Lau J, Trikalinos TA. Vitamin D with or without calcium supplementation for prevention of cancer and fractures: an updated meta-analysis for the US Preventive Services Task Force. *Ann Intern Med* 2011 Dec 20; 155(12): 827–38.

97 Lee JE, Willett WC, Fuchs CS, Smith-Warner SA, Wu K, Ma J, et al. Folate intake and risk of colorectal cancer and adenoma: modification by time. *Am J Clin Nutr* 2011 Apr; 93(4): 817–25.
98 Cole BF, Baron JA, Sandler RS, Haile RW, Ahnen DJ, Bresalier RS, et al. Folic acid for the prevention of colorectal adenomas: a randomized clinical trial. *JAMA* 2007 Jun 6; 297(21): 2351–9.
99 Logan RF, Grainge MJ, Shepherd VC, Armitage NC, Muir KR. Aspirin and folic acid for the prevention of recurrent colorectal adenomas. *Gastroenterology* 2008 Jan; 134(1): 29–38.
100 Stevens VL, McCullough ML, Sun J, Jacobs EJ, Campbell PT, Gapstur SM. High levels of folate from supplements and fortification are not associated with increased risk of colorectal cancer. *Gastroenterology* 2011 Jul; 141(1): 98–105.

ANSWERS TO MULTIPLE-CHOICE QUESTIONS

Case 1

1 A
2 B, C, D

Case 2

1 C
2 A, B, C

CHAPTER 2

Screening for colorectal cancer

Robert JC Steele[1] & Paula McDonald[2]

[1] *Medical Research Institute, Population Health Sciences, Ninewells Hospital & Medical School, Dundee, UK*

[2] *Scottish Bowel Screening Centre, King's Cross Hospital, Dundee, UK*

KEY POINTS

- Population based randomized trials of colorectal cancer screening using guaiac based faecal occult blood testing have consistently demonstrated reductions in disease specific mortality.
- Guaiac based faecal occult blood tests are not specific for human haemoglobin.
- Faecal immunochemical testing (FIT) is specific for human haemoglobin and can be quantified.
- FIT is likely to replace guaiac based faecal occult blood testing as the standard method of screening using faecal testing.
- Randomized trials of flexible sigmoidoscopy have demonstrated both reductions in disease specific mortality and disease incidence owing to removal of adenomas as part of the screening process.
- There is evidence that colonoscopy reduces both mortality and incidence of the disease, but as yet there are no results available from population-based randomized trials of colonoscopy as a screening modality.
- The uptake of screening is affected by gender, deprivation, and ethnic background.
- Novel approaches to screening include using DNA markers in stool and blood tests for proteins and DNA methylation. These are not, however, currently recommended for population screening.

CASE STUDY

A 65-year-old man is invited to participate in a population screening program. He first received a letter in the post from the Screening Centre indicating that he would be sent a faecal occult blood test two weeks later. An explanatory leaflet setting out the pros and cons of screening was included with this pre-notification letter. Two weeks later the

Colorectal Cancer: Diagnosis and Clinical Management, First Edition. Edited by John H. Scholefield and Cathy Eng.

patient received the guaiac based faecal occult blood test in the post. He duly completed this and sent it back to the Screening Centre. A strong positive result was obtained. Four days later he received a letter indicating that the test was positive and a colonoscopy was arranged. This was carried out two weeks later and detected a small cancer in the sigmoid colon. A CT of the chest and abdomen was then performed, which showed no evidence of metastatic disease. He proceeded to a laparoscopic sigmoid colectomy from which he made an uneventful recovery. The pathology report on the resected specimen indicated that the tumor was a moderately differentiated T2 N0 adenocarcinoma (Dukes' Stage A). No further treatment was advised.

TIPS AND TRICKS/KEY PITFALLS

- The sensitivity and specificity of faecal occult blood test screening are dependent on the analytical sensitivity of the test. By increasing the analytical sensitivity, the clinical sensitivity will increase (i.e. more cancers will be diagnosed). However, the specificity will fall, increasing the false/positive rate.
- Interval cancers are an inevitable consequence of a screening program, but are not necessarily associated with a poor prognosis. Increasing the sensitivity of the screening test will reduce the number of interval cancers.
- The clinical sensitivity of faecal occult blood testing is higher in men than in women and this may require a differential cut-off in order to overcome gender inequality.
- Endoscopic screening is more sensitive and specific than faecal occult blood test screening, but is generally associated with a much poorer uptake. A combination of endoscopic and faecal occult blood test screening may be the appropriate way forward.

Introduction

Colorectal cancer continues to be the fourth most commonly diagnosed cancer worldwide [1], and although survival after diagnosis has improved over the last 4 decades [2], the overall 5-year survival remains less than 50%. The most important prognostic factor in colorectal cancer is stage at diagnosis [2] and it follows that the most effective way of improving prognosis is early detection. Unfortunately, symptomatic colorectal cancer tends to be relatively advanced and a recent systematic review and meta-analysis indicates that individual symptoms and symptom complexes have poor sensitivity for colorectal cancer [3]. In a screening population, symptoms are poor predictors of significant neoplastic disease [4]. Screening is therefore the only reliable method of early detection.

Screening is the process whereby theoretically asymptomatic individuals are tested with a view to diagnosing a disease at an early stage of its development, with the aim of improving the outcome of treatment. In cancer, this includes not only detecting early invasive disease but also, where possible, the detection of premalignant disease so that the screening process may have an effect on disease incidence as well as outcome [5]. The criteria for effective population screening were first established by Wilson and Jungner [6], and when these criteria are applied, colorectal cancer is undoubtedly a very suitable candidate for screening. It is an important health problem, especially in the UK [2]. Treatment for colorectal cancer is now largely based on firm evidence [7] and its natural history is well understood; the adenoma-carcinoma sequence is now widely accepted [8] and there is now unequivocal evidence that removal of adenomas can prevent colorectal cancer (q.v.). Finally, it is well documented that the prognosis of colorectal cancer is highly stage dependant [2]. However, the real evidence for colorectal cancer screening comes from population based randomized trials, which are necessary to overcome the inherent biases in the screening process, and these will be examined in the following sections.

Guaiac based faecal occult blood testing (gFOBT)

For many years the technology for detecting blood in faeces relied on the indirect guaiac test. Guaiac reacts with haem by means of its ability to detect peroxidase and is not capable of detecting the degradation products of haem [9]. In addition, when haem is introduced into the gastrointestinal tract, it is modified by microflora thus losing its peroxidase activity. Because of this, guaiac tests rarely detect dietary haem and for the same reason they are more sensitive for bleeding lesions in the colon than in the upper gastrointestinal tract. However, guaiac can react to any peroxidase in the stool, including those of dietary origin. For this reason dietary restriction was originally recommended to exclude peroxidase from the diet prior to gFOBT, but a meta-analysis has indicated that with non-rehydrated guaiac tests, where there is a delay of a few days before testing, this becomes unnecessary [10].

Within a screening context, the sensitivity of guaiac testing for cancer is difficult to estimate, but by using interval cancer data (q.v.), the most commonly used test (Haemoccult II®) seems to detect in the region of 50% of cancers in a population that accepts screening. This low clinical sensitivity is due partly to the relatively low analytical sensitivity of Haemoccult II for blood and due to the fact that cancers bleed intermittently. On the other hand, the specificity (percentage of disease-free individuals with a negative test) is around 98%, but although this seems high, as the majority of the population do not have colorectal cancer, this still results in a high false positive rate. It should also be noted that, although most studies use non-rehydrated Haemoccult II, rehydration increases both its analytical and clinical sensitivity by lysing red cells and exposing more haem to the guaiac reaction. However, the increase in clinical sensitivity has an adverse effect on its specificity; this is an issue with all methods of detecting blood in faeces as a means of detecting colorectal neoplasia.

With the advent of immunological means of detecting blood in faeces (see next section), it can be argued that gFOBT has become obsolete Nevertheless, the original population-based trials of colorectal cancer screening utilized gFOBT and, as the results of these trials proved unequivocally that screening for colorectal cancer is effective, it is worth examining them in detail. They were carried out in the United States, England, Denmark, France and Sweden and all employed the Haemoccult II test.

The study from the United States, which took place in Minnesota, randomized volunteers into three groups: a group offered annual screening with rehydrated Haemoccult II, a group offered biennial screening, and an observation group. A positive test was followed by colonoscopy and colorectal cancer mortality was reduced by 21% in the biennial group and by 33% in the annual group [11]. It should be noted that, uniquely, amongst the randomized studies, the Haemoccult II was rehydrated resulting in a 10% positivity rate and, as a result, in the group offered annual screening, 38% had a colonoscopy on at least one occasion. Importantly, the *incidence* of colorectal cancer in both groups offered screening fell significantly compared with the control group after 18 years of follow-up [12]. This phenomenon has not been observed in any of the other trials of gFOBT screening and is probably the result of the high colonoscopy rate leading to a high rate of polypectomy.

The study carried out in UK took place in Nottingham and 150,000 subjects were randomized by household [13]. The group offered screening were aged between 50 and 74 and were offered biennial non-rehydrated Haemoccult II. Colonoscopy was offered after a positive test result and in the first (prevalence) round, the investigation rate was 2% and in the subsequent (incidence) rounds, it fell to 1.2%. In the course of five screening rounds, 60% of the group that was offered screening completed at least one screening test. The screen-detected cancers were diagnosed at a favorable stage, with 57% at Dukes Stage A, but it should be noted that there were a large number of interval cancers and 50% of the cancers diagnosed in those who had accepted at least one screening test were not screen-detected.

Thus, in this study, gFOBT was associated with a relatively low uptake and relatively poor sensitivity. Nevertheless, the colorectal cancer specific mortality in the group offered screening was statistically significantly reduced by 15% when compared to the control group after a median of 7.8 years of follow-up. At a median of 19.5 years of follow-up, the reduction in colorectal cancer mortality was maintained at 13% and when adjusted for non-compliance, the reduction was found to be 18% [14]. It should be noted, however, that despite the fact that 615 adenomas greater than 10 mm in diameter were removed from individuals in the intervention arm, no significant difference in colorectal cancer incidence could be detected.

Screening programs may have a 'halo' effect and the Nottingham study illustrates this. In the *control* group, the percentage of patients presenting with rectal cancer at Dukes Stage A increased from 9% in the first half of the recruitment period to 28% in the second [15]. Thus, it seems that the very presence of the screening program had an effect on individuals who were not invited for screening and this may be related to increased awareness of the significance of rectal bleeding. On the same theme, significantly fewer emergency admissions for colorectal cancer were seen in the group offered screening when compared to the control group [16], indicating that screening also had the effect of reducing the number of patients presenting as emergencies.

In the Danish study, 61,933 subjects were randomized into a group that was offered screening by means of biennial Haemoccult II testing or into a control group [17;18]. The uptake in the first round was 67% and more than 90% accepted repeated screening invitations, presumably owing to the fact that those who did not accept the first invitation were excluded. As in the Nottingham study, screen detected cancers were detected at a favorable stage with 48% at Dukes Stage A and interval cancers accounted for 30% of all cancers diagnosed in those offered screening at least once. Thus, screening in the Danish study performed in a very similar way to that of the Nottingham study and the disease specific mortality reduction after 5 years was 18%.

In the French study, a randomized approach was not adopted [19]. Rather, small geographical areas were allocated either to be offered screening or to act as controls. Again, the non-rehydrated Haemoccult II test was used on a biennial basis and offered to individuals between the ages of 50 and 74. A total of 91,199 were offered screening, the positivity rate was 1.2% in the first round but increased slightly in further rounds, and uptake in the first round was 52.8% and remained fairly constant thereafter. Reflecting the results of the Nottingham and Danish studies, the mortality reduction seen in those offered screening was 16%.

In Gothenburg, Sweden, 68,308 citizens aged 60 to 64 years were randomized into either a control group or a group that was offered biennial Haemoccult II [20]. Uptake was 70% and those with a positive test result were investigated by means of flexible sigmoidoscopy and a double contrast barium enema. After a mean follow-up period of 9 years from the last screening episode, a statistically significant reduction in colorectal cancer mortality of 16% was seen.

These five studies are of the utmost importance as they are the only controlled studies of population screening compared to no intervention; the consistent reduction in colorectal cancer specific mortality indicates that early detection of colorectal cancer is truly beneficial. In a recent systematic review and meta-analysis, population screening by gFOBT was estimated to reduce colorectal cancer mortality by 16%, going up to 23% when adjusted for uptake [21]. Thus, the principle of screening for colorectal cancer is sound and, although gFOBT may be considered as a sub-optimal test, these results can be used as benchmarks for newer tests.

In the UK, the National Screening Committee advised a demonstration pilot of biennial gFOBT screening to determine whether or not the results of the randomized trials could be reproduced within the UK National Health Service [22]. This pilot was successfully carried out in two areas of the UK, one in Scotland and one in England [23] and as a result, the UK Health Departments have now rolled out screening programs and the initial outcomes indicate that the national programs should produce the expected results [24;25].

Faecal immunochemical testing

As outlined above, gFOBT has significant disadvantages; in particular the fact that it relies on a peroxidase reaction makes it susceptible to false positive results. The solution to this problem has been the introduction of tests employing antibodies raised against human haemoglobin: faecal immunochemical testing (FIT). Not only are these tests specific for human haemoglobin but there are now several manufacturers who produce quantitative FIT that provide a measure of the concentration of haemoglobin in faeces. However, such quantization is not currently accurate nor is it transferrable between different tests. As haemoglobin concentration is usually expressed as ng Hb/ml of the buffer into which the faecal sample is placed, the concentration will, of course, vary according to the ratio of buffer to faeces and the concentration of haemoglobin may be dependent on the composition of the faeces.

Qualitative FIT have been available for many years but their high analytical sensitivity for blood results in poor clinical specificity and a consequently high false positive rate. Despite this, qualitative FIT may be used in concert with gFOBT in order to reduce the false positive rate created by the non-specific nature of the guaiac test. In a study of screening patients awaiting colonoscopy for a positive gFOBT, it was shown that those with a negative high sensitivity FIT (detecting 50 μg Hb/g faeces) had a negligible risk of significant neoplastic disease (cancer or adenoma) [26]. This led to the two-tier reflex approach for faecal occult blood testing where a gFOBT (detecting ~600 μg Hb/g of faeces) is used as the first line test and refined by a second line high sensitivity FIT. This approach has been introduced into the Scottish Bowel Screening Programme [27], but although it reduces the numbers of unnecessary colonoscopies, it does not address the issue of the poor clinical sensitivity of gFOBT. For this reason, there has been major interest in using FIT as the first line screening test.

In two recent studies, a quantitative FIT was compared with the Haemoccult II gFOBT. In the first study, from France, 10,677 individuals undergoing screening were offered both gFOBT and FIT [28]. Using a cut-off of 20 ng Hb/ml, the gain in sensitivity produced by the FIT was 50% for cancer and 256% for high risk adenoma. This was offset by a decrease in specificity, such that the number of extra false positive results needed to detect one extra advanced neoplasm (cancer or high risk adenoma) was 2.17. In the second study, from the Netherlands, 20,623 individuals between 50 and 75 years of age were randomized to either a Haemoccult II gFOBT or a quantitative FIT [29]. For the FIT, a cut-off of 100 ng Hb/ml was used to trigger colonoscopy. The positivity rate of the FIT was 5.5% compared with 2.4% for the gFOBT. However, the number needed to scope to find one cancer was the same between the two tests and the detection rates for advanced adenomas and cancer were significantly higher for FIT than gFOBT. A further study comparing gFOBT with FIT at a cut-off level of 50 ng/ml also examined the effect of varying the cut-off level between 50 and 200 ng/ml (30). The positivity rate of FIT ranged between 8.1% and 3.5%, the detection rate of advanced neoplasia between 3.2% and 2.1%, and the specificity between 95.5% and 98.9%. A cut-off value of 75 ng/ml gave a detection rate two times higher than that with gFOBT and the number needed to scope to find one case of advanced neoplasia was similar. The authors concluded that FIT at a cut-off value of 75 ng per ml provided an acceptable trade-off between detection of advance neoplasia and the number needed to scope.

These comparisons between gFOBT and FIT seem to indicate that FIT is a preferable screening tool. However, all the comparative studies have used FIT at a cut-off level that is much lower than that achieved by the Haemoccult II gFOBT, which equates to around 400 ngHb/ml, so it is not clear whether the enhanced performance is merely a consequence of increased sensitivity for blood or whether the specific nature of the immunological test also enhances its performance.

There are a number of studies in which people undergoing colonoscopic screening have performed a quantitative FIT prior to investigation and these studies provide a measure of the sensitivity and specificity of different haemoglobin concentration cut-off levels. In a study from Israel, 1000 consecutive patients undergoing colonoscopy for screening or symptoms provided three samples for quantitative FIT (31). There were 17 patients with cancer and the sensitivity at a cut-off of 50 ng Hb/ml was 100%. At lower thresholds it did not perform so well; at a cut-off of 150 ng per ml, sensitivity dropped to 82.4%. It should be noted, however, that the specificity operated in the opposite direction and at a cut-off of 50 ng per ml, it was 84.4%, whereas at 150 ng per ml, it was 91.9%. This equated to false positive rates for cancer of 90% and 85% respectively.

In another study carried out as part of the German Colonoscopy Screening Programme, quantitative FIT was carried out in 2324 subjects [32]. Here, the lowest cut-off was described as 2 μg Hb/g and indicted a sensitivity for all adenomas and cancers of 41.6%. Unfortunately, in this study adenomas were not separated from carcinomas. In a further study from Japan, of 1085 asymptomatic individuals undergoing screening colonoscopy, a quantitative FIT offered a sensitivity for cancer of 75%, both at the 25 n/ml and at the 50 ng/ml cut-off levels [33]. Specificity at these two levels was 76% and 86% respectively, suggesting that 50 ng Hb/ml performed better.

From the relatively limited amount of information available from these studies of sensitivity and specificity, it would appear that a low cut-off for quantitative FIT in the region of 50 ng Hb/ml will detect most although not all cancers but will miss a substantial number of adenomas, particularly those of small size. Thus the price for detecting a higher proportion of cancers and adenomas is a higher colonoscopy rate and a higher false positive rate.

Another method of estimating sensitivity is to examine the interval cancer rate after negative tests. In a study from Italy, using a quantitative FIT with a cut-off of 100 ng/ml, the sensitivity for cancer was estimated at 78% [34]. It is also interesting to note that, in studies of quantitative FIT used as a screening test, the faecal haemoglobin concentration below the threshold used to trigger colonoscopy predicts the subsequent risk of interval cancer [35].

Colonoscopy is a precious resource, and the great advantage of quantitative FIT is that a threshold for colonoscopy can be set at any positivity rate that can be accommodated within a health system. There is, however, another fundamental question to be addressed. For all forms of FOBT screening, biennial screening has, by default, become the gold standard. However, there is evidence that, using a quantitative FIT at a cut-off of 50 ng Hb/ml, the total number of advanced neoplastic lesions found at repeat screening is not influenced by interval length within a range of 1 to 3 years [36]. It is therefore possible that using a high sensitivity FIT as a one-off screening test or with an interval much greater of two years may perform as well or better than a low sensitivity test such as Haemoccult II gFOBT carried out every two years without an appreciable increase in colonoscopy rates. This is a complex area to study as it offers an endless permutation of cut-off levels and screening intervals but, in order to move to an optimal screening strategy based on the detection of blood in faeces, it is important that this is addressed in future studies.

Flexible sigmoidoscopy

As 75% of all colorectal cancers and adenomas arise in the rectum or sigmoid colon, the use of flexible sigmoidoscopy (FS) as a primary screening modality would seem reasonable. It was, therefore, proposed that a single FS at around the age of 60 years, with removal of all adenomas would provide effective screening that would reduce the mortality *and* incidence of colorectal cancer [37]. This approach was studied by two multi-center randomized controlled trials, one in Italy (SCORE) [38] and the other in the UK (Flexiscope) [39]. In the UK study, potential participants aged between 60 and 64 from 14 centers were sent a questionnaire to ask if they would be interested in attending for FS screening. Of 354,262 people receiving this questionnaire, 55% responded positively. Of these, 170,432 were randomized using a 2:1 ratio of controls to subjects. FS was performed with removal of all polyps and going onto colonoscopy in those who had high risk adenomas (defined as 3 or more adenomas a villous or more severely dysplastic adenoma or an adenoma greater than 1 cm). Of 57,254 people who were invited 71% attended, and extrapolating from these figures, the population uptake would have been around 30%.

Of those undergoing FS, 12% were found to have adenomas and 0.3% cancer. Subsequent colonoscopy in the high risk groups revealed proximal adenomas in 18.8% and cancer in 0.4%. Long-term follow-up (median 11.2 years) demonstrated a significant reduction in colorectal cancer mortality in the group offered flexible sigmoidoscopy *and* after a period of four years a significant reduction in colorectal cancer incidence was observed, presumably as a result of the removal of adenomas. Interestingly, the reduction in incidence was restricted to left-sided cancers, despite the fact that total colonoscopy was carried out in all those with significant index lesion found at FS (5% of the screened population).

In the SCORE Trial [38], which was similar in design and length of follow-up to the UK study, the rate of colorectal cancer incidence was statistically significantly reduced in the group offered FS screening and the colorectal cancer mortality rate was non-statistically significantly reduced. It should be noted, however, that the uptake was only 58.3% compared with the 71% seen in the UK study, despite the use of a similar pre-randomization strategy. The importance of these two studies is that they demonstrate beyond doubt that endoscopy and polypectomy can reduce the incidence of colorectal cancer and that FS is a credible candidate as a first line screening test. Indeed, in England, a commitment has been made to roll-out 'once only' FS as a screening modality between the ages of 55 and 60 prior to the commencement of FOBT screening.

There remains a significant question around uptake of FS screening. Because the UK Flexiscope and the SCORE trials were performed in volunteers, the population uptake of FS is unknown. In Norway, a population-based randomized trial of FS achieved a participation rate of 67% [40], although it did not demonstrate any mortality or incidence reductions, probably because the analysis had been carried out too early. However, a randomized study from the Netherlands, comparing gFOBT, FIT, and FS, achieved an uptake of 32.4% for FS compared with 49.5% and 61.5% for gFOBT and FIT respectively [41]. In addition, the participants perceived the personal burden of flexible sigmoidoscopy to be greater than that of either type of faecal testing [42]. On the other hand, a study from Italy found a similar participation rate for FIT and FS, although both were low at 32% of those invited [43]. Two small studies conducted in the London area observed an uptake of screening FS of around 50% [44], but a similar study carried out in Tayside, Scotland achieved an uptake of only 24% [45]. It is not clear why there should be such discrepancies in the uptake of FS, but both cultural issues and differences in level of deprivation are likely to be important [46].

The comparative study from the Netherlands [41] demonstrated that the diagnostic yield of advanced neoplasia (cancers and significant adenomas per 100 invitees) was greater for FS than for either of the faecal tests, suggesting that the overall performance of FS may be better than faecal testing, despite a lower participation rate. This introduces an important ethical dimension; namely whether or not it is acceptable to use a population screening tool that reaches a relatively small proportion of the population rather than a test that is associated with a higher participation rate but has an overall poorer performance in terms of disease detection. This is further complicated by the adverse effect of deprivation on uptake of screening. It is known that, in Scotland, the difference in uptake of gFOBT population screening between the most deprived and the least deprived quintile is around 20% [47]. Less in known about the effect of deprivation on uptake of FS, although in the UK Flexiscope Trial, there was a 16% difference in intention to participate and a 20% difference in actual uptake in those invited between the most and least deprived quintiles in Glasgow [46]. Thus, the role of FS in population screening has yet to be fully defined and it may be that a combination of FS and FOBT would be optimal. Indeed, there are studies from the Netherlands and Italy [48;49] that indicate that between 20% and 25% of individuals who do not wish to participate in FS screening may be prepared to undergo FIT screening.

Colonoscopy

Colonoscopy is recognized as the gold standard method of visualizing the large bowel and provides a means whereby adenomas can be removed, thus conferring protection against colorectal cancer. It would therefore seem to be the ideal screening test; as false positive results for neoplasia are not possible, the specificity is 100% and the sensitivity is very high, albeit not 100% [50]. Furthermore, a study comparing colonoscopy with CT colography suggests that, for polyps, the sensitivity of colonoscopy may only be in the region of 90% [51]. Nevertheless, colonoscopy is widely used for opportunistic screening and the epidemiological evidence that colonoscopy and attendant polypectomy can reduce the incidence of colorectal is excellent [52]. However, the use of colonoscopy as a population screening tool remains controversial and although there are currently four randomized trials of colonoscopy screening worldwide, none of these have reported and there are relatively little data from which conclusions can be drawn.

Perhaps the most important study comes from Poland, which analysed the results of screening colonoscopy in 50,148 participants between the ages of 40 and 66 years of age [53]. The yield of pathology and the number of colonoscopies required to detect neoplasia was age dependant but in the 50–66 age group, 0.9% had cancer, 5.9% had advanced neoplasia (cancer or significant adenoma), and 14.9% had any adenoma or cancer. Interestingly, analysis of adenoma detection rates from different endoscopists indicated that the risk of developing colorectal cancer after colonoscopy was significantly associated with the adenoma detection rate, emphasising the importance of careful colonoscopy [54]. Unfortunately, this study did not provide any indication of uptake and it is therefore impossible to estimate how colonoscopy would perform as a population screening tool. A study carried out in US military veterans, between the ages of 50 and 75 years, reported similar detection rates for cancer and adenoma and was associated with an uptake of only 20% [55]. The results of the randomized trials of population screening using colonoscopy will be extremely informative, but the limited evidence that is currently available suggests that colonoscopy is not associated with an uptake that would be compatible with a population screening tool and a study comparing biennial FIT. Once-only flexible sigmoidoscopy and once-only colonoscopy indicated that the uptake for colonoscopy was significantly lower than for either FIT or flexible sigmoidoscopy [56].

It is also interesting to note that the effect of colonoscopy in reducing colorectal cancer mortality and incidence is much stronger for the left side of the colon than for the right side of the colon [57–59]. This is presumably associated with the quality of colonoscopy; bowel preparation is often poorer in the right colon than the left colon and adenomas in the right colon are often flat and subtle when compared with the polypoid lesions seen more commonly on the left. This again emphasises the importance of quality in colonoscopy, and in a study from Germany examining interval cancers occurring 1–10 years after negative colonoscopy, there was a strong association between incompleteness of colonoscopy and the occurrence of interval cancer [55].

Radiology

Evidence relating to the use of barium enema as a screening test is lacking, but there is increasing interest in CT colography. A study from the United States, in which 1,233 asymptomatic individuals around the age of 60 underwent both CT, colography and, colonoscopy on the same day, testifies to the accuracy of this technology [51]. Thus, CT colography would appear to be sufficiently accurate to be used as a screening tool and a recent randomized trial from the Netherlands compared colonoscopy with CT colography in a population screening context [60]. Participation in screening with CT colography (34%) was significantly better than with colonoscopy (22%), but colonoscopy identified significantly more advanced neoplasia per 100 participants than was found in CT colography. However, on an intention to screen basis, the diagnostic yield was similar for both strategies. In this study the uptake of both

CT colography and colonoscopy were far from ideal and it has to be remembered that individuals with a positive CT colography (in the region of 10%) would have to be offered colonoscopy. As is the case with colonoscopy, there is no randomized evidence relating to the effect of CT colography on colorectal cancer mortality or incidence.

Uptake

Adequate uptake is an essential pre-requisite for an effective population screening program. What constitutes adequate uptake, however, is more difficult to quantify. For gFOBT screening, the randomized trials that demonstrated a mortality reduction achieved an uptake of between 50% and 60% but, of course, the uptake required to produce a measurable reduction in death rates or incidence will depend on the sensitivity of the test. Thus, a highly sensitive test such as colonoscopy may produce the same mortality reduction as FOBT screening, even although it may be associated with a much lower uptake.

As demonstrated above, the type of test used has an important effect on uptake, and the most of the evidence quoted earlier indicates that gFOBT or FIT is more acceptable than flexible sigmoidoscopy which, in turn, is more acceptable than colonoscopy. However, there does seem to be considerable national variation.

Socio-demographic factors also have a profound influence on uptake. Experience from the UK shows that uptake of gFOBT screening falls with increasing deprivation and that a non-white ethnic background is associated with low uptake [47;61], and the same observations have been made with flexible sigmoidoscopy screening [46]. Another factor which significantly increases screening uptake is gender. Across the deprivation gradient, women are more likely to accept an invitation for FOBT screening than men [47;61]. Surprisingly, however, this gender difference does not appear to be so pronounced with flexible sigmoidoscopy screening [44]. There is also evidence that being married has a positive effect on uptake [62].

Given the importance of uptake in population screening, there has been great interest in interventions aimed at improving participation in population screening programs. Perhaps the most obvious is to continue to invite individuals for screening, even if they do not accept the first invitation and a recent analysis of prevalence and incidence screening in Scotland demonstrated that the cumulative uptake of the first screening invitation rose from 53% to 63% over 3 biennial rounds [63]. This has important implications, not only for screening tests that are offered repeatedly on a regular basis, but also for 'one off' screening procedures such as flexible sigmoidoscopy or colonoscopy; if the first invitation is not accepted then there may be merit in repeating invitation at regular intervals.

As indicated above, the test itself has an important influence on uptake and different forms of faecal testing also influence uptake and there is good evidence from randomized studies that sampling method has an important effect and FIT seems to be consistently more acceptable than gFOBT [41;64]. This is presumably due to the fact that modern quantitative FIT tests use a probe or a brush to sample the faeces, whereas the gFOBT tests rely on participants smearing faeces onto a card using a spatula.

Two other approaches have been used: endorsement by general practitioners and pre-notification. A qualitative evaluation of strategies to increase colorectal cancer uptake from Canada [65] has identified the importance of receiving the invitation from a family physician, and comparisons of invitations with or without endorsement from a general practitioner carried out in Australia and England showed enhanced participation from general practitioner involvement [66;67]. Pre-notification has also attracted some interest and there have been two randomized studies, one from Australia [68] and one from Scotland [69], demonstrating that an explanatory letter sent prior to the dispatch of the screening test kit increases uptake by almost 10%.

Another important issue is the uptake of colonoscopy after a positive faecal occult blood test. Unlike the screening invitation itself, this does not appear to be strongly associated with either gender or deprivation [47] although, unsurprisingly, geographical remoteness does appear to have an adverse effect [70]. In Scotland, an evaluation of telephone assessment rather than a face-to-face meeting after a positive FOBT demonstrated a marked increase in uptake of colonoscopy [71]. This was presumably related to the fact that a telephone interview was more convenient than travelling to an assessment clinic, and it would appear that once contact with a health professional has been made, people are much more willing to go ahead with colonoscopy.

Adverse effects of screening

Faecal occult blood testing itself is, of course, without hazard but colonoscopy and, to a lesser extent, flexible sigmoidoscopy have the potential to create morbidity and even mortality. In addition to this, testing for blood in faeces is inevitably associated with false negative results and this leads to the development of interval cancers, defined as cancers that are diagnosed after a negative screening test in the interval between that test and the next test date. There is a concern that a negative test result can falsely reassure people to such an extent that they may choose to ignore symptoms and this in turn may lead to diagnostic delay – the so-called 'certificate of health effect'.

This issue has been studied by an analysis of interval cancers in the Scottish gFOBT Programme, which found that, of all cancers diagnosed in the screened population, interval cancers comprised 31.2% in the first round, 47.7% in the second, and 58.9% in the third [72]. Reassuringly, in all three rounds, both overall and cancer specific survival were significantly better for patients diagnosed with interval cancers when compared to an age and sex matched population within Scotland that had not been offered screening [72]. This indicates that interval cancers have a relatively good prognosis when compared with cancers arising in a similar population that has not been offered screening, but it does not detract from the observation that with gFOBT screening, high interval cancer rates occur.

Two other observations from this study have significant implications for gFOBT screening. Firstly, the proportion of both right-sided and rectal cancers was significantly higher amongst those with interval cancers when compared to those with screen-detected or non-screened cancers. Secondly, it was found that the percentage of cancers arising in women was significantly higher in the interval cancer group, when compared with either the screen-detected or the non-screened groups. Thus, it would appear that gFOBT screening tends to miss cancers in both the right side of the colon and the rectum, and it preferentially detects cancers in men rather than women. This gender effect appears to be due to the fact that faecal occult blood testing is less sensitive for cancer in women than in men and in a recent study using a quantitative FIT test, it has been shown that faecal haemoglobin concentrations are higher in men than in women [73]. This begs the question of whether or not differential cut-offs should be employed for male and female participants.

The issue of the effect of screening on 'all cause' mortality has created some controversy recently [74] and it has been suggested that screening programs should be assessed on the basis of their effect on this parameter rather than on disease-specific mortality. It must be appreciated, however, that because colorectal cancer accounts for only 2% of all deaths, a 15% reduction in disease-specific mortality, as demonstrated at the Nottingham study, would only be expected to reduce overall mortality by 0.3%. To demonstrate an effect of this size would require a randomized trial that would be prohibitively large.

One frequently quoted analysis of the Nottingham randomized study found 'all cause' mortality to be increased in the group offered screening [75], but it should be emphasised that this finding was statistically non-significant and likely to be a chance finding.

Finally, there has been some concern over whether or not to investigate patients with false positive FOBT results. To examine this issue, a cohort of 238 FOBT positive cases from the Nottingham study who had a normal colonoscopy were followed up for a median period of five years [76]. Five percent had undergone a gastrointestinal endoscopy because of symptoms and two were found to have gastric cancer. The asymptomatic individuals did not present with serious disease. It would, therefore, appear that if there are no gastrointestinal symptoms, upper gastrointestinal endoscopy is not required after a false positive gFOBT test. This was confirmed by a study carried out in Aberdeen, where a cohort of individuals being screened underwent upper gastrointestinal endoscopy immediately after a negative colonoscopy. In this study, no significant neoplastic pathology was found in the upper gastrointestinal tract [77].

The economics of screening

Analysis of the cost effectiveness of screening has to take into account the sensitivity and specificity of the test, the uptake, the cost of testing and subsequent investigations, differential costs of treating early and late disease, and the possibility of over-diagnosis. A recent study commissioned by the English Bowel Cancer Screening Programme compared various strategies involving both faecal occult blood testing and FS [78]. The conclusion was that, for willingness to pay, thresholds of less than £10,000 per QALY once-only FS at age 60 resulted in the greatest expected benefit. On the other hand, for willingness to pay thresholds greater than £10,000, flexible sigmoidoscopy at age 60 followed by biennial FOBT screening up until the age of 70 resulted in the greatest benefit. The authors also stressed that, when compared with a policy of 'no screening', all approaches involving either flexible sigmoidoscopy or FOBT screening could be expected to produce health gains at an acceptable cost. This model was, however, associated with considerable uncertainty, particularly around population uptake of FS. When FIT and gFOBT were considered, using data derived from a study in France, where 20,322 individuals aged between 50 and 74 performed both FIT and gFOBT, it was concluded that FIT at a cut-off of 75 ng Hb/ml would be more cost effective than gFOBT [79]. In another study, taking into account the rising costs of chemotherapy for advanced colorectal cancer, it was estimated that gFOBT, FIT, and a combination of FS and gFOBT would be cost saving [80], although this was less certain for colonoscopy. These results were based on US data, but would probably be applicable worldwide.

The consensus from economic studies of colorectal cancer screening is that all existing strategies have the potential to confer benefit at a reasonable cost and may indeed be cost saving. This does, however, depend on adequate uptake of screening and appropriate quality control of both the screening test and subsequent investigations.

Novel approaches to screening

Currently, faecal testing for blood and lower gastrointestinal endoscopy are the only credible strategies for colorectal cancer screening, but this may change in the near future. DNA markers in stool have been investigated and a DNA panel involving the measurement of 21 separate mutations in K-RAS APC and P53 genes, as well as the detection of BAT26 and long DNA, has been developed and compared with various forms of faecal occult blood test screening [81]. Although this approach appears to perform somewhat better than tests for faecal blood, it has not been developed into a test that is suitable for population screening. Other approaches that look promising include the measurement of DNA methylation specific RNAs and specific protein panels that are associated with colorectal cancer [76]. In a relatively recent systematic review, it was noted that promising results were reported for assays based on proteomics.

Techniques such as SELDI-TOF and MALDI-TOF mass spectography for proteins including soluble C82. However, current evidence tends to be restricted to small numbers of studies, with limited sample size and further external validation is awaited. One exception is the Septin 9 DNA methylation assay, which has been shown in initial studies to be associated with a sensitivity for colorectal cancer of over 70% while maintaining a specificity of over 90% [83]. It is not clear, however, whether this approach has a viable role in population screening. Finally, a group of Japanese workers have carried out some interesting work where a Labrador retriever was trained to detect colorectal cancer by smelling the breath and watery stool of colorectal cancer patients and controls [84]. Impressive sensitivity (91%) and specificity (99%) were achieved by this approach, suggesting that the detection of cancer specific volatile organic compounds may be important for the development of new colorectal screening tests.

Conclusions

It is clear from the original randomized trials of gFOBT screening, which early detection of colorectal cancer is associated with, improved outcomes and colorectal cancer screening has been embraced enthusiastically worldwide. Although gFOBT screening is being overtaken by more sophisticated quantitative FIT tests and, indeed by endoscopic screening, it is no longer essential to carry out population based randomized trials with a group that is not offered screening. The results achieved by the randomized trials can be used as benchmarks, whereby new screening modalities can be evaluated. In order to achieve this, it is important to standardize the key performance indicators for colorectal cancer screening on an international basis and, through the international colorectal cancer screening network, this is now being achieved [85].

MULTIPLE-CHOICE QUESTIONS

1 Guaiac based faecal occult blood testing is:
- **A.** Specific for human haemoglobin
- **B.** Based on the detection of peroxidase
- **C.** Employs immunochemical technology
- **D.** Has a clinical sensitivity for colorectal cancer of 90%
- **E.** In population screening is associated with an uptake of less than 20%

2 Colonoscopy screening:
- **A.** Has been shown to be associated with a reduction in colorectal cancer incidence
- **B.** Has been tested in population-based randomized control trials
- **C.** Is associated with an uptake of over 70%
- **D.** Is effective in reducing the incidence of right-sided cancer
- **E.** Has been shown to be cost effective in a population screening context

3 Uptake of colorectal cancer screening is:
- **A.** Higher in men than in women
- **B.** Falls with increasing deprivation
- **C.** Higher with endoscopic screening than with faecal occult blood test screening
- **D.** Not affected by endorsement by General Practitioners
- **E.** Not be modified by pre-notification

References

1 Cancer Research Campaign. *Cancer Stats*: *Cancer Worldwide*, September 2011.
2 Cancer Research Campaign. *Cancer Stats*: *Large bowel cancer – UK*, June 2006.

3 Jellema P, van der Windt DAWM, Bruinvels DA, et al. Value of symptoms and additional diagnostic tests for colorectal cancer in primary care; systematic review and meta-analysis. *BMJ* 2010; 340: c1269. doi:10.1136/bmj.c1269.
4 Ahmed S, Leslie A, Thaha M, Carey FA, Steele RJC. Lower gastrointestinal symptoms do not discriminate for colorectal neoplasia in a faecal occult blood screen-positive population. *Br J Surg* 2005; 92: 478–81.
5 Winawer SJ, Zauber AG, Fletcher AG, et al. Guidelines for colonoscopy surveillance after polypectomy: a consensus update by the US Multi-Society Task Force on colorectal cancer and the American Cancer Society. *Gastorenterology* 2006; 130: 1872–85.
6 Wilson JM, Jungner F. Principles and practice of screening for disease. *Public Health Papers No. 34.* Geneva WHO 1968.
7 IGN (Scottish Intercollegiate Guidelines Network). Diagnosis and management of colorectal cancer. Edinburgh: SIGN; 2011 (SIGN publication no.126) [December 2011]. Available from: *http://www.sign.ac.uk*
8 Leslie A, Carey FA, Pratt NR, Steele RJC. The colorectal adenoma-carcinoma sequence. *Br J Surg* 2002; 89: 845–60.
9 Young GP, Macrae FA, St John DJB. Clinical methods for early detection: basis, use and evaluation. In: Young GP, Rozen P, Levin B (eds), *Prevention and Early Detection of Colorectal Cancer*, WB Saunders, London 1996.
10 Pignone M, Campbell MK, Carr C, Phillips C. Meta-analysis of dietary restriction during faecal occult blood testing. *Eff Clin Pract* 2001; 4: 150–6.
11 Mandel JS, Bond JH, Church JR, Snover DC, Bradley GM, Schuman LM, et al. Reducing mortality from colorectal cancer by screening for faecal occult blood. *N Engl J Med* 1993; 328: 1365–71.
12 Mandel JS, Church TR, Bond JH, Ederer F, Geisser MS, Mongin SJ, et al. The effect of fecal occult-blood screening on the incidence of colorectal cancer. *N Engl J Med* 2000; 343: 1603–7.
13 Hardcastle JD, Chamberlain JO, Robinson MHE, Moss SM, Amar SS, Balfour TW, et al. Randomized controlled trial of faecal occult blood screening for colorectal cancer. *Lancet* 1996, 348: 1472–7.
14 Scholefield JH, Moss S, Mangham CM, Whynes DK, Hardcastle JD. Nottingham trial of faecal occult blood testing for colorectal cancer: a 20-year follow-up. *Gut* 2012; 61: 1036–40. doi: 10.1136/gutjnl-2011-300774.
15 Robinson MHE, Thomas WM, Hardcastle JD, Chamberlain J, Mangham CM. Change towards earlier stage at presentation of colorectal cancer. *Br J Surg* 1993; 80: 1610–12.
16 Scholefield JH, Robinson MH, Mangham CM, Hardcastle JD. Screening for colorectal cancer reduces emergency admissions. *Eur J Surg Oncol* 1998; 24: 47–50.
17 Kronborg O, Fenger C, Olsen J, Jorgensen OD, Sondergaard O. Randomised study of screening for colorectal cancer with faecal occult blood test. *Lancet* 1996; 348; 1467–71.
18 Jorgensen OD, Krongborg O, Fenger C. A randomised study of screening for colorectal cancer using faecal occult blood testing: results after 13 years and seven biennial screening rounds. *Gut* 2002; 50: 29–32.
19 Faivre J, Dancourt V, Lejeune C, Tazi MA, Lamour J, Gerard D, et al. Reduction in colorectal cancer mortality by fecal occult blood screening in a French controlled study. *Gastroenterology* 2004; 126: 1674–80.

20 Lindholm E, Brevinge H, Haglind E. Survival benefit in a randomised clinical trial of faecal occult blood screening for colorectal cancer. *Br J of Surg* 2008; 95: 1029–36.

21 Hewitson P, Glasziou P, Watson E, Towler B, Irwig L. Cochrane systematic review of colorectal cancer screening using the faecal occult blood test (hemoccult): an update. *Am J Gastroenterol* 2008; 103: 1541–9.

22 Steele RJC, Parker R, Patnick J et al. A demonstration pilot for colorectal cancer screening in the United Kingdom: a new concept in the introduction of health care strategies. *J Med Screen* 2001; 8: 197–202.

23 UK Colorectal Cancer Screening Pilot Group. Results of the first round of a demonstration pilot of screening for colorectal cancer in the United Kingdom. *BMJ* 2004; 329: 133–5.

24 Steele RJC, McClements PL, Libby G, Black R, Morton C, Birrell J, et al. Results from the first three rounds of the Scottish demonstration pilot of FOBT screening for colorectal cancer. *Gut* 2009; 58: 530–5.

25 Logan RFA, Patnick J, Nickerson C, et al. Outcomes of the Bowel Cancer Screening Programme (BCSP) in England after the first 1 million tests. *Gut* 2012; 61: 1439–46. doi: 10.1136/gutjnl-2011–300843.

26 Fraser CG, Matthew CM, Mowat NAG, Wilson JA, Carey FA, Steele RJC. Immunochemical testing of individuals positive for guaiac faecal occult blood test in a screening programme for colorectal cancer: an observational study. *Lancet Oncol* 2006; 7: 127–31.

27 Fraser CG, Digby J, McDonald PJ, Strachan JA, Carey FA, Steele RJC. Experience with a two-tier reflex gFOBT/FIT strategy in a national bowel screening programme. *J Med Screen* 2012; 19: 8–13.

28 Guittet L, Bouvier V, Mariotte N, et al. Comparison of a guaiac based and an immunochemical faecal occult blood test in screening for colorectal cancer in a general average risk population. *Gut* 2007; 56: 210–14.

29 Van Rossum LG, van Rijn AF, Laheij RJ, et al. Random comparison of guaiac and immunochemical fecal occult blood tests for colorectal cancer in a screening population. *Gastroenterology* 2008; 135: 82–90.

30 Hol L, Wilschut JA, van Ballegooijen M, van Vuuren AJ, van der Valk H, Reijerink JCIY, et al. Screening for colorectal cancer: random comparison of guaiac and immunochemical faecal occult blood testing at different cut-off levels. *Br J Cancer* 2009; 100: 1103–10.

31 Levi Z, Rozen P, Hazazi R, Vilkin A, Waked A, Maoz E, et al. A quantitative immunochemical fecal occult blood test for colorectal neoplasia. *Ann Internal Med* 2007; 146: 244–55.

32 Brenner H, Haug U, Hundt S. Sex differences in performance of fecal occult blood testing. *Am J Gastroenterol* 2010; 105: 2457–64.

33 Omata F, Shintani A, Isozaki M, Masuda K, Fujita Y, Fukui T. Diagnostic performance of quantitative fecal immunochemical test and multivariate prediction model for colorectal neoplasms in asymptomatic individuals. *Eur J Gastroenterology & Hepatology* 2011, 23: 1036–41.

34 Zorzi M, Fedato C, Grazzini G, et al. High sensitivity of five colorectal screening programmes with faecal immunochemical test in the Veneto Region, Italy. *Gut* 2011; 60: 944–9.

35 Chen L-S, Yen AM-F, Chiu S Y-H, Liao C-S, Chen H-H. Baseline faecal occult blood concentration as a predictor of incident colorectal neoplasia: longitudinal follow-up of a Taiwanese population-based colorectal cancer screening cohort. *Lancet Oncol* 2011; 12: 551–8. doi: 10.1016/S1470-2045(11)70101-2.
36 Van Roon AHC, Goede SL, van Ballegooijen M, van Vuuren AJ, Looman CWN, et al. Random comparison of repeated faecal immunochemical testing at different intervals for population-based colorectal cancer screening. *Gut* 2013; 62: 409–15. doi: 10.1136/gutjnl-2011-301583.
37 Atkin WS, Edwards R, Wardle J, Northover JM, Sutton S, Hart AR, et al. Design of a multicentre randomised trial to evaluate flexible sigmoidoscopy in colorectal cancer screening. *J Med Screen* 2001; 8: 137–44.
38 Segnan N, Armaroli P, Bonelli L, Risio M, Sciallero S, Zappa M, et al. and the SCORE Working Group. *JNCI* 2011; 193: 1310–22.
39 Atkin WS, Edwards R, Kralj-Hans I, et al. Once-only flexible sigmoidoscopy screening in prevention of colorectal cancer: a multicentre randomised controlled trial. *Lancet* 2010; 375: 1624–33.
40 Hoff G, Grotmol T, Skovlund E, Bretthauer M, for the Norwegian Colorectal Cancer Prevention Group. Risk of colorectal cancer seven years after flexible sigmoidoscopy screening: randomised controlled trial. *BMJ* 2009; 338: b1846.
41 Hol L, van Leerdam ME, van Ballegooijen M, et al. Screening for colorectal cancer: a randomised trial comparing guaiac-based and immunochemical faecal occult blood testing and flexible sigmoidoscopy. *Gut* 2010; 59: 62–8.
42 Hol L, de Jonge V, van Leerdam ME, et al. Screening for colorectal cancer: comparison of perceived test burden of guaiac-based faecal occult blood test, faecal immunochemical test and flexible sigmoidoscopy. *Eur J Cancer* 2010; 46: 2059–66.
43 Segnan N, Senore C, Andreoni B, et al. Comparing attendance and detection rate of colonoscopy with sigmoidoscopy and FIT for colorectal cancer screening. *Gastroenterology* 2007; 132: 230.
44 Robb K, Power E, Kralj-Hans I, Edwards R, Vance M, Atkin W, et al. Flexible sigmoidoscopy screening for colorectal cancer: uptake in a population-based pilot programme. *J Med Screen* 2010; 17: 75–8.
45 Gray M. Screening sigmoidoscopy: a randomised trial of invitation style. *Health Bulletin* 2000; 58: 137–40.
46 McCaffery Wardle J, Nadel M, Atkin W. Socioeconomic variation in participation in colorectal cancer screening. *J Med Screen* 2002; 9: 104–8.
47 Steele RJC, Kostourou I, McClements P, Watling C, Libby G, Weller D, et al. Effect of gender, age and deprivation on key performance indicators in a FOBT based colorectal screening programme. *J Med Screen* 2010; 17: 68–74.
48 Hol L, Kuipers EJ, van Ballengooijen M, van Vuuren AJ, Reijerink JCIY, Habbema DJF, et al. Uptake of faecal immunochemical test screening among nonparticipants in a flexible sigmoidoscopy screening programme. *Intl J Cancer* 2012; 130: 2096–102.
49 Senore C, Ederle A, Benazzato L, Arrigoni A, Silvani M, Fantin A, et al. Offering people a choice for colorectal cancer screening. *Gut* 2013; 62: 735–40. doi: 10.1136/gutjnl-2011-301013.
50 Rex DK, Cutler CS, Lemmel GT et al. Colonoscopic miss rates of adenomas determined by back-to-back colonoscopies. *Gastroenterology* 1997; 112: 24–8.

51 Pickhardt PJ, Choi JR, Hwang I, Butler JA, Puckett ML, Hildebrand HA, et al. Computed tomographic virtual colonoscopy to screen for colorectal neoplasia in asymptomatic adults. *N Engl J Med* 2003; 349: 2191–200.
52 Zauber AG, Winawer SJ, O'Brien MJ, Landsdorp-Vogelaar I, van Ballegooijen M, Hankey BF, et al. Colonoscopic polypectomy and long-term prevention of colorectal-cancer deaths. *N Eng J Med* 2012; 366: 687–96.
53 Regula J, Rupinski M, Kraszewska E, Polkowski M, Pachlewski J, Orlowska J, et al. Colonoscopy in colorectal-cancer screening for detection of advanced neoplasia. *N Eng J Med* 2006; 355: 1863–72.
54 Kaminski M F, Regula J, Kraszewska E, Polkowski M, Wojciechowska U, M, Rupinski M, et al. Quality indicators for colonoscopy and the risk of interval cancer. *N Engl J Med* 2012; 362: 1795–803.
55 Muller AD, Sonnenberg A. Protection by endoscopy against death from colorectal cancer. A case-control study among veterans. *Arch Intern Med* 1995; 155: 1741–8.
56 Segnan N, Senore C, Andreoni B, Azzoni A, Bisanti L, Cardelli A, et al. and the SCORE3 Working Group – Italy. *Gastroenterology* 2007; 132: 2304–12.
57 Baxter NN, Goldwasser MA, Paszat LF, Saskin R, Urbach DR, Rabeneck L. Association of colonoscopy and death from colorectal cancer. *Ann Intern Med* 2009; 150: 1–8.
58 Brenner H, Hoffmeister M, Arndt V, Stegmaier C, Altenhofen L, Haug U. Protection from right- and left-sided colorectal neoplasms after colonoscopy: population-based study. *JNCI* 2010; 102: 89–95.
59 Singh H, Nugent Z, Demers AA, Kliewer EV, Mahmud SM, Bernstein CN. The reduction in colorectal cancer mortality after colonoscopy varies by site of the cancer. *Gastroenterology* 2012; 139: 1128–37.
60 Stoop EM, de Haan MC, de Wijkerslooth TR, Bossuyt PM, van Ballegooijen M, Nio CY, et al. Participation and yield of colonoscopy versus non-cathartic CT colonography in population-based screening for colorectal cancer: a randomised controlled trial. *Lancet Oncol* 2012; 13: 55–64.
61 Von Wagner C, Baio G, Raine R, Snowball J, Morris S, Atkin W, et al. Inequalities in participation in an organised national colorectal cancer screening programme: results from the first 2.6 million invitations in England. *Intl J Epidem* 2011; 40: 712–8. doi: 1093/ije/dyr008.
62 Von Euler-Chelpin M, Brasso K, Lynge E. Determinants of participation in colorectal cancer screening with faecal occult blood testing. *J Public Health* 2009; 32: 395–405.
63 Steele RJC, Kostourou I, McClements P, Watling C, Libby G, Weller D, et al. Effect of repeated invitations on uptake of colorectal cancer screening using faecal occult blood testing: analysis of prevalence and incidence screening. *BMJ* 2010: 341: c5531. doi:10.1136/bmj.c5531.
64 Young GP, St John DJB, Cole SR, Bielecki BE, Pizzey C, Sinatra MA, et al. Prescreening evaluation of a brush-based faecal immunochemical test for haemoglobin. *J Med Screen* 2003; 10: 123–8.
65 Tinmouth J, Ritvo P, McGregor SE, Claus D, Pasut G, Myers RE, et al. A qualitative evaluation of strategies to increase colorectal cancer uptake. *Can Fam Physician* 2011; 57: e7–15.
66 Zajac IT, Whibley AH, Cole SR, Byrne D, Guy J, Morcom J, et al. Endorsement by the primary care practitioner consistently improves participation in screening for colorectal cancer: a longitudinal analysis. *J Med Screen* 2010; 17: 19–24.

67 Hewitson P, Ward AM, Heneghan C, Halloran SP, Mant D. Primary care endorsement letter and a patient leaflet to improve participation in colorectal cancer screening: results of a factorial randomised trial. *Br J Cancer* 2011; 105: 475–80.

68 Cole SR, Smith A, Wilson C, Turnbull D, Esterman A, Young GP. An advance notification letter increases participation in colorectal cancer screening. *J Med Screen* 2007; 14: 73–5.

69 Libby G, Bray J, Champion J, Brownlee LA, Birrell J, Gorman DR, et al. Pre-notification increases uptake of colorectal cancer screening in all demographic groups: a randomized controlled trial. *J Med Screen* 2011: 18: 24–9.

70 Dupont-Lucas C, et al. Socio-geographical determinants of colonoscopy uptake after faecal occult blood test. *Dig Liver Dis* 2011; 43: 714–20. doi: 10:1016/j.dld.2011.03.003.

71 Rodger J, Steele RJC. Telephone assessment increases uptake of colonoscopy in a FOBT colorectal cancer-screening programme. *J Med Screen* 2008; 15: 105–7.

72 Steele RJC, McClements P, Watling C, Libby G, Weller D, Brewster DH, et al. Interval cancers in a FOBT-based colorectal cancer population screening programme: implications for stage, gender and tumour site. *Gut* 2012; 61: 576–81.

73 MacDonald PJ, Strachan JA, Digby J, Steele RJC, Fraser CG. Faecal haemoglobin concentrations by gender and age: implications for population-based screening for colorectal cancer. *Clin Chem Lab Med* 2011; 50: 935–40. doi: 10.1515/CCLM.2011.815.

74 Steele RJC, Brewster D. Should we judge cancer screening programmes by their effect on total mortality rather on cancer specific mortality? *BMJ* 2011; 343: 938–9 (d6397).

75 Black WC, Haggstrom DA, Welch HG. All-cause mortality in randomised trials of cancer screening. *JNCI* 2002; 94: 167–73.

76 Thomas WM, Hardcastle JD. Role of upper gastrointestinal investigations in a screening study for colorectal neoplasia. *Gut* 1990; 31: 1294–7.

77 Hisamuddin K, Mowat NAG, Phull PS. Endoscopic findings in the upper gastrointestinal tract of faecal occult blood-positive, colonoscopy-negative patients. *Dig Liver Dis* 2006; 38: 503–7.

78 ScHARR. Colorectal cancer screening options appraisal. *Report to the English Bowel Cancer Screening Working Group*, September 2004.

79 Berchi C, Guittet L, Bouvier V, Launoy G. Cost-effectiveness analysis of the optimal threshold of an automated immunochemical test for colorectal cancer screening. *Intl J Tech Assess Health Care* 2010; 26: 48–53.

80 Lansdorp-Vogelaar I, van Ballegooijen M, Zauber AG, Habbema JDF, Kuipers EJ. Effect of rising chemotherapy costs on the cost savings of colorectal cancer screening. *JNCI* 2009; 101: 1412–22.

81 Duffy MJ, van Rossum LGM, van Turenhout ST, Malminiemi O, Sturgeon C, Lamerz R, et al. Use of faecal markers in screening for colorectal neoplasia: a European group on tumor markers position paper. *Intl J Cancer* 2011: 3–11.

82 Hundt S, Haug U, Brenner H. Blood markers for early detection of colorectal cancer: a systematic review. *Biomarkers Prev* 2007; 16: 1935–53.

83 Grützmann R, Molnar B, Pilarsky C, Habermann JK, Schlag PM, Saeger HD, et al. Sensitive detection of colorectal cancer in peripheral blood by Septin 9 DNA methylation assay. *Plos One* 2008; 3: e3759.

84 Sonoda H, Kohnoe S, Yamazato T, et al. Colorectal cancer screening with odour material by canine scent detection. *Gut* 2011; 60: 814–9. doi:10.1136/gut2010.218305.

85 Benson VS, Atkin WS, Green J, Nadel MR, Patnick J, Smith RA, et al. on behalf of the International Colorectal Cancer Screening Network. Toward standardizing and reporting colorectal cancer screening indicators on an international level: the International Colorectal Cancer Screening Network. *Int. J. Cancer* 2012; 130: 2961–73.

ANSWERS TO MULTIPLE-CHOICE QUESTIONS

1 B
2 A
3 B

CHAPTER 3

Management of adenomas

Sunil Dolwani[1], Rajvinder Singh[2], Noriya Uedo[3] & Krish Ragunath[4]

[1] *Cardiff University School of Medicine, Cardiff, Wales*

[2] *University of Adelaide, Adelaide, Australia*

[3] *Osaka Medical Center for Cancer and Cardiovascular Diseases, Osaka, Japan*

[4] *Nottingham University Hospitals NHS Trust, Nottingham, UK*

KEY POINTS

- Assessment of colonic polyps benefits from a structured approach using the Paris classification for overall morphology and assessment of surface structure after contrast dye staining using the Kudo pit patterns or electronic enhancement of capillary vascular patterns
- Careful assessment of polyps facilitates diagnosis of depth of involvement and consequent potential risk of lymph node involvement
- Depressed type lesions (Paris type IIc), Non-Granular laterally spreading polyps, and Kudo type V pit pattern may indicate an advanced lesion
- Thick stalked pedunculated polyps have a higher risk of post-polypectomy bleeding and benefit from pre-treatment of the stalk
- The Non-Lifting sign during attempted endoscopic mucosal resection (EMR) may indicate deep submucosal invasion or submucosal fibrosis due to previous biopsy or diathermy
- Large sessile or flat polyps may be resected piecemeal by EMR but carry a 10–15% risk of recurrence of adenoma, which with further treatment reduces overall recurrence to below 5%

Introduction

Adenomas account for the vast majority of polyps resected in the colon that are thought to be precursor lesions for colorectal cancer. Appropriate management of colonic adenomas potentially reduces the incidence of colorectal cancer [1]. This chapter will focus on the detection, accurate characterization, and appropriate resection of colonic adenomas.

Colorectal Cancer: Diagnosis and Clinical Management, First Edition. Edited by John H. Scholefield and Cathy Eng.

Detection

Colonoscopy is the current gold standard test to detect colonic polyps, though radiological modalities such as CT Colonography (CTC) have been shown to achieve high levels of detection of colonic polyps. However, CTC continues to have limitations in detection of polyps with a flat morphology with a size of more than 5 mm [2], as well as being a purely diagnostic modality in overall management of adenomas. Chromoendoscopy or the use of contrast dye has been demonstrated to improve the detection of colorectal adenomas as compared to standard white light colonoscopy [3]. Recent advances in optical imaging have resulted in high definition colonoscopy that can obtain clear views of the colon, thereby detecting subtle mucosal abnormalities. In addition, other electronic image enhancement techniques, such as Narrow Band Imaging (NBI), Autofluorescence imaging (AFI), I-scan, and Flexible Spectral Imaging Color Enhancement (FICE), are being evaluated to enhance adenoma detection. However, at present there is no clear evidence of any advantage over standard white light colonoscopy [4] for detection of adenomas, although they do seem to confer some advantage in accurate characterization of polyps [5]. Good bowel preparation has proven to be a significant factor and key to any advanced imaging technique being successful. In addition, other interventions such as patient position change, routine retroversion in the rectum, and adequate colonoscope withdrawal time of ≥6 minutes can also improve adenoma detection [6].

Characterization

Accurate characterization of polyps is crucial to appropriate further management. This is ideally performed in a systematic manner, initially with assessment of morphology in a standardized description, as outlined in the Paris classification, followed by a more detailed assessment of surface architecture including granularity (smooth or nodular) and the Kudo pit pattern (KPP). Chromoendoscopy (dye spray) using indigocarmine or methylene blue is used to aid this. In addition, the vascular patterns can be assessed with some of the newer electronic image enhancement techniques described. The aim of lesion characterization is to differentiate neoplastic from non-neoplastic lesions, outline the margins of the lesion accurately in order to plan the most appropriate method of removal, estimate the probability of deep submucosal invasion and or lymph node involvement (based on morphological and surface architectural characteristics), and assist in decision making for removal.

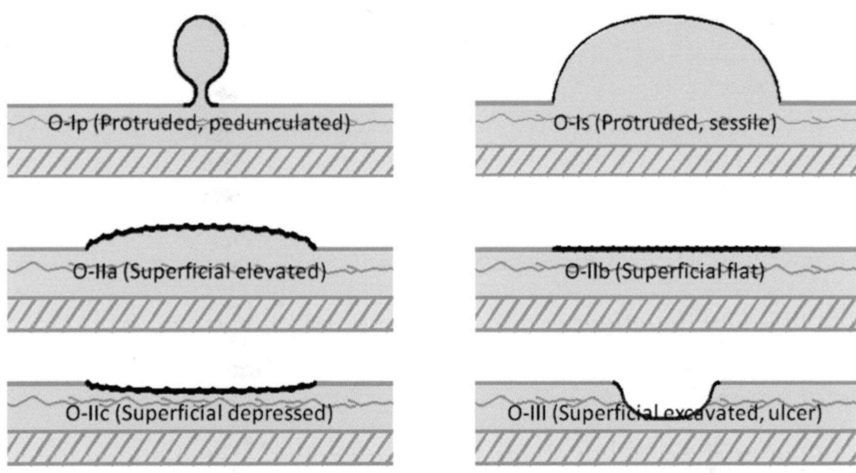

Figure 3.1 The Paris classification of polyp morphology.

Lesion assessment – morphology

A. Paris classification

The Paris classification (Figure 3.1) is especially important, not only for standardization but also allows the endoscopist to predict the risk of submucosal invasion [7].

Polyps can be divided into:

1 **Protruding lesions**
   a) Ip (pedunculated)
   b) Is (sessile) ≥2.5 mm in height from the base of the polyp (surrounding mucosa)

2 **Flat lesions**
   a) Type IIa: Slightly elevated (<2.5 mm in height)
   b) Type IIb: True flat lesion
   c) Type IIc: Mildly depressed lesion

The 2.5 mm limit is used to differentiate sessile (Is) from flat (0–IIa) lesions and approximates the diameter of a closed biopsy forceps.

3 **Excavated lesions**
   a) Type III: ulcerated

Flat colorectal lesions account for 56% of all colorectal polyps [8], while depressed lesions are less frequent, occurring in up to only 1.2% of all polyps [9]. Excavated lesions (ulcerated) are rare but almost always represent invasive cancer. However, the prevalence of high grade dysplasia (HGD) or invasive cancer increases as the lesion becomes more depressed. In Rembacken's landmark study, up to 59% of all Paris type IIc lesions harbored HGD and half of all flat and depressed lesions demonstrated submucosal invasion (SMI) [10].

Relatively large colorectal lesions (measuring >20 mm in size) account for approximately 4% of all polyps (11), although, to some extent, this does depend on the population or cohort under study. However, size of the lesion alone does not necessarily appear to matter when lesions are assessed for submucosal invasion. In a recent ongoing multi-center Australian study, looking at large sessile lesions measuring more than 20 mm, submucosal invasion was detected in 33 of 680 polyps. The mean size of these polyps was 37 mm in comparison to 35 mm when no submucosal invasion was detected ($p = 0.53$) [12].

B. Granularity

Flat lesions of more than 20 mm should be further evaluated based on the granularity of the surface. They can be divided into granular (G), non-granular (NG), or a mixed pattern containing both morphologies (Figures 3.2A and B). The surface of G lesions appears ragged, nodular, and almost polypoid, whereas NG lesions are smooth. The NG lesions in combination with flat and depressed Paris type IIc morphology compared to granular, flat non-depressed Paris type IIa morphology, tend to have a relative risk of 54.0 for SMI [12].

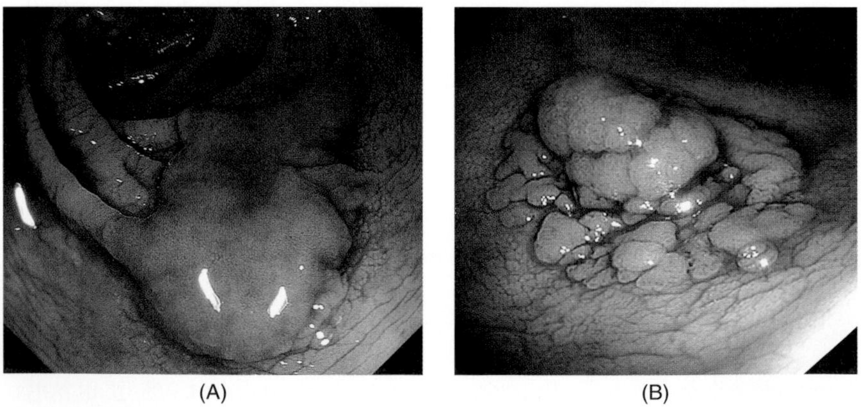

Figure 3.2 (A) Smooth laterally spreading polyp; and (B) granular laterally spreading polyp.

Lesions assessment – surface architecture

A. Kudo pit pattern

Shin ei Kudo introduced the Kudo pit pattern (KPP) classification in his seminal paper in 1994 (13). Some of the commonly used dyes include Indigo carmine (0.2%–0.5%), which is a surface contrast agent; Methylene blue (2 mls in 40–50 mls of water), a dye which is absorbed actively into the mucosa; or crystal violet (0.2%: 10 mls in 40 mls of water), which is generally used in exceptional cases where pit pattern type V needs to be defined further. The KPP is best visualized subsequent to washing off all debris and mucous and application of contrast dye with aspiration of excess dye (Figure 3.3) [14].

Briefly the KPP classification can be divided into:

1 Type I: Pits appear round- normal colonic mucosa
2 Type II: Pits appear star-like or onion-skin-like – hyperplastic polyps
3 Type III: Elongated pits – adenomas
4 Type IV: Cerebriform pits – adenomas
5 a) Type V_I: Irregular (I) asymmetrical pits indicating malignancy confined to the mucosa (suitable for endoscopic resection)
   b) Type V_N: Pit patterns disappears, non-structured (N) or 'structure less' – advanced or signifying invasive cancer (surgery)

Subramanian et al. looked at more than 27,000 polyps in 30 studies comparing the accuracy of standard white light endoscopy, chromoendoscopy,

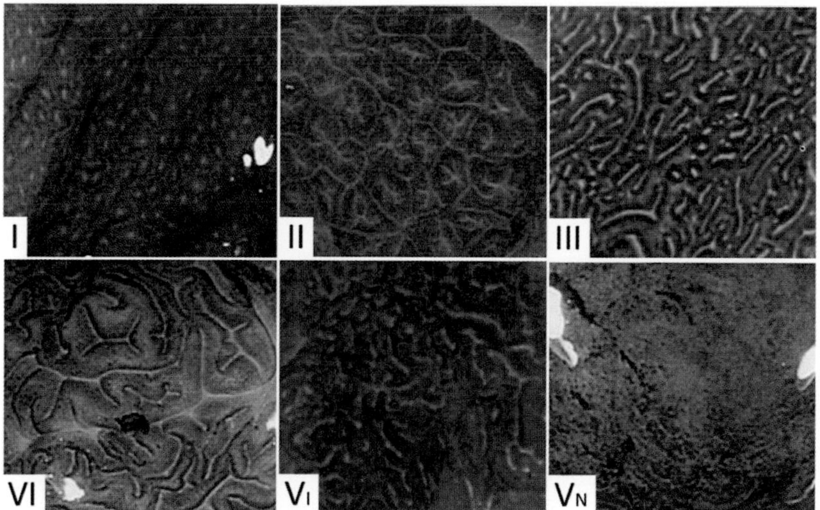

Figure 3.3 The Kudo pit pattern classification of polyps.

white light endoscopy with magnification, chromoendoscopy with magnification, and NBI with magnification in the prediction of colorectal polyp histology [15]. The authors found that using chromoendoscopy and NBI, both with optical magnification, was the most effective method in predicting polyp histology resulting in an area under the ROC of more than 0.90.

B. Electronic chromoendoscopy

Some of the electronic chromoendoscopy techniques widely available now include Narrow Band Imaging (NBI, Olympus), I scan (Pentax), or the Flexible Spectral Imaging Color Enhancement (FICE, Fujinon). All these imaging modalities can assist in defining the micro-vascular architecture in colorectal polyps, although they differ in their mechanism of optical characterization (Pre-image processing for NBI and Post Image acquisition for I-scan and FICE). There have been numerous classifications utilized, which at times can be confusing. With NBI, the modified Sano's classification appears to be the most 'user friendly' (Figure 3.4) [16;17]:

1 Type I: absent cn (hyperplastic polyp),
2 Type II: regular cn present, surrounding mucosal glands (adenoma)
3 Type IIIA: high density cn with tortuosity and lack of uniformity (intramucosal cancer)
4 Type IIIB: nearly avascular cn (invasive cancer)

In a preliminary feasibility study, the sensitivity (Sn), specificity (Sp), positive (PPV), and negative predictive values (NPV) in differentiating neoplastic from non-neoplastic lesions with high confidence was 98%, 89%, 93%, and 97%, respectively, while the Sn, Sp, PPV, and NPV in predicting endoscopic resectability (type II, IIIa vs. type I, IIIb) was 100%, 90%, 93%, and 100%, respectively (18). The interobserver agreement between assessors (k value) was also substantial at 0.89.

A pragmatic approach before polypectomy

The step-by-step methodological approach described above can often aid in the characterization of colorectal polyps before a decision is made to proceed onto endoscopic resection. This includes assessing the lesion where the gross morphology is determined using the Paris classification and the granularity followed by assessing the pit pattern and if possible (and available) the vasculature using some of the newer electronic chromoendoscopy techniques. Consideration must also be given to the location of the polyp, the ease of access to the lesion, and the manoeuvrability of the colonoscope, as well as

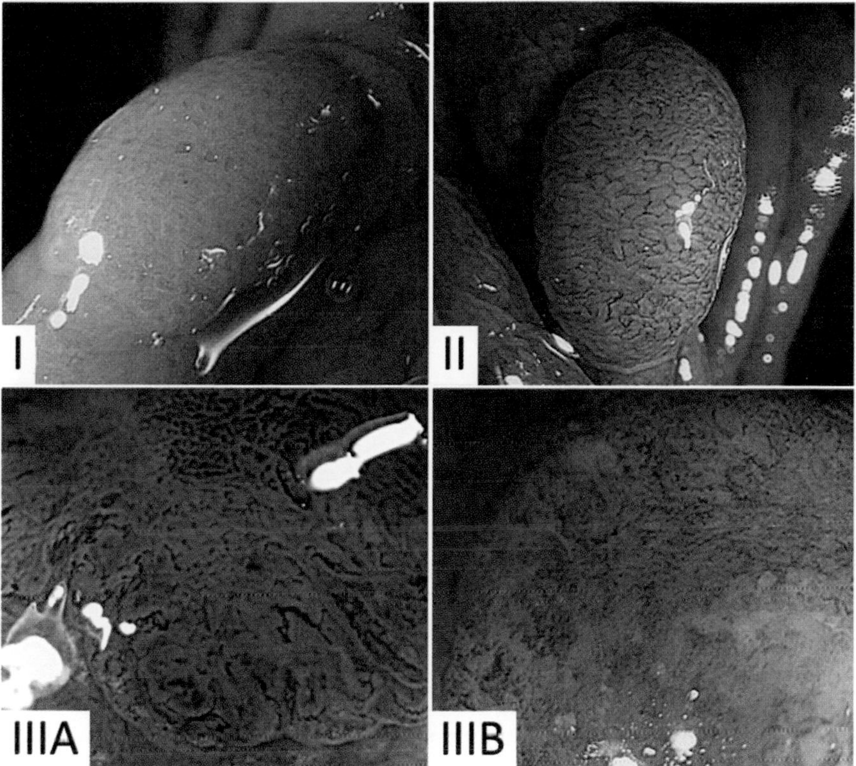

Figure 3.4 The NBI modified Sano classification of polyps.

previous attempts at resection before resection is performed. An assessment of potential risk of resection through an endoscopic approach versus alternative surgical approaches, bearing in mind the above factors as well as others such as thickness of the stalk of a pedunculated polyp and location of the polyp at flexures or in a peri appendiceal location, is essential to plan strategy as well as obtain informed consent from the patient.

Technique for resection of diminutive (<5 mm) and small polyps (6–10 mm in size)

Most diminutive polyps, unless exhibiting morphological appearances of advanced lesions as described above, may be removed with cold biopsy or cold snare, though some prefer to use hot biopsy forceps in the left colon. We would not recommend the use of hot biopsy forceps in the right colon, due to the potential risk of conduction of heat diathermy and unnoticed diathermy injury in a relatively thin walled structure. While it is interesting to note that cold biopsy, even when targeted precisely, may not remove all adenomatous tissue, this has not resulted in any demonstrable difference in outcomes for diminutive polyps [19]. For small polyps up to 1 cm in size, the preferred modalities would seem to be hot snare polypectomy if pedunculated, and EMR if sessile or flat, as described above, as this has the greatest chance of complete resection.

Technique for resection of larger pedunculated polyps

Pedunculated polyps, particularly those with a thick stalk or pedicle, need consideration of the risk of post-polypectomy bleeding and may thus need pre-treatment of the stalk to reduce or avoid this risk. Pre-treatment modalities include use of clips, loops, and/or adrenaline prior to polypectomy. Important considerations during snare polypectomy are:

- familiarity with diathermy settings depending on location, size, and type of polyp (some operators prefer to use greater coagulation current or effect size in blended current during polypectomy of thick stalked polyps);
- distance from the head of the polyp or margin or adenomatous tissue, in order to achieve complete resection balanced against the risk of resection of the stalk too low or in proximity to a clip or loop, which can result in greater diathermy injury;
- strategy in case of complications such as post polypectomy bleeding in an area of difficulty, such as a narrow segment of sigmoid diverticular disease.

Technique of EMR for resection of larger sessile and flat lesions

The technique of EMR involves injection of fluid in the submucosal layer, in order to lift mucosal lesions away from the muscle layer in the colonic wall. The submucosal injection solution is often saline or a mixture of saline and a contrast dye with or without adrenaline for smaller lesions, though more often a more viscous fluid is mixed with a contrast dye and often very dilute adrenaline to achieve a longer lasting lift [20], particularly for larger lesions. This technique is much safer as it enables a better grip of the snare onto the lesion, in effect converting flat lesions into more elevated areas as well as moving the lesion and plane of resection away from the muscle layer – the usual plane of resection being in the superficial submucosal layer. Larger lesions (>20 mm) may need a piecemeal resection, as attempting to remove these *en bloc* does increase the risk of complications.

The principles of large piecemeal resection of colonic polyps are to resect starting from a margin and resect in continuity without leaving residual islands of adenomatous tissue. Excellent results have been achieved in terms of overall success for complete resection and relatively low complication rates even for quite large lesions. However, the recurrence rates for EMR of lesions larger than 20 mm in size that are removed piecemeal are usually between 10 and 15% and, though subsequent procedures and further endoscopic intervention reduce this to below 5%, overall this may need consideration during counselling and planning for such procedures. It may also be extremely difficult to achieve accurate histopathological characterization of lesions removed piecemeal, due to the fragmented nature of the specimen, unless painstakingly mapped and pieced together prior to sending to the laboratory. The non-lifting sign, when the lesion does not appear to lift despite apparently accurate injection within the submucosal plane, may indicate deeper invasion and or a degree of submucosal fibrosis such as that due to previous diathermy or biopsy, which usually makes subsequent attempts at endoscopic removal more difficult. Due to some of the above, endoscopic submucosal dissection (ESD) has been proposed as a modality for *en bloc* resection of these larger and often more complex lesions.

Endoscopic submucosal dissection (ESD) for colorectal lesions

As the endoscopic submucosal dissection (ESD) technique has primarily been used widely in Japan, the best results are from Japanese centers, though careful case selection and training in selected European and American centers has resulted in slower adoption throughout the world. The ESD technique consists of recognition of the tumor boundary with chromoendoscopy (Figure 3.5A) injection of a solution around the lesion (Figure 3.5B); mucosal incision outside the lesion with an electrosurgical knife inserted through working channel of an endoscope (Figure 3.5C); additional injection into the submucosa underneath the lesion to achieve sufficient mucosal elevation; submucosal dissection with the electrosurgical knife (Figures 3.5D and E); and retrieval of the specimen (Figure 3.5F). The great advantage of ESD over EMR is

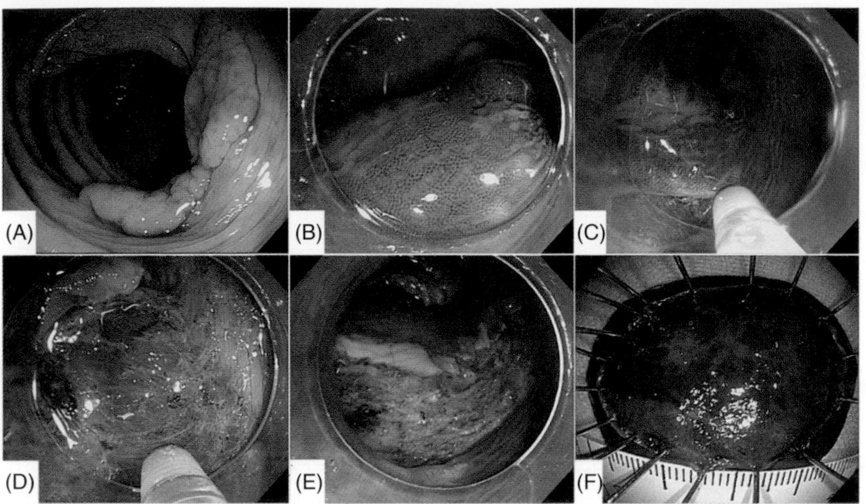

Figure 3.5 (A) to (F) ESD of a flat polyp in the colon.

enablement of achieving high *en bloc* resection rate for even large sessile and flat tumors. The Japanese large-scale data of 1111 procedures showed 88% of *en bloc* resection rate with a mean (±SD) tumor size of 35 ± 18 mm [21]. It allows not only complete removal of the tumors but also full pathological evaluation of the histological type, depth of tumor invasion, presence of lymphatic and venous involvement, and tumor involvement to the horizontal (mucosal) and vertical (submucosal) margins. Drawbacks of ESD include requirement of high expertise, long procedure time, and relatively high complication rate. However, refinement in techniques and equipment is likely to improve outcomes [22]. ESD may offer an important alternative to surgery in the therapy of large sessile and flat polyps [23].

Complications and follow-up

The majority of complications become apparent during or immediately post-resection of the polyp, though it is important for patients, endoscopists, and departments to be aware of the small but potentially significant risks of delayed complications, sometimes up to two weeks after the procedure. The two major complications are bleeding and perforation, with rates of these varying widely, depending on the cohorts studied and types of lesions as well as operator expertise. These are usually quoted as 5–10% for bleeding during polypectomy or EMR of lesions greater than 3 cm in size and 0.5–1.0%

for perforation [24]. Follow-up is extremely important and surveillance often determined by histology, nature of resection (piecemeal vs. *en bloc*), and size and number of polyps [25].

Characteristics and surveillance of advanced adenomas

Most studies agree that on the basis of outcome and management, advanced adenomas are defined as greater than 1 cm in size, having a significant villous component on histology and high grade dysplasia on biopsy or resection specimen histology. Data from the National Polyp study and other similar cohorts also indicate that individuals with greater than three concurrent adenomas have a relatively higher risk of further metachronous lesions and therefore require closer follow-up.

Serrated colorectal polyps

In recent years there has been increasing recognition of polyps with 'serrated' histology that seem to follow an alternative pathway to colorectal cancer. The prevalence and detection of these seems variable and possibly at least partly dependent on the quality of colonoscopy [26]. There may be an increased prevalence of these sessile serrated polyps in the proximal colon and they are more commonly associated with a 'flat' morphology as compared to conventional adenomas. Certain features, such as the presence of a mucus cap overlying the surface of the polyp, make them difficult to detect as well as define the surface morphology. Contrast enhancement, either digital or with dye, is often helpful in detection. Though studies in this area have largely been retrospective and in different settings, there is general agreement that serrated polyps may contribute to the development of interval colorectal cancers post colonoscopy [27;28]. Despite there being agreement regarding the need for their removal at colonoscopy due to the malignant potential, recommendations on surveillance are currently uncertain at best [29]. There is also recognition of the syndrome of serrated polyposis with specific criteria for diagnosis. Individuals with hyperplastic or serrated polyposis and their first-degree relatives are at increased risk for colorectal cancer. The two major WHO criteria for diagnosis are:

1. either greater than 20 such polyps throughout the colon; or
2. at least 5 hyperplastic or serrated polyps in the proximal colon with two ≥10 mm in size [30].

Multiple polyps or polyposis syndrome

A pertinent issue in clinical practise is when a colonoscopist should consider the possibility of an underlying polyposis syndrome in the absence of an obviously suggestive family history when faced with multiple colorectal polyps (most often adenomas). There is a reasonable degree of consistency in the phenotype of syndromes, such as classical familial adenomatous polyposis (FAP), with often hundreds to thousands of carpeting and easily recognizable polyps [31]. However a fairly wide variation in the numbers of polyps associated with other syndromes, such as Attenuated FAP (AFAP) and MutYH associated polyposis (MAP), may make the diagnosis difficult. As a broad guide, consideration must be given to the possibility of an underlying polyposis syndrome in the presence of greater than 10 colorectal adenomas or the diagnosis of synchronous or metachronous colorectal cancer, particularly if diagnosed at a relatively young age. Due to the recessive inheritance in the case of MAP, the classical dominant history of involved family members in every generation may not be obtained and an effort should be made to elicit a history of multiple polyps or early onset cancer in siblings [32]. Input from Cancer Genetics services with corroboration of detailed family history is usually of benefit. In many such cases a discussion with the patient is required regarding the need for surgery either prophylactically or in order to manage long-term complications once the diagnosis has been clarified. Current evidence also suggests that in specific individuals and families, a program of surveillance of the upper gastrointestinal tract as well as extra-intestinal sites may be required [33].

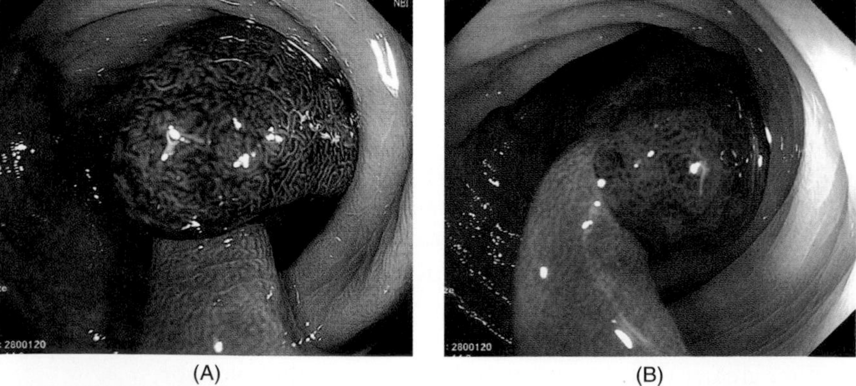

Figure 3.6 Case study.

CASE STUDY AND MULTIPLE-CHOICE QUESTIONS

Case

A 75-year-old gentleman undergoes colonoscopy for symptoms of altered bowel habit. A large polyp was noted in the sigmoid colon (Figures 3.6A and B).

Question 1

With regard to the endoscopic management of a thick stalked polyp all the following statements may be true except?

A. There is an increased risk of post-polypectomy bleeding

B. Polypectomy should be performed after pre-injection of the stalk with adrenaline

C. The stalk may be pre-clipped prior to polypectomy to reduce incidence of complications

D. The deployment of an endo-loop around the stalk often makes subsequent polypectomy safer

E. Use of pure cutting current at high wattage is the safest technique for polypectomy in this situation

Question 2

The Paris classification of this polyp is:

A. Paris 0-IIa

B. Paris 0-Ip

C. Paris 0-Is

D. Paris 0-IIb

E. Paris 0-IIc

Question 3

The histo-pathological correlation of this type of pit pattern is usually:

A. Tubular adenoma

B. Villous adenoma

C. Hyperplastic polyp

D. Carcinoma with deep invasion

E. Serrated adenoma

References

1 Zauber AG, Winawer SJ, O'Brien MJ, et al. Colonoscopic polypectomy and long-term prevention of colorectal cancer deaths. *N Engl J Med* 2012; 366: 687–96.

2 Heresbach D, Djabbari M, Riou F, et al. Accuracy of computed tomographic colonography in a nationwide multicentre trial, and its relation to radiologist expertise. *Gut* 2011; 60: 658–65.

3 Brown SR, Baraza W. Chromoscopy versus conventional endoscopy for the detection of polyps in the colon and rectum. *Cochrane Database Syst Rev* 2010; (10) Review.
4 Dinesan L, Chua TJ, Kaffes AJ. Meta-analysis of narrow band imaging versus conventional colonoscopy for adenoma detection. *Gastrointest Endosc* 2012; 75: 604–11.
5 Wada Y, Kashida H, Kudo SE, et al. Diagnostic accuracy of pit pattern and vascular pattern analyses in colorectal lesions. *Dig Endosc* 2010; 22: 192–9.
6 Barclay RL, Vicari JJ, Greenlaw RL. Effect of a time dependant colonoscopic withdrawal protocol on adenoma detection during screening colonoscopy. *Clin Gastroenterol Hepatol* 2008; 6: 1091–8.
7 Endoscopic Classification Review Group. Update on the Paris Classification of superficial neoplastic lesions in the digestive tract. *Endoscopy* 2005; 37: 570–8.
8 Rex DK, Helbig CC. High yields of small and flat adenomas with high definition colonoscopes using either white light or narrow band imaging. *Gastroenterology* 2007; 133: 42–7.
9 Soetikno RM, Kaltenbach T, Rouse RV, et al. Prevalence of nonpolypoid (flat and depressed) colorectal neoplasms in asymptomatic and symptomatic adults. *JAMA* 2008; 299: 1027–1035.
10 Rembacken BJ, Fujii T, Cairns A, et al. Flat and depressed colonic neoplasms: a prospective study of 1000 colonoscopies in the UK. *Lancet* 2000; 355: 1211–14.
11 Kudo SE, Lambert R, Allen J, et al. Non polypoid neoplastic lesions of the colorectal mucosa. *Gastrointest Endosc* 2008; 68: 4: S3–47.
12 Moss A, Bourke MJ, Williams SJ, et al. Endoscopic mucosal resection outcomes and prediction of submucosal cancer from advanced colonic mucosa. *Gastroenterology* 2011; 140: 1909–18.
13 Kudo S, Hirota S, Nakajima T, et al. Colorectal tumours and pit patterns. *J Clin Pathol* 1994; 47: 880–5.
14 Singh R, Owen V, Shonde A, et al. White Light Endoscopy, Narrow Band Imaging and Chromoendoscopy with magnification in diagnosing colorectal neoplasia. *World J Gastrointest Endosc* 2009; September 15; 1: 45–50.
15 Subramaniam V, Mannath J, Hawkey CJ, et al. Utility of Kudo Pit Pattern for Distinguishing adenomatous from non-adenomatous colonic lesions *in vivo*: meta analysis of different endoscopic techniques. *Gastrointest Endosc* 2009; 69(5): AB277.
16 Ikematsu H, Matsuda T, Emura F, et al. Efficacy of capillary pattern type IIIA / IIIB by magnifying narrow band imaging for estimating depth of invasion of early colorectal neoplasms. *BMC Gastroenterol* 2010; 10: 33.
17 Singh R, Kaye PV, Ragunath K. Distinction between neoplastic and non-neoplastic colorectal polyps utilizing Narrow Band Imaging with magnification: A novel technique to increase the efficacy of colorectal cancer screening? *Scand J Gastroenterol* 2008; 43: 380–1.
18 Singh R, Nordeen N, Mei SL, et al. West meets East: Preliminary results of Narrow Band Imaging with optical magnification in the diagnosis of colorectal lesions: A multicentre Australian study using the modified Sano's classification. *Dig Endosc* 2011; 23(Suppl 1), 126–30.
19 Froehlich F. Is cold biopsy forceps resection of diminutive polyps really so inadequate? *Endoscopy* 2011; 43: 1015.
20 Turner J, Green J, Dolwani S. Use of Gelofusine for endoscopic mucosal resection. *Gut* 2010; 59: 1446–47.
21 Saito Y, Uraoka T, Yamaguchi Y, et al. A prospective, multicenter study of 1111 colorectal endoscopic submucosal dissections (with video). *Gastrointest Endosc* 2010; 72: 1217–25.

22 Takeuchi Y, Uedo N, Ishihara R, et al. Efficacy of an endo-knife with a water-jet function (Flushknife) for endoscopic submucosal dissection of superficial colorectal neoplasms. *Am J Gastroenterol.* 2010; 105: 314–22.
23 Kiriyama S, Saito Y, Yamamoto S, et al. Comparison of endoscopic submucosal dissection with laparoscopic-assisted colorectal surgery for early-stage colorectal cancer: a retrospective analysis. *Endoscopy* 2012; 44: 1024–30.
24 Chukmaitov A, Bradley CJ, Dahman B, Siangphoe U, Warren JL, Klabunde CN. Association of polypectomy techniques, endoscopist volume, and facility type with colonoscopy complications. *Gastrointest Endosc* 2013; 77:436–46.
25 Cairns SR, Scholefield JH, Steele RJ, et al. Guidelines for colorectal cancer screening and surveillance in moderate and high risk groups (update from 2002). *Gut* 2010; 59: 666–89.
26 Kahi CJ, Hewett DG, Norton D, Eckert G, Rex D. Prevalence and variable detection of proximal colon serrated polyps during screening colonoscopy. *Clin Gastroenterol Hepatol* 2011; 9: 42–6.
27 Schreiner M, Weiss D, Lieberman D. Proximal and large hyperplastic and non-dysplastic serated polyps detected by colonoscopy are associated with neoplasia. *Gastroenterology* 2010; 139: 1497–502.
28 Cooper GS, Xu F, Barnholtz-Sloan JS, Schluchter M, Koroukian S. Prevalence and predictors of interval colorectal cancers in Medicare beneficiaries. *Cancer* 2012; 118: 3044–52.
29 Rex D, Ahnen D, Baron J, et al. Serrated lesions of the colorectum: review and recommendations from an expert panel. *Am J Gastroenterol* 2012; 107: 1315–29.
30 Rosty C, Buchanan D, Walsh M, et al. Phenotype and polyp landscape in serrated polyposis syndrome: a series of 100 patients from genetics clinics. *Am J Surg Pathol* 2012; 36: 876–82.
31 Jass JR. Colorectal polyposis: from phenotype to diagnosis. *Pathol Res Pract* 2008; 204: 431–47.
32 Sampson J, Dolwani S, Jones S, et al. Autosomal recessive colorectal adenomatous polyposis due to inherited mutations of MYH. *Lancet* 2003; 362: 39–41.
33 Vasen HF, Moslein G, Alonso A, et al. Guidelines for the clinical management of familial adenomatous polyposis (FAP). *Gut* 2008; 57: 704–13.

ANSWERS TO CASE STUDY AND MULTIPLE-CHOICE QUESTIONS

1 E
2 B
3 B

PART 2

Histopathology

CHAPTER 4

How histopathology affects the management of the multidisciplinary team

Dipen Maru

Department of Pathology, and Translational Molecular Pathology, The University of Texas MD Anderson Cancer Center, Houston, TX, USA

KEY POINTS

- Invasion into submucosa or beyond is necessary for diagnosing invasive adenocarcinoma in the colorectum.
- Appropriate pathological staging of colorectal carcinoma requires knowledge of anatomical variations in different segments of the colon and rectum, meticulous examination of specimens, and effective communication with clinicians.
- Histological sub-typing is important to select appropriate adjuvant chemotherapy and to predict microsatellite instability status in colorectal cancer.
- Histopathological response to neoadjuvant chemotherapy in rectal cancer and hepatic colorectal metastases is a strong predictor of patient outcome and increasingly becoming a valid endpoint for biomarker assessment.

CASE STUDY

An 84-year-old woman without a significant family history of cancer underwent colonoscopy due to blood in her stool. An exophytic mass in the right colon was detected by colonoscopy. Her metastatic work-up was negative. She underwent right hemicolectomy. There was a 4 × 4 × 3 cm mass in the right colon with grossly positive lymph nodes in pericolic soft tissue. The histopathology review showed adenocarcinoma with variegated histology with mucinous and signet ring cell differentiation, an undifferentiated carcinoma component, and increase in intraepithelial lymphocytosis. Tumor cells extended up to the serosa and 16 of 32 regional lymph nodes were positive for metastatic adenocarcinoma. The tumor showed lymphovascular and extensive perineural invasion.

Colorectal Cancer: Diagnosis and Clinical Management, First Edition. Edited by John H. Scholefield and Cathy Eng.

Criteria of malignancy

Colorectal adenocarcinoma arises from an adenomatous polyp or flat dysplasia on a background of inflammatory bowel disease. High grade dysplasia in an adenomatous polyp has higher likelihood of progression to invasive adenocarcinoma. Invasion of the lamina propria and muscularis mucosae is almost never associated with regional lymph node metastases in colorectal cancer and invasion into or beyond the submucosa is required to diagnose invasive adenocarcinoma. Due to a very low likelihood of lymph node metastases with intramucosal carcinoma, high grade dysplasia and intramucosal carcinoma can be used interchangeably as carcinoma *in situ*. It can be challenging to diagnose submucosal invasion in an endoscopic biopsy or a polypectomy sample. Presence of desmoplasia, association of highly dysplastic glands without lamina propria associated with thick walled blood vessels, and ulceration are the findings indicative of submucosal invasion in a biopsy or polypectomy specimens of colorectal cancer. In biopsy samples, where all these features are not present, correlation of the pathological findings in a multidisciplinary setting, with endoscopic and other clinical findings, will clarify whether a repeat biopsy is necessary. If the lesion is an exophytic/ulcerated mass strongly suspicious of adenocarcinoma by endoscopy, a repeat biopsy may not be required to document unequivocal submucosal invasion. A repeat biopsy may be required to document submucosal invasion if the lesion is clinically and endoscopically indeterminate.

A polypectomy/endoscopic mucosal resection is routinely used for initial treatment of early (T1) adenocarcinoma. Presence of poorly differentiated histology, lymphovascular invasion, and distance of the deep margin of less than 1 mm are associated with a higher likelihood of regional lymph node metastases in these tumors. The College of American Pathologist requires these three parameters to be included in the pathology report on the polypectomy specimens [1].

Pathology Staging

Staging of colorectal cancer was first described by Dr Duke in 1932. This was based on depth of tumor infiltration into various layers of the colorectal wall, regional lymph node involvement, and distant metastasis. Subsequently Modified Astler Collins and Tumor (T), Node (N), and Metastasis (M) staging systems were developed based on the principles of the Duke System. The first

Table 4.1 Pathologic staging (pTNM) of colorectal carcinoma as per the guidelines of the AJCC 7th edition staging system.

Primary tumor (T):
TX: Primary tumor cannot be assessed
T0: No evidence of primary tumor
Tis: Carcinoma *in situ*, intraepithelial, or invasion of lamina propria
T1: Tumor invades submucosa
T2: Tumor invades muscularis propria
T3: Tumor invades through the muscularis propria into pericolorectal tissues
T4a: Tumor penetrates to the surface of visceral peritoneum (applicable to peritonealized segment of large bowel, including cecum, sigmoid colon, transverse colon, and anterolateral surface of ascending, descending colon, and upper rectum
T4b: Tumor directly invades or is adherent to other organs or structures (presence of tumor cells and not fibrosis or mucin in the adherent organ is required)

Regional lymph nodes (N):
NX: Regional lymph nodes cannot be assessed
N0: No regional lymph node metastasis
N1: Metastasis in 1–3 regional lymph nodes
N1a: Metastasis in one regional lymph node
N1b: Metastasis in 2–3 regional lymph nodes
N1c: Tumor deposit (s) in subserosa, mesentery, non-peritonealized pericolic, or perirectal tissues without regional lymph node metastasis
N2: Metastasis in 4 or more regional lymph nodes
N2a: Metastasis in 4–6 regional lymph nodes
N2b: Metastasis in 7 or more regional lymph nodes

Distant metastasis (M):
M0: No distant metastasis
M1: Distant metastasis
M1a: Distant metastasis in one organ or site
M1b: Distant metastasis in more than one organ/site or peritoneum

pocketbook of Union for International Cancer Control (UICC) TNM was published in 1968. UICC and the American Joint Committee on Cancer (AJCC) joined together and published the 4th edition of the TNM staging book in 1987. Since then, TNM stage has been updated three times and the most recent 7th edition was published in 2010 (Table 4.1, Figure 4.1) [2]. The major changes included in the 7th edition are expansion of stage II and III categories, primarily due to subdivision of the T4 stage, introduction of the N1c category for satellite soft tissue tumor deposits with negative nodes, and expansion of the sub-classification of N and M stages based on the number of lymph nodes and sites of distant metastases involved. This expansion is supported by survival differences in these groups based on expanded outcome in SEER data

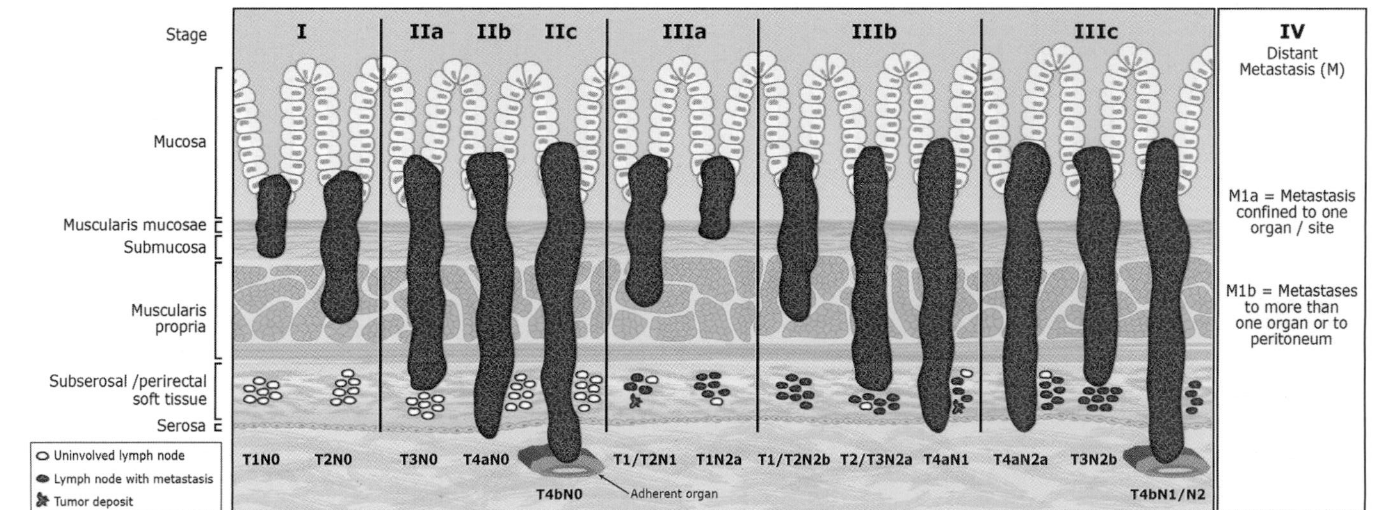

Figure 4.1 Diagram demonstrating layers of colorectal wall and pericolonic tissue with different T, N, and M stages, as per the AJCC/UICC 7th edition staging system for colorectal carcinoma.

analyses [3]. Figure 4.1 demonstrates various T, N, and M stages and their combination at the final pathological stage.

Appropriate pathology staging of the colorectal resection specimens requires that the pathologist or pathology assistant are familiar with anatomical variations in different segments of the colorectum and are meticulous in gross examination of the specimen, with particular focus on the extent of the tumor in the colorectal wall, distance from the resection margins, generous sampling for the regional lymph nodes, and are aware of unique situations such as tumor associated perforation, tumor extending into the adherent organ, multiple tumors, preoperative neoadjuvant therapy, and patients with polyposis or non-polyposis syndromes. Reviewing the clinical history, endoscopic findings, and operative notes makes it easier for the pathologist to identify, appropriately describe, and sample the tumor.

The serosal (visceral peritoneal) cover is variable in different segments of the colon and rectum. The cecum, transverse colon, and sigmoid colon are entirely intraperitoneal. The ascending colon, descending colon, and upper rectum are partly covered by the visceral peritoneum, with the posterior surface being retroperitoneal. The mid-rectum is covered by the peritoneum only anteriorly, with the lateral and posterior surfaces being retroperitoneal. The lower rectum is entirely retroperitoneal. These variations in the serosal covering influences the T stage of the tumor. A tumor present at the deep surface of the cecum, transverse colon, or sigmoid colon is classified as T4a. For tumors in the ascending colon, descending colon, or upper rectum, the tumor is classified as T3 if tumor cells are present at the deep surface (non-peritonealized surface) posteriorly, and T4a if tumor cells are present at the deep surface (peritonealized surface) anteriorly. The lower rectum is entirely retroperitoneal and a tumor in the lower rectum is classified as T3 if tumor cells are present at the deep surface anteriorly or posteriorly. It is often difficult to differentiate peritonealized from non-peritonealized surfaces and the pathologist needs to identify these surfaces in every colorectal resection specimen and if necessary ask for input from the surgeon. It is critical to appropriately pT stage patients with stage II disease because patients with stage II pT4 disease are considered to be at high risk of disease recurrence and may be offered postoperative adjuvant therapy [4].

The pathology stage is the single most important guide in deciding on the postoperative chemotherapy in primary colon cancer, as all node positive (stage III) patients receive postoperative chemotherapy. Therefore it is critical to perform meticulous lymph node sampling and histopathology review. The AJCC recommends that at least 10–14 lymph nodes should be examined for carcinoma in a colon/rectal resection specimen. Since the N stage is dependent on the number of metastatic lymph nodes, and a higher number of negative lymph nodes predicts better survival, it is recommended to sample as many lymph nodes as possible. In specimens with more than one tumor, lymph nodes corresponding to each tumor should be sampled separately, with a minimum number of 10–14 for each tumor.

Tumor deposits in pericolonic and perirectal soft tissue, away from the leading edge of the tumor without residual lymph nodes, are classified as tumor deposits (TD). They either represent entirely replaced lymph nodes or large vessel or nerve invasion. They should be reported separately and in cases of the T stage being T1 or T2, the tumor deposits with negative regional lymph nodes are assigned to the N1c category.

An increasing number of patients with distant oligometastatic colorectal cancer are offered resection of the metastatic tumor. This is the standard practise for colorectal metastases to liver, lung, ovary, or non-regional lymph nodes. Due to this, the distant metastasis (M) category has been classified as M1a and M1b in the 7th edition of AJCC staging. M1a is designated to oligometastatic disease and M1b is designated as metastasis to more than one viscera or to peritoneal disease.

The staging system for residual tumor after neoadjuvant therapy or recurrent tumor at the anastomotic site is similar to a primary tumor, except the prefix *y* is applied to the former and prefix *r* is applied to the latter.

Resection margins

Circumferential resection margin (radial) corresponds to the surgically dissected non-perotinealized surface of the specimen. This includes the posterior surface of the ascending colon, descending colon, upper rectum, the posterior and lateral surface of mid-rectum, and all deep surfaces of the rectum. The distance of the tumor from the circumferential mesorectal margin is required to be included in the pathology report. The tumor cells at or within 1 mm of the circumferential mesorectal margin indicates this margin to be positive, with higher likelihood of local recurrence.

The mesenteric margin is relevant, particularly in segments of the colon that are entirely intraperitoneal. The mesenteric margin in these segments should be reported independently of serosal involvement. In other segments of the colon, the highest vascular pedicle, which is composed of neurovascular tissue and possibly lymph nodes, is critical. A metastatic lymph node or vascular invasion at the transected margin of highest vascular pedicle makes it an incomplete resection and so a higher risk of recurrence. This site should be marked by the surgeon with a stitch or other identifier and sampled in a separate tissue block.

The distance of the distal margin from the tumor is critical, particularly in lower rectal tumor resection specimens, in deciding the patient outcome and quality of surgery. In rectal tumors, it is recommended to have 2 cm between the tumor and the distal margin in the low anterior resection. A distance of 1 cm is acceptable in T1/T2 tumors.

In some cases of T4b colorectal cancers, there is a need for multivisceral resection. The latter poses a significant challenge for the pathologist in demonstrating extension of tumors in adherent organs and assessment of additional margins. Advanced lower rectal tumors can extend into the pelvic organs such as the prostate, urinary bladder, vaginal wall, and pelvic bone. This may be identified on preoperative imaging or intraoperatively. The pathology sampling is very much facilitated if the surgeon separately identifies the area/areas which are clinically most relevant, including the soft tissue margin and the site of intraoperative radiotherapy.

Resection specimens for anastomotic recurrence and regional lymph node recurrence are infrequent. Appropriate gross examination and sampling of these specimens require identifying the tumor location with the help of preoperative imaging. In cases of nodal recurrence, the radial/mesenteric margin can be important and should be marked and sampled for microscopy review.

Histological subtyping

The majority of colorectal adenocarcinomas are gland-forming well to moderately (low grade) differentiated adenocarcinomas. They are composed of large to intermediate size glands lined with columnar epithelium with stratified columnar or rounded nuclei with or without goblet cells. Many of these tumor show necrosis.

Most of the microsatellite instability high (MSI-H) colorectal cancers show unique histological features [7]. These tumors have variegated histology with a mixture of moderately differentiated adenocarcinomas, poorly differentiated adenocarcinomas, mucinous adenocarcinomas, carcinomas with dominant cribriform architecture, carcinomas with serrated architecture, signet ring cell adenocarcinomas, and undifferentiated medullary carcinomas. In some of these tumors only one of these components is seen (Figure 4.2). Intraepithelial lymphocytosis, defined as three or more per high power fields on Hematoxylin and eosin sections, is the most specific marker in predicting microsatellite instability (MSI) status in colorectal cancer [8] (Figure 4.3).

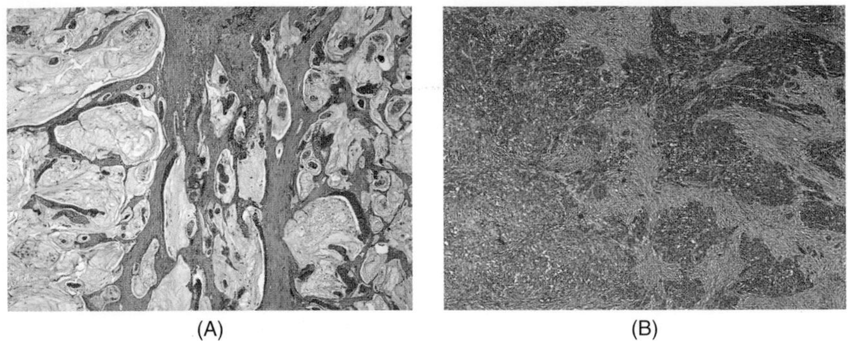

Figure 4.2 Histological features of microsatellite instability high colon cancer: (A) well to moderately differentiated mucinous adenocarcinoma; (B) poorly differentiated/ undifferentiated carcinoma.

Intraepithelial lymphocytosis is also present in adenomatous polyps from patients with hereditary non-polyposis colon cancer syndrome. Other histological features seen in the MSI-H colorectum are a pushing tumor border and an increase in peritumoral Crohn's-like lymphoid aggregates. Pathologists and clinicians should be aware of these unusual histological features of MSI-H colorectal cancer and not mistakenly diagnose them as metastatic carcinoma. These histological features should prompt clinicians to request

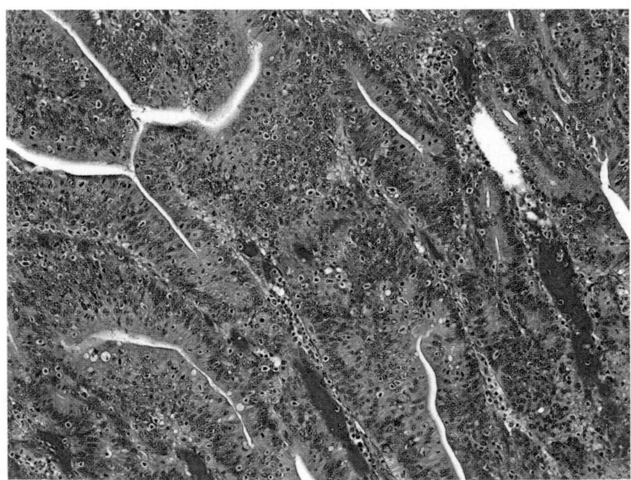

Figure 4.3 Marked intraepithelial lymphocytosis in microsatellite instability high colon cancer.

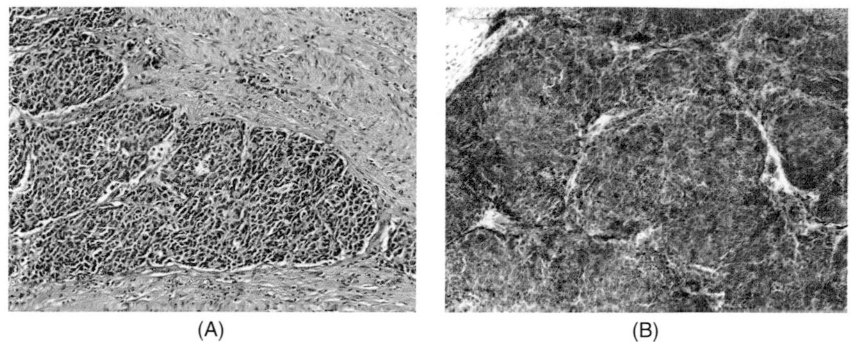

Figure 4.4 High-grade neuroendocrine carcinoma: (A) HE; and (B) Synaptophysin immunostaining.

immunohistochemistry and molecular testing of microsatellite instability to confirm or exclude unsuspected hereditary non-polyposis colon cancer syndrome or sporadic MSI-H colorectal cancer with *h-MLH1* promoter methylation.

High grade neuroendocrine carcinomas (Figure 4.4) are classified into small cell carcinomas and large cell neuroendocrine carcinomas. These tumors are more frequent in the rectum followed by the cecum and other parts of the colon. Similar to other sites, these tumors are aggressive, with 70% of patients presenting with distant metastases and 3-year survival being 13% [9]. In addition, due to rarity of these tumors, there is no consensus on type of chemotherapy agents to be used. Many oncologists prefer to use cisplatin and etoposide to treat this tumors. Data on high grade neuroendocrine carcinomas seen as a component of mixed adenocarcinomas and neuroendocrine carcinomas is very limited and at present these tumors are treated no differently from conventional adenocarcinomas.

Carcinomas with more than 50% signet ring cells are classified as signet ring cell adenocarcinomas. They are more frequently associated with MSI-H tumors and inflammatory bowel disease. In a biopsy specimen of the colorectum, signet ring cell histology should prompt the pathologist to consider these two associations. In addition, metastatic adenocarcinoma from the appendix, stomach, and lobular carcinoma of the breast should also show similar histological features and should be excluded by reviewing medical records and image findings, and if necessary by immunohistochemistry.

Adenocarcinomas with more than 50% mucinous component are classified as mucinous adenocarcinomas. Microsatellite stable well-differentiated mucinous adenocarcinomas are rare in the colon. They show similarities to appendiceal mucinous tumors in histology and pattern of spread within and beyond the colon wall. They are composed of abundant acellular mucin admixed with well differentiated mucinous epithelium. The pattern of invasion in the colonic wall shows abundant acellular mucin without any stromal reaction and sometimes it is difficult to differentiate them from colitis cystica profunda.

Other rare histological subtypes include serrated adenocarcinomas, carcinomas with cribriform architecture with comedo necrosis, micropapillary carcinomas, adenosqumaous carcinomas, and spindle cell carcinomas. Serrated adenocarcinomas are reported to be associated with the MSI-H phenotype with BRAF mutation and CpG island hypermethylation. Cribriform carcinomas with comedo necrosisare are reported to be of the microsatellite stable CpG island hypermethylator type. Adenocarcinomas with a micropapillary component are reported to have aggressive behavior, with high likelihood of regional lymph node metastases.

Histopathological response to neoadjuvant therapy

Tumor regression and tumor down staging after preoperative chemoradiotherapy are primary reasons for improvement in patient outcome and in achieving complete surgical resection in rectal cancer. Extensive sampling of the tumor is necessary to appropriately assess tumor regression. Table 4.2 shows the College of American Pathologists (CAP)/AJCC recommended four-tier grading system for assessing tumor regression rectal cancer [2].

Preoperative chemotherapy followed by liver resection is the standard of care in many patients with colorectal liver metastases. Resected colorectal liver metastases after preoperative chemotherapy are a relatively new addition to the type of specimens resected for colorectal cancer. For these specimens it is

Table 4.2 Tumor regression system of response to neoadjuvant chemoradiation in rectal cancer

TRG grade	Histological features
0 (complete response)	No viable cancer cells
1 (moderate response)	Single cells or small groups of cancer cells
2 (minimal response)	Residual cancer cells outgrown by fibrosis
3 (poor response)	Minimal or no tumor kill. Extensive residual cancer

necessary to report the number of tumor nodules, largest size of the tumor, and status of the margin. Pathological response to preoperative chemotherapy is one of the predictors of patient outcome in these patients and should be included in the pathology report [6].

Other histological prognostic factors

The histological grade has shown independent prognostic significance in multivariate analyses of colorectal cancer patients and should be reported in biopsy and resection specimens. The College of American Pathologists recommends a two-tier system of histological grading. Tumors with more than a 50% gland forming component are classified as low grade and tumors with less than a 50% gland forming component are classified as high grade.

Venous (large vessel) invasion is an independent predictor of patient outcome and distant (hepatic) metastases in the colorectum. Extramural venous invasion is particularly associated with a higher likelihood of distant metastases. Similar to large vessel invasion, invasion of small thin-walled vessels (lymphatic or post-capillary venules), and perineural invasion are independent predictors of poor prognosis. The challenge with interpretation of small vessel invasion is high inter-observer variations among pathologists. The recommended histological criteria in identifying lymphovascular invasion are rounded clusters of tumor cells identified in spaces lined with endothelium with cells adherent to the endothelium. Immunohistochemical stains of vascular markers (CD34, C31) to identify lymphovascular invasion are not recommended for routine use to confirm or exclude lymphovascular invasion.

Perforations at the tumor site or proximal to the tumor are associated with poor patient outcome. A perforated tumor is an indicator of a higher risk of recurrence in stage II colon cancer and patients with a perforated tumor may be considered for postoperative adjuvant chemotherapy [4]. Review of intraoperative findings and assessing the resected specimen for perforation before opening the specimen are the most effective ways to identify and sample the site of perforation. Histological findings indicative of perforation are transmural inflammation and necrosis with serositis.

In rectal resection specimens, quality of the mesorectal excision is one of major determinants of quality of surgery. The quality of mesorectal excision is assessed by examination of the bulk of the mesorectum and presence and depth of defects in the radial margin, and smoothness of the radial margin after serial sectioning of the rectum. Optimal assessment of mesorectal excision is performed if the surgeon and pathologist are in communication at the time of initial examination of the specimen.

Immunohistochemistry and role of histopathology in molecular analysis

Immunohistochemistry identifies the specific DNA mismatch protein, which is abnormally lost in *MSI-H* cancer (Figure 4.5), and further guides testing. Immunohistochemistry also contributes to sub-typing of the *MSI-H* colorectal cancer into hereditary or sporadic types. Most common mismatch repair genes lost in hereditary non-polyposis colon cancer syndrome due to germ line mutation are *MSH-2* and *MLH-1*. In sporadic *MSI-H* cancer, *MLH-1* is lost in almost all cases (Figure 4.5). The mechanism of loss of *MLH-1* in sporadic cancer is through promoter hypermethylation. Loss of *MLH-1* in sporadic colorectal cancer suggests additional testing for *h-MLH1* hypermethylation and *BRAF* mutation studies. *MSH-2* is diamerized with *MSH-6* and *MLH-1* is diamerized with PMS-2. This loss of *MSH-2* is associated with loss of *MSH-6*. However, *MSH-6* loss is not always associated with loss of *MSH-2*. Similarly, loss of *MLH-1* is associated with loss of *PMS-2* but not vice versa.

Immunohistochemistry and polymerase chain reaction (PCR)-based mircosatelillite, instability, have similar analytic sensitivity. However, neither of the two methods can identify all tumors with mismatch repair genes deficiency. In a very small percentage of cases with missense mutation, particularly for *MLH-1*, immunohistochemistry shows intact expression of

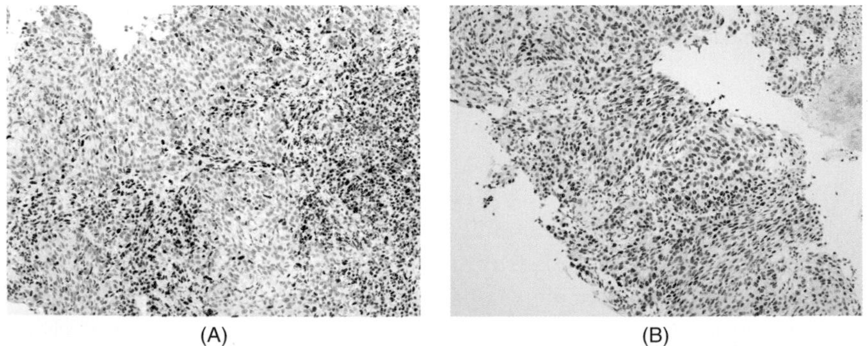

Figure 4.5 Immunohistochemistry staining showing loss of *MLH-1* nuclear expression in tumor cells with intact expression in inflammatory and other stromal cells and intact nuclear staining for *MSH-2* in tumor cells, inflammatory and other stromal cells.

MLH-1 due to intact antigenicity, but with microsatellite instability high tumor by PCR-based assay due to functional loss of *MLH-1*. False negative results are most likely due to technical issues with specimen fixation and staining technique. A patchy staining is common with *PMS-2* and *MSH-6*. A small subset of tumors with only in *MSH-6* loss is shown to be microsatellite stable.

Immunohistochemistry also helps in differential diagnosis of metastasis from primary colorectal cancer. In biopsy samples, metastasis from mullerian, upper gastrointestinal, and breast primaries can mimic colorectal cancer and should be excluded by clinical correlation and if necessary immunohistochemistry staining.

Histopathology is a critical pre-analytical step in various molecular tests performed on extracted nucleotides from the tissue samples. The advancement in molecular testing for clinical care demands that histopathology practise should be optimized for high-quality molecular testing. These require reduction of the ischemia time before the specimen is opened and fixed, appropriate fixation protocol, optimal quantization of tumor cells in a tissue block, and deciding the type of specimen required for molecular test. Tests such as microsatellite instability by PCR and loss of heterozygosity need tumor and normal control DNA. The latter can be procured from blood if normal tissue is not available.

TIPS AND TRICKS

- TNM staging as per the 7th edition of AJCC book has expanded T and N categories and it is important to know the variations in peritoneal covering of different segments of the colorectum.
- Microsatellite instability high colorectal cancers have unique histopathological features.
- Age and family history are very important in guiding the tests for microsatellite instability high colorectal cancers.

MULTIPLE-CHOICE QUESTIONS (Correct answer marked with *)

1 What is the pT and pN stage of this tumor, as per the 7th edition of the AJCC staging system?

A. pT4aN1b (IIIB)
B. pT4aN2b (IIIC)
C. pT4bN2a (IIIC)
D. pT4bN2b (IIIC)

2 Among the features described below, which feature is most sensitive in predicting microsatellite instability high status in colorectal cancer?

A. Signet ring cell histology
B. Mucinous histology
C. Increase in intraepithelial lymphocytosis
D. Right-sided tumor

3 The histological features described below suggest a possibility of microsatellite instability high colon cancer. Based on the clinical history provided, which group of laboratory findings are most likely present in this patient?

A. Immunohistochemistry for DNA mismatch repair genes shows loss of *MLH-1* with secondary loss of *PMS-2,* positive promoter methylation of *h-MLH1* gene, and *BRAFV600E* mutation
B. Immunohistochemistry for DNA mismatch repair genes shows loss of MLH-1 with secondary loss of PMS-2, due to germline mutation in *h-MLH-1* and negative *BRAFV600E* mutation
C. Immunohistochemistry for DNA mismatch repair genes shows loss of *PMS-2* with secondary loss of *MLH-1* and positive *BRAFV600E* mutation
D. Immunohistochemistry for DNA mismatch repair genes shows loss of *MSH-2* with secondary loss of *MSH*-6, positive promoter methylation of *h-MSH2*, and positive *BRAFV600E* mutation

4 Which of the following histopathological findings is seen in microsatellite instability high colon cancer?

A. Neuroendocrine carcinoma
B. Tumor budding
C. Peritumoral nodular lymphoid aggregates
D. Extensive perineural invasion

References

1 Washington K, Berlin J, Branton P, et al. Protocol for the examination of specimens from patients with primary carcinoma of the colon and rectum. Available from: *http://www.cap.org/apps/cap.portal*

2 *American Joint Committee on Cancer Staging Atlas,* 7th edn. New York: Springer; 2010: 140–3.

3 Gunderson LL, Jessup JM, Sargent DJ, et al. Revised TN categorization for colon cancer based on national survival outcomes data. *J Clin Oncol* 2010 Jan 10; 28(2): 264–71.

4 Benson AB 3rd, Schrag D, Somerfield MR, et al. American Society of Clinical Oncology recommendations on adjuvant chemotherapy for stage II colon cancer. *J Clin Oncol.* 2004 Aug 15; 22(16): 3408–19.

5 Sargent DJ, Marsoni S, Monges G, et al. Defective mismatch repair as a predictive marker for lack of efficacy of fluorouracil-based adjuvant therapy in colon cancer. *J Clin Oncol* 2010 Jul 10; 28(20): 3219–26.

6 Blazer DG 3rd, Kishi Y, Maru DM, et al. Pathologic response to preoperative chemotherapy: a new outcome end point after resection of hepatic colorectal metastases. *J Clin Oncol* 2008 Nov 20; 26(33): 5344–51.

7 Alexander J, Watanabe T, Wu TT, et al. Histopathological identification of colon cancer with microsatellite instability. *Am J Pathol* 2001 Feb; 158(2): 527–35.
8 Smyrk TC, Watson P, Kaul K, et al. Tumor-infiltrating lymphocytes are a marker for microsatellite instability in colorectal carcinoma. *Cancer* 2001 Jun 15; 91(12): 2417–22.
9 Bernick PE, Klimstra DS, Shia J, et al. Neuroendocrine carcinomas of the colon and rectum. *Dis Colon Rectum* 2004 Feb; 47(2): 163–9.

ANSWERS TO MULTIPLE-CHOICE QUESTIONS

1 B
2 C
3 A
4 C

PART 3

Surgical

CHAPTER 5

Radical colonic resection

Kenichi Sugihara[1], Yusuke Kinugasa[2] & Shunsuke Tsukamoto[2]

[1] *Department of Surgical Oncology, Graduate School, Tokyo Medical and Dental University, Tokyo, Japan*

[2] *Division of Colon and Rectal Surgery, National Cancer Center Hospital, Shizuoka, Japan*

KEY POINTS

- A tumor should be resected with draining of the lymphatics, lymph nodes, and blood vessels, through which the tumor may disseminate, by dissecting along embryologic tissue planes in an intact peritoneal and fascial lined package.
- D3 lymph nodes dissection comprises removal of epicolic nodes within 10 cm of the tumor margin, plus removal of the intermediate and main nodes.
- Laparoscopic surgery for colorectal cancer has the advantages of less pain, lower invasiveness, and better cosmetic outcomes, in addition to better postoperative recovery compared to open surgery. However, there may be no differences in survival rates between laparoscopic and open surgery.

Introduction

In radical surgery for colon cancer, first reports were from Reybard [1] on sigmoidectomy in 1844 and Maydl [2] on right hemicolectomy in 1885. Cheever [3], Grinnell [4], as well as Mayo [5], emphasized the significance and necessity of lymph node dissection. However, surgical resection of colon cancer continues to lack international standardization, unlike rectal cancer, for which total mesorectal excision (TME) is considered the optimal operation.

Anatomy for colonic resection

Arteries

The marginal artery runs along the colon, from which the vasa recta are delivered towards the colon. The number of vasa recta is less than that of the small

Colorectal Cancer: Diagnosis and Clinical Management, First Edition. Edited by John H. Scholefield and Cathy Eng.

intestine. The trunks connecting the marginal artery with the aorta are multiple colic arteries originating from the superior mesenteric and inferior mesenteric arteries.

The three colic branches of the superior mesenteric arteries are distinguished as the ileocolic, right colic, and middle colic arteries. The ileocolic artery feeds the ileum, cecum, and ascending colon, which is divided into the ileal, cecal, ascending, and appendicular arteries. Though the right colic artery is the dominant artery of the ascending colon, its origin is unstable, with only one-third originating from the superior mesenteric artery, and often forming a common trunk with the ileocolic artery or middle colic artery. The middle colic artery is the dominant artery of the transverse colon, its first branch originating from the right edge of the superior mesenteric artery at the lower edge of the body of the pancreas, and sometimes forming a common trunk with the inferior pancreaticoduodenal artery. The accessory middle colic artery originates from the left edge of the superior mesenteric artery and travels towards the left half of the transverse colon or the left colic flexure. The anastomosis tends to form between this artery and the left colic artery, originating from the inferior mesenteric artery towards the inside rather than the marginal artery (Riolan's anastomosis).

The inferior mesenteric artery branches from the abdominal aorta 1–3 cm caudal to the bottom edge of the third portion of the duodenum. The left colic artery and sigmoid artery are colic branches of the inferior mesenteric artery. The left colic artery originates 1–3 cm distal to the inferior mesenteric artery root as the first branch of the inferior mesenteric artery, is sometimes divided into an ascending branch and a descending branch, and is distributed to the descending colon. In some cases the branches separated from the ascending branch travel along the inferior mesenteric vein and form an anastomosis with the accessory middle colic artery. Several sigmoid colon arteries originate from the inferior mesenteric artery. The number and form of distribution varies according to the length of the sigmoid colon.

Michels et al. indicated several cases in which the marginal artery is very narrow or defective in the ileocecum, splenic flexure, and Sudeck point (critical points) [6]. In particular, there are many variations in the anastomosis of the superior/inferior mesenteric artery in splenic flexure; this is considered to be an area requiring maintenance of blood flow and is known as the Griffiths's point.

Veins

The venous return from the colon generally accompanies the arterial supply. The difference is that it does not drain to the inferior vena cava, but enters the liver via the portal vein. The right gastroepiploic vein also flows into the superior mesenteric vein, often forming a common trunk with the middle colic vein, known as the gastro-colic trunk.

Lymphatics

The lymphatic vessels of the colon fundamentally accompany the arteries. Pericolic lymph nodes are present in the surroundings of the marginal artery and vasa recti; these are the frontier lymph nodes. Most lymphatic vessels exiting the colonic wall travel along the vasa recta and marginal artery, from the pericolic lymph nodes to the intermediate lymph nodes, by gradually increasing in thickness, and finally reaching the main lymph nodes. The lymphatic vessels of the colon converge at three sections of the right inferior (the origin of ileocolic artery), center (the origin of the middle colic artery/right colic artery), and left inferior (the origin of the left colic artery/sigmoid artery), subsequently continuing to the aortic lymph nodes.

The range of bowel resection and lymph node dissection

In Western countries, studies on colon cancer, from the late 1950s to early 1960s, showed tumor cells over a wide range inside the intestinal tract. In 1954, Cole proposed extended bowel resection, in which the colon was blocked at an early period of surgery and broadly resected in order to prevent anastomotic recurrence due to dispersion of tumor cells in the intestinal lumen [7]. However, central lymph node dissection along the feeding vessels was not recommended. In 1950, Barnes proposed blocking the blood flow and lymph flow initially during surgery, in order to prevent liver metastasis [8]. In 1967, Turnbull et al. reported that the 5-year survival rate of a conventional group (232 cases) was 34.8%, while that of the non-touch isolation technique (NTIT) group (664 cases), using early clamp of both the bowel and drainage vessels, was 50.9% from the retrospective study, and so proposed NTIT as optimal surgery for colon cancer [9]. The randomized controlled trial (RCT), comparing NTIT with the conventional method by Wiggers et al., failed to demonstrate statistically significant differences in the recurrence rate, liver recurrence rate, and survival rate between the two groups [10]. It is believed that the better outcome in the NTIT group, by Turnbull et al., was not due to the NTIT, but due to the fact that the feeding vessel was ligated at the root; and central lymph node dissection was done in the NTIT group.

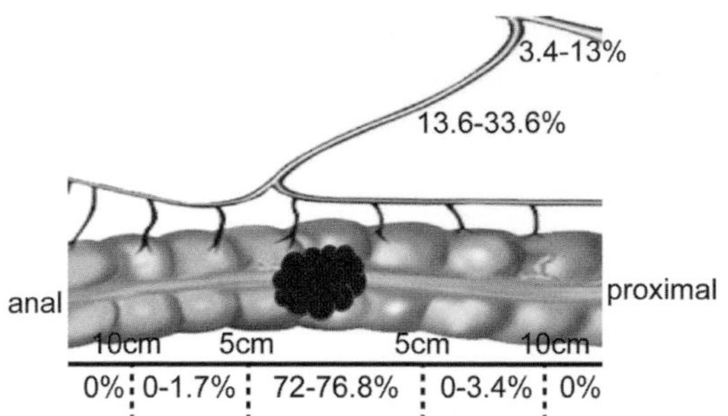

Figure 5.1 Distribution of positive lymph nodes of colon cancer [11–13].

In Japan, several studies of the distribution of positive lymph nodes in colon cancer, by using the surgical specimens, were conducted in the 1980s (Figure 5.1). Kimura et al. analyzed the distribution of 127 positive lymph nodes of 36 stage III colon cancer cases with clearing methods [11]. Metastasis to the pericplic lymph nodes adjacent to the tumor (up to 5 cm from tumor margins) was the most common at 72%, followed by metastasis to the intermediate lymph nodes at 15.7%, and to the main lymph nodes at 3.9%. However, metastasis was not found in the pericolic nodes more than 5 cm (proximal or distal) along the bowel from the tumor. Izumimoto et al. also studied the distribution of positive lymph nodes: 58 positive nodes from 20 stage III right-sided colon cancers and 125 positive nodes from 40 stage III left-sided colon cancers [12]. Forty-five percent of positive lymph nodes were located in the pericolic nodes within 5 cm from the tumor margin in right-sided colon cancer and 76.8% within 5 cm from the tumor margin in left-sided colon cancer. The intermediate nodes situated along the feeding artery of right-sided and left-sided colon cancer, were 15.5% and 13.6% of the positive lymph nodes, respectively; 3.4% and 8% were situated in the main node area of right-sided and left-sided colon cancer, respectively. No tumor cells were found in pericolic nodes located more than 10 cm along the bowel from the tumor. Koyama et al. reported that no patients had positive pericolic nodes more than 10 cm from the tumor margin in a clinicopathological study of 41 stage III right-sided colon cancers and 89 stage III left-sided colon cancers [13].

Some studies have reported flow heading towards the lymph nodes along the gastroepiploic vein from the hepatic flexure, towards the splenic hilum from near the splenic flexure along the inferior mesenteric vein to the pancreatic vein, and directly to the aortic lymph node from the superior rectal artery. Such lymphatic pathways are probably only found in palliative resection cases

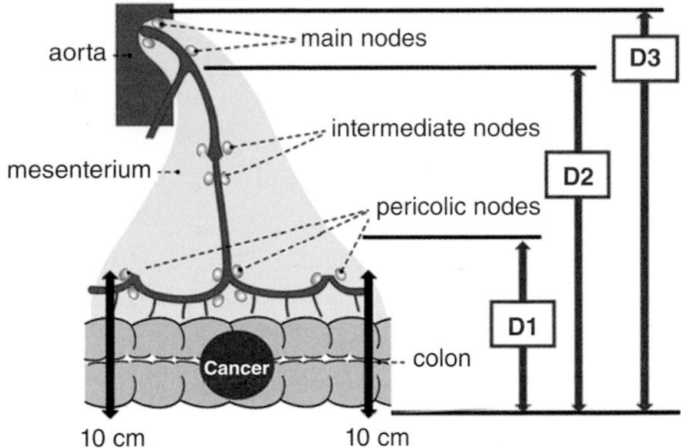

Figure 5.2 Japanese grading of lymph node dissection. D1 means removal of the pericolic nodes within 10 cm from tumor edges, D2 is D1 plus removal of the intermediate nodes, and D3 is D2 plus removal of the main nodes.

with wide lymphatic spread of tumor cells and so may not be relevant in curative surgery. From these research outcomes, the Japanese guidelines for the treatment of colorectal cancer, published by the Japanese Society for Cancer of the Colon and Rectum (JSCCR) in 2005, classify the grade of regional lymph nodes dissection as D1, D2, and D3. D1 dissection is removal of the epicolic nodes within 10 cm from tumor margins, D2 dissection is D1 dissection plus removal of the intermediate modes along the feeding artery, and D3 dissection is D2 dissection plus removal of the main nodes, which lie along the superior mesenteric vein in right-sided colon cancer or along the inferior mesenteric artery in left-sided colon cancer. The guidelines recommend D3 dissection for clinical stage II and stage III colon cancer [14] (Figure 5.2).

Recent studies on colon cancer surgery

West et al. retrospectively studied the surgical specimens in 399 cases, who had undergone surgery for colon cancer at Leeds General Infirmary between 1997 and 2002, reporting that 98 cases (24%) were observed with the muscularis propria plane (little bulk to mesocolon with disruptions extending down to the muscularis propria) and 177 cases (44%) were observed with the intramesocolic plane (moderate bulk to mesocolon with irregularity, but the incisions do not reach down to the muscularis propria) [15]. It has been shown that colon cancer resection in the mesocolic plane (intact mesocolon with a smooth peritoneal-lined surface) was associated with a 15% improvement in the 5-year overall survival rate compared to cases with the muscularis propria plane, with the difference rising to 27% in stage III disease.

Hohenberger et al. introduced complete mesocolic excision (CME) with central vascular ligation (CVL), by following the same sound principles of total mesoretal excision (TME) for rectal cancer [16]. CME with CVL attempted to remove the tumor and the entire mesocolon by dissecting along embryologic tissue planes in an intact peritoneal and fascial lined package. CME with CVL surgery removed more tissue compared with conventional surgery in terms of the distance between the tumor and the high vascular tie, the length of large bowel and ileum removed, and the area of mesentery removed. In addition, CME with CVL surgery was associated with more mesocolic plane resections and a greater lymph node yield [17].

Japanese D3 dissection surgery is based on similar principles to CME with CVL, apart from extended bowel resection, and impressive outcomes have been reported. Both in CME with CVL, and Japanese D3 resection, an intact mesocolic plane resection was achieved in 88% and 73% of cases, respectively [18]. Due to the differing concept of surgical approach regarding the axial direction of the bowel resection, Japanese D3 specimens were significantly shorter, thus resulting in a smaller amount of mesentery resected and less nodes harvested. However, there was no difference in central lymph node dissection, because the distance from the bowel wall to the high vascular tie and the number of tumors involving nodes were equivalent.

Surgery for colon cancer

The principle of surgery for colon cancer is that the tumor should be resected with the draining lymphatics, lymph nodes, and blood vessels through which the tumor may disseminate, using careful anatomic dissection along embryologic tissue planes in an intact peritoneal and fascial lined package. Central lymph node dissection with a high vascular tie is recommended to prevent local recurrence. Attention to the blood supply to the segments of anastomosis and the creation of anastomosis without tension are essential to prevent anastomotic problems.

Exploration of the abdominal cavity and assessment of resectability

On first opening the abdominal cavity, careful examination of tumor spread in the abdominal and pelvic cavity is made and resectability is evaluated. Small tumor deposits on the liver surface and peritoneal surface may not be visualized by preoperative CT.

Surgery for sigmoid colon cancer

Mobilization of the left colon

The peritoneal white line is incised by diathermy while retracting the sigmoid colon to the right side, and dissection between the mesosigmoid and the anterior layer of the renal fascia in dividing the Toldt's fusion fascia is carried out. When the dissection is along anatomic embryonic tissue planes, the left ureter, spermatic, or ovarian vessels are automatically preserved behind the retroperitoneum and there is little bleeding. Mobilization of the sigmoid colon and mesosigmoid is mostly conducted to the left edge of the aorta, to the left common iliac artery, and to the lower pole of the left kidney. Mobilization of the splenic flexure is not necessary in Japanese D3 dissection because of the shorter bowel resection. The sigmoid colon and mesosigmoid are retracted ventrolaterally to expose the left base of the mesosigmoid, and the autonomic nerve fibers running longitudinally on the aorta are visible. The nerve branches from the superior hypogastric plexus to the superior rectal vessels are cut by diathermy, resulting in preservation of the superior hypogastric plexus.

Central lymph node dissection (D3 dissection) (Figure 5.3)

The sigmoid colon is retracted left and the base of the mesosigmoid is incised; subsequently, this is connected to the dissected area from the left side in front of the aorta. Isolation of the mesosigmoid from the retroperitoneum is extended to the cranial side while preserving the superior hypogastric plexus, and when the root of the inferior mesenteric artery is exposed, it is ligated and divided at the root. The inferior mesenteric vein is divided at the same level. Blood flow to the segments of anastomosis, that is the rectum or rectosigmoid colon as the distal segment and the distal descending colon as the proximal segment, is supplied via the marginal arteries from the internal iliac arteries and from the middle colic artery, respectively.

A topological relationship of the tumor and the sigmoid arteries and veins is confirmed, and the mesosigmoid between a dividing point of the bowel 10 cm from the tumor margin and the root of the inferior mesenteric artery is divided. The distal mesosigmoid between a dividing point of the bowel 10 cm away from the tumor margin and the superior rectal vessels is also divided. After exposure of the bowel wall, the bowel is divided.

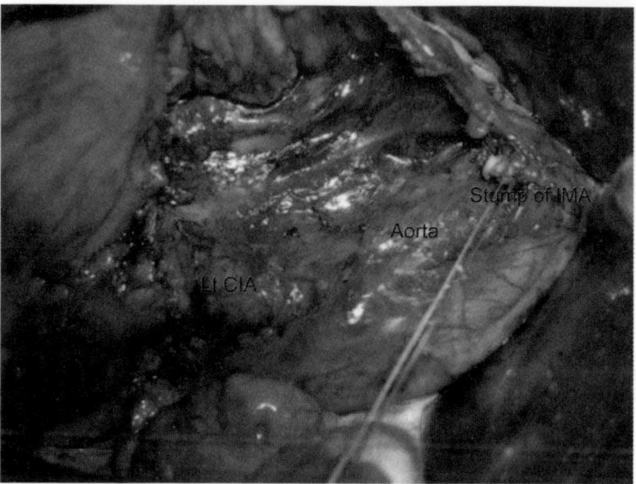

Figure 5.3 D3 dissection for sigmoid colon cancer. CIA: common iliac artery; IMA: inferior mesenteric artery.

Anastomosis

When it is confirmed that there is no ischemia or tension at the anastomotic site, anastomosis is complete. There are several types of stapling of anastomosis, including single stapling technique, double stapling technique, and functional end-to-end anastomosis, or hand-sewn anastomosis, which is chosen according to surgeon's preference. The authors preference is for a hand-sewn anastomosis by an interrupted, single-layer, layer-to-layer anastomosis (Gambee anastomosis) for all colonic anastomosis.

Surgery for right colon cancer

Mobilization of the right colon

The small bowel is retracted into the left half of the abdominal cavity, and mobilization of the cecum and ascending colon is started by incising the peritoneum along the paracolic gutter near the cecum. The right colon and terminal ileum are elevated and freed from the retroperitoneum by dissecting anatomically along the embryologic tissue planes between the mesocolon and the retoroperitoneum, resulting in the right ureter, spermatic, or ovarian vessels being automatically preserved behind the retroperitoneum. Care must be taken to avoid injury to the duodenum or to not go behind the duodenum. After isolation of the greater omentum from the ascending colon and transverse colon, the hepatic flexure is freed by advancing dissection from the ascending colon. Most surgeons divide the gastrocolic omentum and enter into the lesser sac, but the authors prefer to preserve the greater omentum by isolating it from the colon if tumor has not invaded it. Dissection along anatomic planes is continued medially, and after the duodenum and pancreatic head is sufficiently exposed, the superior mesenteric vein is also exposed.

Central lymph node dissection (D3 dissection) (Figure 5.4)

Once the colon has been fully mobilized, the mesentery and colic vessels are divided. The ascending colon is retracted to the right side, the peritoneum at the left edge of the distal superior mesenteric vein is incised, and the superior mesenteric vein is exposed. The ileocolic artery and veins are isolated at the roots and divided. Exposure of the superior mesenteric vein is continued cranially, and the right colic artery and vein (when present), as well as the middle colic artery, are isolated at the roots and divided. In most cases, the middle colic vein forms a common trunk with the right gastroepiploic vein and/or the pancreaticoduodenal vein near the pancreas head, with care not to damage any of these.

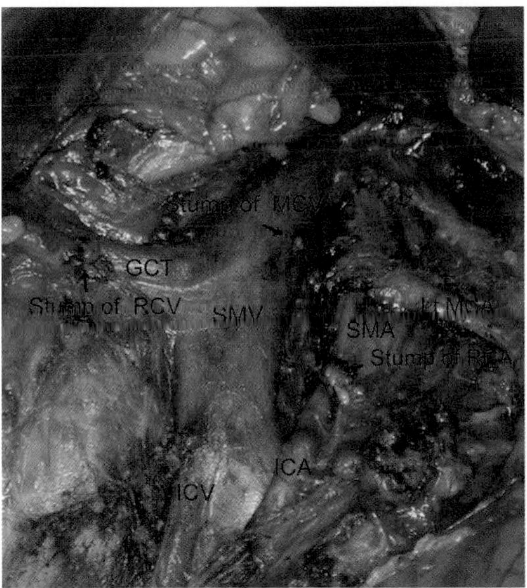

Figure 5.4 D3 dissection for right colon cancer. GCT: gastrocolic trunk; ICA and V: ileocolic artery and vein; MCA and V: middle colic artery and vein; RCA and V: right colic artery and vein; SMA and V: superior mesenteric artery and vein.

Anastomosis

The colon is divided 10 cm distal to the tumor margin in Japanese D3 dissection, and the ileum is divided 5 cm proximal to the ileocolic junction. An anastomosis is created using either stapled or hand-sewn techniques. The authors prefer a hand-sewn end-to-side anastomosis using an interrupted, single-layer, layer-to-layer anastomosis.

Laparoscopic surgery for colon cancer

Since the first report of laparoscopic colectomy by Jacobs in 1991 [19], laparoscopic surgery for colorectal cancer has been broadly accepted due to the advantages of less wound pain, lower invasiveness, and better cosmesis, in addition to better postoperative recovery compared to open surgery. Large-scale RCTs comparing the oncological and surgical outcomes between open and laparoscopic surgery are listed in Table 5.1 [20–23].

The Barcelona trial was a RCT conducted at a single institution, and was the first report on the short-term and long-term oncological outcomes comparing laparoscopic surgery with open surgery. The Clinical Outcomes of Surgical Therapy (COST) trial investigated 863 cases of colon cancer in 48 institutions across the United States and Canada. There were no differences in the 3-year and 5-year overall survival rates, as well as relapse-free survival. The Colon Cancer Laparoscopic or Open Resection (COLOR) trial investigated 1079 cases of colon cancer in 29 institutions across Europe. Although the non-inferiority of laparoscopic surgery to open surgery failed to be proven, there were no statistical differences in the overall survival and disease-free survival between the two groups. The Conventional versus Laparoscopic-Assisted Surgery in Colorectal Cancer (CLASICC) trial was conducted at 27 institutions across England. In this trial, rectal cancer was included. No differences in the 3-year relapse-free survival rate and 3-year overall survival rate between open and laparoscopic surgery were reported.

All of these four RCTs reported no differences in survival rates between laparoscopic and open surgery. However, these results need to be interpreted cautiously as in these trials transverse colon cancer was not included, and there was a high conversion rate of laparoscopic surgery to open surgery from 11% to 29%. Furthermore, radical surgery for colon cancer as CME with CVL or Japanese D3 dissection was not employed. West et al. disclosed that central vascular ligation was not employed in the CLASICC trial from the observation that the median distance from the tumor to the high vascular ties was 80 mm in laparoscopic surgery and 90 mm in open surgery, which was similar to that

Table 5.1 Randomized controlled trials comparing laparoscopic and open colorectal surgery.

	Barcelona Trial	**COST**	**COLOR**	**CLASICC**	**JCOG0404**
Institution (n)	Spain (1)	North America (48)	Europe (29)	UK (27)	Japan(30)
Tumor location	Right/left/sigmoid	Right/left/sigmoid	Right/left/sigmoid	Right/left/sigmoid/rectosigmoid/rectum	Right/sigmoid/rectosigmoid
No. of pts	219	863	1248	794	1057
Conversion rate (%)	11	21	17	29	5.4
Adjuvant chemotherapy	FU/LV (Stage II, III)	Unregulated	Unregulated	Unregulated	FU/LV (Stage III)
Morbidity	LAC<OC	NS	NS	NS	NS
Survival	NS	NS	NS	NS	NE

NS: not significant

NE: not evaluated yet

of colon specimens of Leeds General Infirmary, where high vascular tie was not done [17].

The JCOG0404 trial is a randomized trial in Japan, investigating non-inferiority of laparoscopic surgery to open surgery for stage II and stage III colon cancers. In this trial, Japanese D3 dissection is prescribed in protocol as a standard surgery both in laparoscopic and open surgery. Between 2004 and 2009, a total of 1057 patients were enrolled and the results will be available in 2014.

Outcome

According to the CONCORD [24] and OECD Health Quality Indicators data, which analyzed the cancer registration data of countries around the world, the survival rate of colon cancer patients largely differs among the countries. The 5-year survival rate of stage I, IIA, IIB, IIC, IIIA, IIIB, and IIIC colon cancers in Surveillance Epidemiology and End Results (SEER) data, according to TNM Classification (7th edition), were 74.0%, 66.5%, 58.6%, 37.3%, 73.1%, 46.3%, and 28.0%, respectively [25]. Both stage II and stage III consisted of the subgroups with a wide variety of prognoses. The same trends are observed in the Japanese study. The multicenter retrospective study of 3148 colon cancers in the 18 centers, who underwent curative surgery between 1997 and 2000, were prospectively followed; the 5-year survival rates were: stage I 93.5%, IIA88.8%, IIB81.7%, IIC82.1%, IIIA91.3%, IIIB77.4%, and IIIC 55.5% (Figure 5.5).

In adjuvant chemotherapy, this wide variety of prognoses in stage II and stage III is considered. A RCT investigating non-inferiority of UFT (tegafur

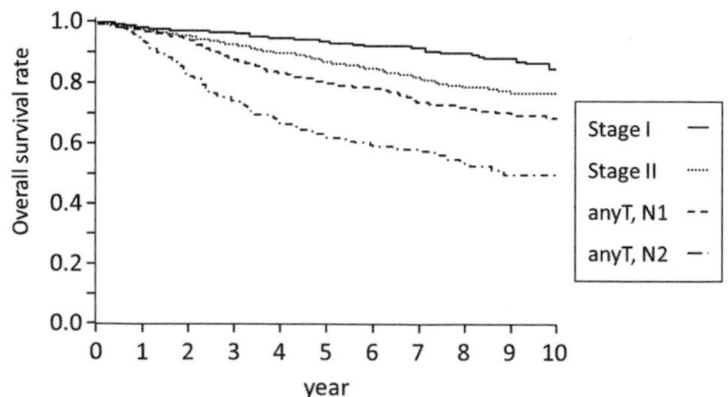

Figure 5.5 Kaplan-Meier curves for the overall survival of colon cancer patients who underwent radical colonic resection in Japan.

plus uracil) + oral leucovorin to fluorouracil (5FU) + leucovorin (RPMI regimen) as adjuvant chemotherapy in stage III colon cancer, was conducted in Japan (JCOG0205 trial). A total of 1101 colon cancer patients were enrolled from February 2003 to October 2006. In this trial, Japanese D3 dissection was carried out in 75.5% of cases and D2 dissection in 24.5% of cases. The 3-year disease free survival and 5-year overall survival of the UFT group and the 5FU group were 77.8%, 87.5%, 79.3%, and 88.4%, respectively. Non-inferiority of UFT + oral leucovorin to 5FU + leucovorin as adjuvant therapy for stage III colon cancer after Japanese D3 dissection was confirmed.

Adjuvant chemotherapy using 5FU/leucovorin + oxaliplatin is a standard treatment for stage III colon cancer, based on the three well designed RCTs (MASAIC, NSABP C-07, and XEROXA trials), which reported similar results; the oxaliplatin group showed significantly improved disease-free survival with a hazard ratio from 0.78 to 0.80 compared with the 5FU/leucovorin group [26–28]. However, survival benefit was observed only in the MOSAIC trial: the difference of the 6-year survival rate in stage III colon cancer was 4.2%. Figure 5.6 shows the 5-year survival rate of the NSABP C-07, XEROXA, and JCOG0205 trials and the 6-year survival rate of the MOSAIC trial. The survival rate of the JCOG0205 trial is better by around 10% than that of other trials

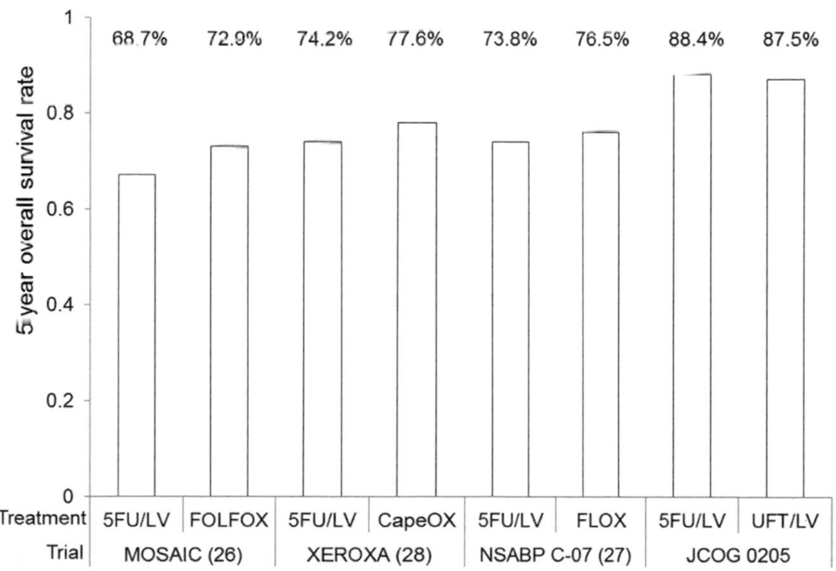

Figure 5.6 The 5-year overall survival rate of stage III colon cancer in XEROXA trial [28], NSABP C-07 trial [27] and JCOG0205 trial and the 6-year overall survival rate of stage III colon cancer in MOSAIC trial [26].

treating with oxaliplatin, and the same tendency is observed in the 3-year disease-free survival rate: 72.2% in the FOLOX group of the MOSAIC trial, 70.9% in the XEROX group of the XEROXA trial, and 79.3% in the 5FU group and 77.8% in the UFT group of the JCOG0205 trial. The differences in survival may be due to the differences in surgical treatment: 75.5% of patients in the JCOG0205 trial underwent Japanese D3 dissection. Hohenberger et al. also reported that use of CME with CVL decreased locoregional recurrence from 6.5% to 3.6% [16].

Conclusion

Introduction of TME in many countries has led to decreased local recurrence and improves the survival of patients with rectal cancer; however, optimization and standardization of surgery for colon cancer have not been achieved. CME with CVL or Japanese D3 dissection, which follows the oncological concept of TME and shows improved outcomes, may become the standard surgery for colon cancer.

CASE STUDY

A 62-year-old male presented to your clinic because a screening test for fecal occult blood was positive. Physical examination revealed no abnormality, and blood tests disclosed anemia to a slight degree. He did not have any medical history. Colonoscopy revealed an ulcerated tumor 40 mm in diameter on the sigmoid colon. You make plans for radical colonic resection following CT for staging.

TIPS AND TRICKS/KEY PITFALLS

- In only one-third of cases, the right colic artery originates from the superior mesenteric artery.
- The veins of the colon are not drained to the inferior vena cava, but flow into the liver via the portal vein.
- Lymph node metastasis along the axial direction of the bowel is confined within a limited range (<10 cm), but lymph node metastasis along the central direction is dominant.
- Attention to blood supply to the segments of anastomosis and creation of anastomosis without tension are essential to prevent anastomotic problems.

MULTIPLE-CHOICE QUESTIONS

1 The first and second most common sites to be involved with colon cancer via the blood stream are:

A. Lung-Ovary
B. Liver-Brain
C. Lung-Brain
D. Lung-Liver
E. Liver-Lung

2 Laparoscopic surgery for colon cancer is considered based on the following criteria, except:

A. The serum creatinine level was 1.8 mg/dl.
B. Acute bowel obstruction by primary tumor
C. T3 tumor by CT
D. Enlarged lymph node near the tumor by CT
E. No previous abdominal major surgery

3 The minimum number of lymph nodes examined to confirm stage II colon cancer in the NCCN guidelines is:

A. 8
B. 10
C. 12
D. 14
E. 16

References

1 Reybard J-F. Memoire sucunetumer cancereuse affectant l'Silliague du colon. *Bull Acad Natl Med* 1844; 9: 1031–2.

2 Maydl C. EinBeitrayzur Dannschrurgie. *Zbl Chir* 1883; 10: 487–8.

3 Cheever D. The choice of operation in carcinoma of the colon. *Ann Surg* 1931; 94: 705–16.

4 Grinnell RS. Lymphatic metastases of carcinoma of the colon and rectum. *Ann Surg* 1950; 131: 494–506.

5 Mayo CW, Lee MJ, Jr., Davis RM. A comparative study of operations for carcinoma of the rectum and rectosigmoid. *Surg Gynecol Obstet* 1951; 92: 360–4.

6 Michels NA, Siddharth P, Kornblith PL, et al. The variant blood supply to the descending colon, rectosigmoid and rectum based on 400 dissections. Its importance in regional resections: a review of medical literature. *Dis Colon Rectum* 1965; 8: 251–78.

7 Cole WH, Packard D, Southwick HW. Carcinoma of the colon with special reference to prevention of recurrence. *J Am Med Assoc* 1954; 28: 1549–53.

8 Barnes JP. Physiologic resection of the right colon. *Surg Gynecol Obstet* 1952; 94: 722–6.

9 Turnbull RB, Jr., Kyle K, Watson FR, et al. Cancer of the colon: the influence of the no-touch isolation technique on survival rates. *Ann Surg* 1967; 166: 420–7.
10 Wiggers T, Jeekel J, Arends JW, et al. No-touch isolation technique in colon cancer: a controlled prospective trial. *Br J Surg* 1988; 75: 409–15.
11 Kimura O, Mizusawa S, Sugasawa A, et al. Comparative studies on the distribution of the lymph node metastases from colorectal cancer between modified clearing and conventional procedures. *Nihon Shokaki Geka Gakkai zasshi* 1987; 20: 865–70.
12 Izumimoto G, Hata M, Nishiyama S, et al. Studies on the lymph node metastases of the colon cancer by the modified clearing method. *Nihon Daicho Komon byo Gakkai zasshi* 1983; 36: 523–31.
13 Koyama Y, Moriya Y, Hojyo K. Anatomy in colorectal cancer surgery. *Nipponn Rinnshou* 1981; 39: 2137–49.
14 Watanabe T, Itabashi M, Shimada Y, et al. Japanese Society for Cancer of the Colon and Rectum (JSCCR) guidelines 2010 for the treatment of colorectal cancer. *Int J Clin Oncol* 2012; 17: 1–29.
15 West NP, Morris EJ, Rotimi O, et al. Pathology grading of colon cancer surgical resection and its association with survival: a retrospective observational study. *Lancet Oncol* 2008; 9: 857–65.
16 Hohenberger W, Weber K, Matzel K, et al. Standardized surgery for colonic cancer: complete mesocolic excision and central ligation–technical notes and outcome. *Colorectal Dis* 2009; 11: 354–64; discussion 64–5.
17 West NP, Hohenberger W, Weber K, et al. Complete mesocolic excision with central vascular ligation produces an oncologically superior specimen compared with standard surgery for carcinoma of the colon. *J Clin Oncol* 2010; 28: 272–8.
18 West NP, Kobayashi H, Takahashi K, et al. understanding optimal colonic cancer surgery: comparison of Japanese D3 resection and European complete mesocolic excision with central vascular ligation. *J Clin Oncol* 2012 Apr 2; 30: 1763–9.
19 Jacobs M, Verdeja JC, Goldstein HS. Minimally invasive colon resection (laparoscopic colectomy). *Surg Laparosc Endosc* 1991; 1: 144–50.
20 Lacy AM, Garcia-Valdecasas JC, Delgado S, et al. Laparoscopy-assisted colectomy versus open colectomy for treatment of non-metastatic colon cancer: a randomised trial. *Lancet* 2002; 29: 2224–9.
21 Clinical Outcomes of Surgical Therapy Study Group. A comparison of laparoscopically assisted and open colectomy for colon cancer. *N Engl J Med* 2004; 13: 2050–9.
22 The Colon Cancer Laparoscopic or Open Resection Study Group. Survival after laparoscopic surgery versus open surgery for colon cancer: long-term outcome of a randomized clinical trial. *Lancet Oncol* 2009; 10: 44–52.
23 Jayne DG, Guillou PJ, Thorpe H, et al. Randomized trial of laparoscopic-assisted resection of colorectal carcinoma: 3-year results of the UK MRC CLASICC Trial Group. *J Clin Oncol* 2007; 25: 3061–8.
24 Coleman MP, Quaresma M, Berrino F, et al. Cancer survival in five continents: a worldwide population-based study (CONCORD). *Lancet Oncol* 2008; 9: 730–56.
25 Edge SB, Byrd DR, Carducci MA, et al. *American Joint Committee in Cancer. AJCC Cancer Staging Manual*, 7th edn, New York, Springer, 2010.
26 Andre T, Boni C, Navarro M, et al. Improved overall survival with oxaliplatin, fluorouracil, and leucovorin as adjuvant treatment in stage II or III colon cancer in the MOSAIC trial. *J Clin Onol* 2009; 27: 3109–16.

27 Yothers G, O'Connell MJ, Allegra CJ, et al. Oxaliplatin as adjuvant therapy for colon cancer: updated results of NSABP C-07 trial, including survival and subset analyses. *J Clin Oncol* 2011; 29: 3768–74.

28 Haller DG, Tabernero J, Maroun J, et al. Capecitabine plus oxaliplatin compared with fluorouracil and folic acid as adjuvant therapy for stage III colon cancer. *J Clin Oncol* 2011: 29: 1465–71.

ANSWERS TO MULTIPLE-CHOICE QUESTIONS

1 E
2 B
3 C

CHAPTER 6

ExtraLevator AbdominoPerineal Excision (ELAPE) for advanced low rectal cancer

Brendan J. Moran[1] & Timothy J. Moore[2]

[1] *Basingstoke and North Hampshire Hospital, Basingstoke, UK*

[2] *Royal Hampshire County Hospital, Winchester, UK*

KEY POINTS

- Conventional APE has poorer oncological outcomes than low AR.
- ELAPE offers improved outcomes.
- There are two excision planes for low rectal cancer:
  a) The TME and intersphicteric plane; or
  b) The extralevator plane.
- MRI should be used for local staging and preoperative planning.
- Conventional APE leads to a 'surgical waist'.
- In the abdominal phase of ELAPE, the mesorectum should not be dissected from the levator ani muscles.
- Patient positioning should be based on individual surgeon preference and experience, and include consideration of tumor position.
- The ELAPE technique should include perineal reconstruction with either myocutaneous flap or biological mesh.
- Quality of life is similar following either APE or low AR.
- Precision surgery alone can achieve excellent oncological outcomes.

Introduction

The description and propagation of total mesorectal excision (TME) has led to dramatic improvements in outcome for patients with rectal cancer and involves precise dissection in a relatively avascular anatomical defined plane [1;2]. TME has resulted in reduced local recurrence and improved survival in

Colorectal Cancer: Diagnosis and Clinical Management, First Edition. Edited by John H. Scholefield and Cathy Eng.

patients undergoing anterior resection for upper and mid-rectal cancer, but there are ongoing challenges in low rectal cancer where many patients are not amenable to restorative resection and undergo abdominoperineal excision (APE) with a permanent stoma.

It is pertinent to be aware that for much of the 20th century the gold standard treatment for rectal cancer was APE, first popularized by Miles in 1908 [3]. Over the course of the latter part of the last century, surgical and medical advances meant that restorative resection by colorectal anastomosis became a feasible and acceptable option and anterior resection increased in popularity. At the end of the 20th century, the proponents of TME surgery began to question the validity of the APE operation, and in 1997 Heald et al. published the results of 'an extreme policy of sphincter conservation' for the treatment of low rectal cancer. In this series of 136 patients with cancer of the low rectum (tumors <5 cm from the anal verge), 77% were treated by low anterior resection, with a 6-year local recurrence rate of 4%. The results for the remaining 23% of cancers treated by APE were far worse, with a local recurrence rate of 47% [4].

Similarly, Phil Quirke and colleagues from Leeds reported inferior outcomes associated with conventional APE compared with anterior resection (AR) in 2005. They reported a significantly higher local recurrence rate (22.3% vs. 13.5%, P = 0.002) and poorer prognosis (survival 52.3% vs. 65.8%, P = 0.003) in patients who had APE compared with those who had AR [5]. Adverse outcomes were associated with an increased incidence of circumferential resection margin (CRM) involvement and intra-operative specimen perforation. Using tissue morphometric studies, they reported that adverse outcomes were related to the surgical removal of less tissue at the level of the tumor in the APE specimens; the so-called 'surgical waist' of the conventional APE specimen. Similarly worse outcomes in patients who had APE compared with those who had AR were reported in a histopathological audit from the Dutch TME study [6], Magnetic Resonance Imaging and Rectal Cancer European Equivalence (MERCURY) study [7], and Conventional versus Laparoscopic-Assisted Surgery in Colorectal Cancer (CLASICC) study [8;9], all having a higher proportion of incomplete APE specimens compared with AR TME specimens.

These reports have led to renewed focus on the treatment of low rectal cancer, with increasing calls for a change in approach to APE surgery towards an extended operation similar to the original Miles procedure [10]. In particular, a number of European surgeons advocate what has been termed 'extended' or 'cylindrical' APE to reduce the 'waisting' effect on the surgical specimen and have published results showing a reduction in the involved CRM rate and specimen perforations compared with conventional APE (49.6% to 20.3%, $P < 0.001$ and 28.2% to 8.2%, $P < 0.001$, respectively) [11].

This chapter focuses on what was initially termed 'cylindrical APE' and now best described as an ExtraLevator AbdominoPerineal Excision (ELAPE), whereby the rectum is excised *en-bloc* with the levator complex [12]. With a standardized anatomical approach, early reports suggest a reduction in local recurrence rates and improved survival in patients with low rectal cancers [13–15].

Historical aspects of rectal cancer surgery

The first documented rectal resection for cancer was performed by Jacques Lisfanc in 1826 via a perineal approach [16]. Kocker and then Kraske introduced some modifications to include a coccygectomy [17] and the perineal approach was adopted as the preferred route of excision for the next 70–80 years, but with only a limited exposure of the operative field possible, radical removal of tumors was virtually impossible. Morbidity and mortality were high with recurrence rates of 95–100% and a poor quality of life prior to death for most.

Towards the end of the 19th century, advances in anaesthesia, including muscle relaxants, and the development of Lister's aseptic principles led to the feasibility of laparotomy. Carl Gaussenbauer was the first surgeon to perform a bowel resection through an abdominal approach in 1879. The French surgeon, Henri Hartmann, went on to propagate this method for high rectal cancers [18], with the eponymous 'Hartmann' procedure still in practice today. In 1884, Vincent Czerny employed the first combined abdominal and perineal approach to remove a rectal cancer; however, this was an emergency manoeuvre carried out to resolve catastrophic bleeding encountered during a sacral resection for a proximal tumor. The patient did not survive, and although further attempts were made, it was more than 20 years later before the concept of an abdominoperineal approach began to be accepted as a treatment for rectal cancer.

In 1908, after 7 years of using the perineal approach whereby he noted a 95% recurrence rate, Ernest Miles reported his initial experience with a planned two stage approach, combining laparotomy with perineal resection [3]. Miles felt this would facilitate resection of 'the zone of upward spread' as he had recorded upward disease dissemination at post-mortem examination of his patients with local recurrence.

In Miles' initial series of 12 patients, 5/12 (42%) died from perioperative complications, but in 1912 he reported that 3 of the 7 survivors were disease free at 4 years [19]. These survivors inspired him to persevere and in 1923 he reported a recurrence rate of 29.5% and a perioperative mortality rate of 15% [20].

This abdominoperineal procedure became the gold standard for the resection of rectal tumors and, with advances in anaesthesia and critical care, was refined into a one stage procedure by Lloyd-Davis et al. [21]. Miles originally described the operation as a two stage procedure, moving the patient from the supine to the right lateral position for the perineal part [3]. Subsequently, further reports outlined a move towards the lithotomy position and two teams of surgeons working simultaneously from both the perineal and abdominal approaches, the so-called combined abdominoperineal approach [21].

Miles had suggested division of the vascular pedicle below the left colic branch, but Moynihan initiated a higher ligation of the inferior mesenteric artery, near its origin from the aorta, to allow for excision of the atypical high lymph nodes that could potentially be a source of recurrence [22].

Abdominoperineal excision continued to be the method of choice until the middle of the last century, when anterior resection began to be reported. In 1948, Claude Dixon reported results of 400 patients treated at the Mayo clinic with anterior resection, with restoration of bowel continuity [23]. Restorative anterior resection had been described previously by Balfour, amongst others, in 1910 [24], but due to a high morbidity and mortality had not become popular. The development and propagation of intestinal stapling, in combination with the description and propagation of TME in the 1980s, resulted in a shift towards anterior resection and away from APE for rectal cancer [4]. Similarly and simultaneously, the recognition that the CRM was a more frequent cause of failure and recurrence than the distal resection margins [25] meant that surgeons began to push the limits of anterior resection and ultra-low anterior resection became an accepted oncological approach for mobile early low rectal cancer [26]. Thus APE rates diminished, from 90% of rectal cancer excisions in the 1970s to 37% by the 1990s [27], and currently APE is generally only performed for locally advanced low rectal tumors and in patients where bowel continuity is not deemed appropriate, for example where sphincter function is deficient. Continued improvements in outcomes from anterior resection were not mirrored by APE results [4], refocusing a re-look at the approach to APE. From this has emanated the concepts variously described as 'extended APE', 'cylindrical APE' and more latterly and precisely 'Extralevator APE' as outlined in a recent editorial [12].

What is a low rectal tumor?

The distal gastrointestinal tract is composed of two parts, the rectum and anal canal. The junction of the rectum and the 'surgical' anal canal is at the pelvic floor and corresponds to the level where the puborectalis portion of the levator ani encircles the bowel and angles it forward [28]. The anal canal is about 4 cm long in men and 2.5–3 cm in women [28]. The rectum varies in length but is normally between 12 cm [29] and 15 cm [30] in length and can be conveniently divided into upper, middle, and lower. A lower third, or low rectal cancer is best categorized on a Magnetic Resonance Imaging (MRI)-based anatomical definition as an adenocarcinoma with its lower edge at, or below, the origin of the levators, at the pelvic sidewall and this usually corresponds as a measurement within 6 cm of the anal verge [31].

Indications for ELAPE

Despite advances in reconstruction and a desire for less permanent stomas, abdominoperineal excision remains the optimal technique in selected cases of low rectal cancer where the tumor involves the pelvic floor or external sphincter complex and restorative procedures are technically impossible, oncologically unsound, or where a restorative technique would result in an unfavorable functional result.

The relationship of the sphincter complex and the pelvic floor to the tumor defines the appropriate surgical plane needed to achieve the optimum oncological outcome. Current thinking is that there are two key planes for low rectal cancer management (Figure 6.1). One is the TME plane, which continues distally into the intersphincteric plane. This dissection can continue as an 'intersphincteric APE' or be terminated and allow a colo-anal anastomosis, usually by a hand-sewn technique. The alternative strategy is the extralevator plane. The plane is usually determined by a combination of clinical assessment by an experienced surgeon combined with a good-quality pelvic MRI. Some have suggested that MRI could be used as a preoperative 'route map' to help plan the surgical approach, accurately predicting the required plane of excision [32].

In the majority of low rectal cancers the TME plane, and if necessary extension into the intersphincteric plane, is oncologically safe and the acceptable treatment is a low anterior resection. Indeed, in selected cases, tumors involving the anal canal can be treated with restorative ultra-low anterior excision

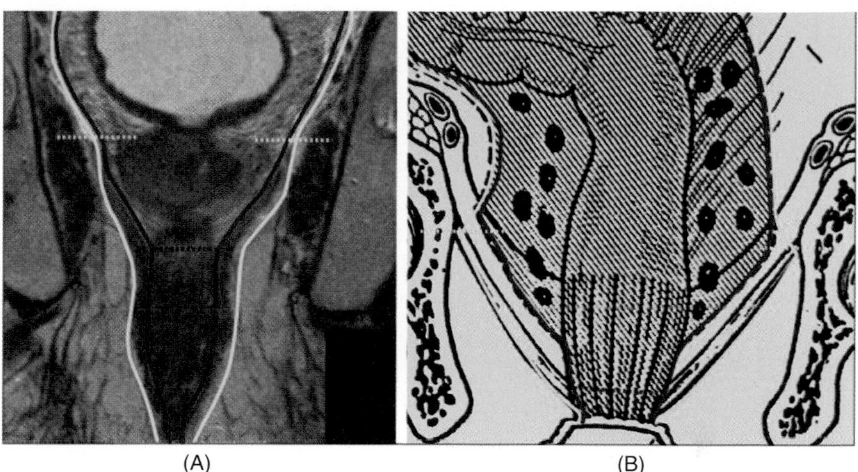

Figure 6.1 Coronal MRI (A) and modification of Miles' drawing (B), showing the intersphincteric/TME plane (red) and the extralevator plane (yellow) [32]. Reproduced with permission of Elsevier.

using the intersphincteric plane. However, if the tumor encroaches to less than 1 cm from the dentate line, or a low rectal tumor is poorly differentiated, then APE should be performed.

An intersphincteric APE may be appropriate for early stage tumors, as it is a less complex procedure [13], but this decision or one to perform ELAPE should be made preoperatively based on the radiological staging and an experienced clinical assessment. Intraoperative 'trial dissection' to the pelvic floor along the TME plane is not recommended, as there is a risk of compromising the circumferential resection margin and also a high risk of specimen perforation.

Preoperative preparation

Assessment and staging

The management of cancers of the low rectum presents many challenges and preoperative preparation is essential; 'to fail to plan is to plan to fail'. There are anatomical complexities at the level of the low rectum, such as the narrow confines of the bony pelvis, the tapering of the mesorectum near the pelvic floor, and the proximity of the pelvic organs and sphincter complex that make operating in this area challenging.

The clinical details, radiological investigations and pre-operative histology should be discussed at a colorectal multidisciplinary team (MDT) meeting to optimize the management strategy and appropriately tailor the surgery to the cancer and patient.

Every low rectal tumor should be assessed by the operating surgeon, who should perform a digital rectal examination and rigid proctosigmoidoscopy. The height of the lower edge of the tumor should be measured in centimeters from the anal verge using a rigid scope with the patient awake in the left lateral position. The surgeon should assess the integrity of the anal canal and, if possible, assess the mobility, or otherwise, of the tumor. The tumor should be biopsied to confirm the diagnosis and to exclude other rare lesions such as squamous carcinoma, infiltrating prostatic carcinoma, or lymphoma, whose management would differ from that of adenocarcinoma. It may be helpful to re-examine the patient 'under sedation' at colonoscopy and, occasionally, an examination under anaesthetic (EUA) is required to fully assess the tumor's relationship to surrounding structures. This assessment should be augmented with local radiological staging using high spatial resolution MRI, as discussed below.

The remainder of the colon should be assessed to identify synchronous neoplasia (present in 3–4%) or other colonic pathology by either colonoscopy, computed tomography (CT) colonography, or a barium enema. Colonoscopy has the advantage of allowing biopsy or removal of synchronous lesions and is currently the gold standard. CT colonography and barium enema are useful in imaging the proximal bowel in patients with stenotic distal lesions or in whom colonoscopy may not be feasible. Current best practise also incorporates staging for systemic disease by chest and abdominal CT scan.

Preoperative anaesthetic assessment should be undertaken for all patients undergoing rectal surgery, in order to identify and optimize co-morbidities, as well as help plan perioperative and postoperative care. Counselling by a stoma nurse specialist and marking for stoma sites should also be mandatory prior to ELAPE.

Radiological staging

Stage assessment is of vital importance in the preoperative planning for rectal cancer, providing information to help tailor the type of operation and the need for neo-adjuvant therapies. Three principal imaging techniques, endoluminal ultrasound, endorectal MRI, and pelvic phased array MRI, have been evaluated in the local staging of rectal cancer. The purpose of local staging is to assess the potential resection margin and select patients who might benefit from neoadjuvant (pre-operative) therapy. In many patients with low rectal cancer, endoluminal probes cannot be inserted, or tolerated by the patient, such that advances in surface coil MRI has been a major advance. Therefore high spatial resolution MRI is optimal, as unlike endoluminal ultrasound and endorectal MRI, surface coil MRI has been shown to consistently depict the mesorectal fascia and anatomical structures that relate to total mesorectal excision surgery for rectal cancer [33;34;35]. The technique enables accurate measurement of depth of extramural spread, identification of tumor deposits within the mesorectum, and hence the prediction of positive CRM. It is also very helpful in the preoperative assessment of low rectal tumors in defining the tumor relationship with the pelvic floor and sphincter complex and hence to help plan the ideal 'plane' of surgery.

Definition of ELAPE; anatomical planes, when to stop the TME, specimen waist and the CRM

There are a number of descriptions and confusion about the terminology associated with APE and indeed references to the same procedure using the terminology abdominoperineal resection (APR), as discussed [12]. Techniques vary, for instance patient positioning prone or supine, abdominal or perineal component first, laparoscopic versus open, etc, which will be discussed below. However, the basis of an extralevator approach is the concept and technique of perineal dissection on the caudal surface of the levators and removing variable amounts of the levators wrapped around the specimen culminating in the removal of a cylindrical specimen without, or with a reduced waist.

Conventional Abdominoperineal Excision

In performing a synchronous combined APE, the surgeon commonly follows the mesorectal plane down to the pelvic floor and the top of the anal canal, and the mesorectum is mobilized from the levator ani muscles, as described in TME dissection. The perineal part of the operation is performed from below, and at the same time in the terrible concept of a 'synchronous' approach. The perineal dissection involves excision of the anal canal including the surrounding skin, ischioanal fat, and the lower portions of the levator ani/external sphincter complex. When APE is thus performed (Figure 6.2) there is usually a 'waist' effect of the excised specimen, narrowing at the lower border of the mesorectum, at the level of the levator sling, which at this point is at one with the external sphincter. The maximum area of surgical 'waisting' is 35–42 mm above the anal verge at the level of the puborectalis muscle where the abdominal and perineal phases of the APE commonly meet [36].

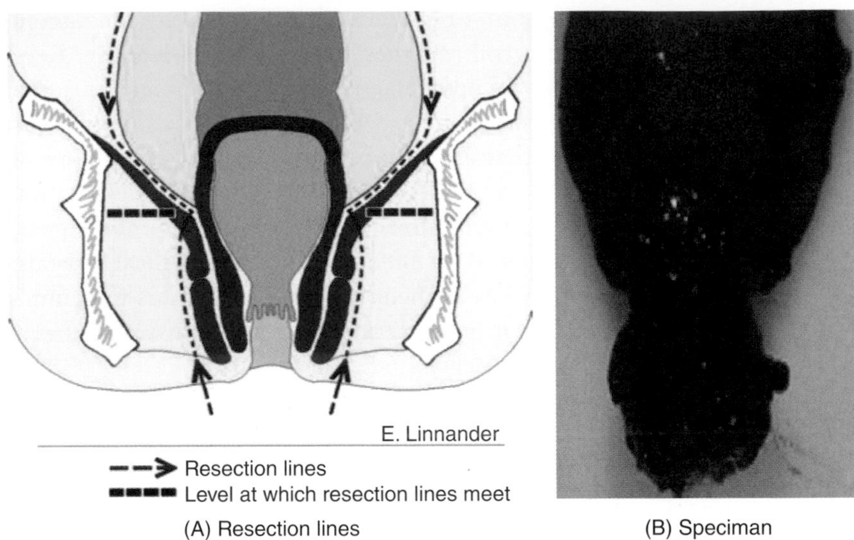

Figure 6.2 Conventional APE: (A) Dissection from above and below meet above the anal canal; (B) This creates a 'waist' on the surgical specimen [13]. Reproduced with permission of John Wiley & Sons, Inc.

At this point, the mesorectum tapers and disappears. A low rectal cancer at the 2–5 cm level will only have the surrounding muscle tube as the circumferential resection margin and an advanced tumor or a waist at this level will result in an involved CRM. The extralevator concept aims to protect the CRM at this level.

ExtraLevator Abdominoperineal Excision [13;37]

The abdominal part of the operation is performed as in the conventional APE, with an important modification: the mesorectum should not be dissected from the levator ani muscle. Thus, after traditional mobilization of the left colon with vascular and bowel division, the rectum and mesorectum are dissected in the extramesorectal fascial plane. The abdominal dissection should stop posteriorly at the sacrococcygeal junction, laterally just below the autonomic nerves and anteriorly just below the seminal vesicles in men or the cervix uteri in women.

The perineal phase commences with an elliptical incision around the anus (there is no necessity to take a wide margin of skin for low rectal adenocarcinoma) and extended cranially to the coccyx. The anus should be closed to reduce spillage, either with a purse string suture before the incision or an inverting running suture after the skin incision. The lateral dissection continues in the subcutaneous fat, just outside the subcutaneous portion of the external anal sphincter. Following this plane, the levator ani muscle is identified on both sides and the dissection is continued along the outer surface of the levator ani muscles proximally until the insertion of the levator on to the pelvic sidewall. In this way, a 'U-shaped' incision is performed exposing the pelvic floor. It is important to expose the levator ani muscles all around the circumference before entering the pelvis. It is important to be aware of the main pudendal blood vessels and nerves [n. pudendus] at the far lateral sides of this dissection.

The lateral dissection is continued dorsally until the position of the coccyx can be clearly palpated and the dissection proceeds on to the coccyx. If coccygectomy is planned, the coccyx is disarticulated from the sacrum and the pelvis is entered by dividing Waldeyer's fascia. This should correspond to the point where intra-abdominal dissection has stopped.

The levators are divided laterally on both sides, from posterior to anterior, until the mesorectum becomes visible at the dorsal and lateral sides. The inferior rectal nerves and vessels, derived from the pudendal nerve and vessels, are transected.

If a 'pull through technique' is favored, then the prone position of the patient for the perineal dissection and routine coccygectomy are helpful, and the specimen can be gently brought out and dissected from the prostate or the posterior vaginal wall in a cranial to caudal direction.

In the case of an anterior tumor, a portion of the prostate, or the posterior vaginal wall may be resected *en bloc* and again, positioning the patient in the prone position facilitates this. Finally, the remaining pelvic floor muscle fibers are divided just posterior to the transverse perineal muscles and the specimen is excised. The resulting specimen (Figure 6.3) is somewhat 'cylindrical', ideally without a waist, owing to the fact that the levator ani muscle is still attached to the mesorectum, forming a cuff around the rectoanal muscle tube.

Surgical technique

Patient positioning

Miles originally described APE as a two-stage procedure, with the patient initially supine and then turned into the semi-prone, right lateral position, for perineal dissection. Over the last century, this has been refined into a synchronous combined perineal and abdominal procedure, facilitated by the patient being in the lithotomy position. A recent trend has been to promote

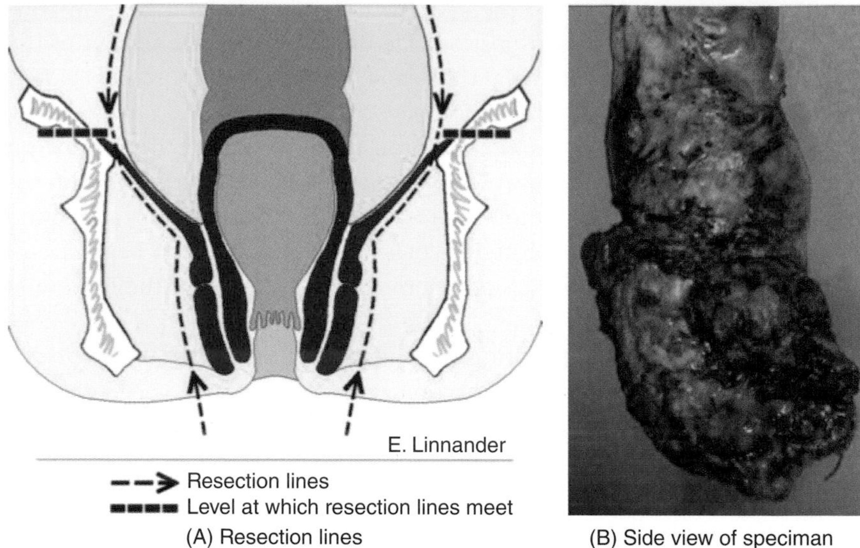

Figure 6.3 ExtraLevator APE (ELAPE): (a) Dissection from above and below meets at the top of the levator muscle; (b) creating a 'cylindrical' surgical specimen (13). Reproduced with permission of John Wiley & Sons, Inc.

ELAPE, with the patient in the prone jack-knife position for the perineal component [12;13].

Outcome related to position

The improved results associated with ELAPE have led to debate regarding whether patient positioning influences surgical and oncological outcomes. Debate persists as to the benefits of prone versus supine, and even whether to commence with the perineal or abdominal phase.

A European study to compare the extralevator with conventional 'standard' APE was published in 2010; this study reported that CRM involvement was 49.6% with 'standard' APE versus 20.3% with ELAPE, and that incidence of intraoperative bowel perforations was 28.2% compared with 8.2% in those who had ELAPE [11]. West et al. also reported in a subset analysis of the ELAPE group (n = 176), that the intraoperative bowel perforation rate was significantly lower with the patient in the prone jack-knife position (n = 127) rather than in the lithotomy or Lloyd-Davies position (n = 30) (6% vs. 20%; $P = 0.027$). However, these numbers are small and in 19 patients the position was unstated.

Others have questioned the need for the prone position, in particular the Cleveland clinic published data in 2011 from a 10-year period (1997–2007), during which period 15 experienced colorectal surgeons had employed both lithotomy (n = 87) and prone (n = 81) positioning for APE in 168 patients [38]. This resulted in iatrogenic bowel perforation rates of 2.4% in the lithotomy and 4.6% in the prone position, and the proportion of patients with an involved CRM (<1 mm) was 13.8% and 8.6% respectively. This corresponded to local recurrence rates at 5 years of 5.7% in the lithotomy and 14.4% in the prone groups; however, this difference was not statistically significant.

A Dutch national referral center for advanced low rectal cancer published data in the same year, also from a 10-year study period (2000–2010), highlighting the impact of a quality improvement program, in which the importance of the perineal dissection was emphasized, on the surgical and oncological outcomes following APE. The program, introduced in 2005, involved standardizing the procedure with emphasis on a perineal first dissection incorporating the extended excision planes already described. All the operations, pre- and post-program, were performed with the patient in the supine position with the legs in dynamic stirrups. The data showed a significant difference in positive resection margins compared with historical controls, 6.8 to 2.2% in T1–3 tumors and 30.2 to 5.7% in T4 tumors, following the introduction of the program. Local recurrence rates and overall cancer survival were also shown to improve with the enhanced perineal dissection [39].

It appears that commitment to a standardized and reproducible surgical technique, based on a sound anatomical and oncological approach, is the key to the improved published outcomes, rather than the patient position during surgery. Mathis et al. add further support to this hypothesis [12] in a 2012 publication from the Mayo clinic over a 16-year period (1990–2006) for rectal cancers treated by surgery alone [30]. In the 246 patients treated with an APE, the local recurrence rate was 5.5%; they employed extended tissue excision planes similar to those described in ELAPE, but all of the patients were operated on in the modified Lloyd-Davies position.

Choice of position and sequence for perineal dissection

The prone position may well allow better perineal access for advanced cases, in particular to the anterior plane in the male pelvis, and may improve visualization. This may facilitate teaching and demonstration [12]. Similarly, coccygectomy may further enhance both access and visualization. The disadvantages are having to physically turn the patient intra-operatively and once the patient is in a prone position, it is not then possible to access the abdomen.

The supine/lithotomy/lloyd-davies position, however, allows bimodal (both abdominal and perineal) assessment of advanced tumors and the time involved and potential risks of turning the patient are avoided. There is an increase in hydrostatic venous pressure in the prone position, but that can be somewhat counteracted by 'Trendelenburg' table adjustment.

The benefits of starting with the perineal dissection means that the dissection planes are easily recognized during the abdominal phase, thus reducing the risk of inadvertently dissecting below the desired anatomical landmarks of the upper TME dissection. However, it means the abdominal cavity cannot be assessed for metastatic disease before the excision is commenced.

Laparoscopic versus open

Laparoscopic surgery for colonic cancer is now widely practised and has been shown to be oncologically equivalent to open surgery with short-term benefits, such as reduced postoperative pain, quicker recovery, reduced hospital stay, and less scarring [41;42]. Concerns regarding the technical difficulties of laparoscopic rectal cancer surgery, and therefore the oncological efficacy, meant most of the initial laparoscopic trials did not include patients with rectal cancer.

However, the MRC CLASICC study included 381 patients with rectal cancer, 97 of whom were treated by APE (34 open and 63 laparoscopically). Early results reported a non-significant increased rate of involved CRM in patients undergoing laparoscopic (12.4%) versus open (6.3%) anterior resection, but in the APE group there was no difference in CRM positivity (20% vs. 26%). There was a significant reduction in time to first bowel activity and hospital stay but an increased operative time [9]. The 5-year follow-up results were published in 2010 and reported no difference in local recurrence rates, or disease free survival, between the laparoscopic and open techniques in anterior resection or APE. The report concludes that, 'the use of laparoscopic surgery to maximize short-term outcomes does not compromise long-term oncological results' [8].

A 2006 meta-analysis, by Aziz et al., found 20 suitable studies (mostly non-randomized) to compare laparoscopic versus open rectal cancer procedures. Specific to APE, they found that there was no significant difference in oncological outcomes (CRM involvement, lymph node harvest, etc.) between the groups. For the laparoscopic approach, they found a significant reduction in time to stoma function, time to oral feeding, and length of hospital stay. There was also a reduction in the incidence of wound infection, but no difference in perineal wound complications or urinary retention. The disadvantage of the laparoscopic approach was a significantly longer operating time [43].

One of the few randomized controlled trials directly comparing laparoscopic with open APE was published by Ng et al. [44] and reported faster return of bowel function, earlier mobilization, and reduced analgesic requirements within the laparoscopic group; however, there was no difference in overall morbidity, hospital stay, or blood loss. Operating time and costs were increased in the laparoscopic group.

Despite TME and nerve sparing surgical techniques, bladder and sexual dysfunction are still recognized complications following excision of the rectum and, although limited, there is some evidence that the incidence of dysfunction is increased with a laparoscopic approach [45;46].

Laparoscopic excision of the rectum has been shown to achieve adequate oncological tumor clearance, with long-term outcomes equivalent to that of an open approach, and includes the potential benefits already recognized in colonic resection. However, rectal cancer surgery is more technically challenging and most reports have been from expert centers and must be interpreted with caution. The benefits are not substantial and experience and case selection are crucial.

Perineal wound closure

The rate of perineal wound complications, including infection and dehiscence, after conventional APE with primary perineal closure varies between 24% and 41% [47;48]. Factors that increase the rate of perineal complications include obesity, diabetes, the use of preoperative radiotherapy, and the extralevator approach [11;48].

The increased risk in ELAPE probably results from more extensive pelvic floor removal, with a larger defect than conventional APE. Most now recommend reconstruction either by myocutaneous flaps or biological tissue grafts after ELAPE.

Myocutaneous flaps

There are three main types of myocutaneous flap commonly described for perineal reconstruction: rectus abdominus, gracilus, and gluteus maximus. A vertical rectus abdominus muscle (VRAM) flap can be mobilized from the anterior abdominal wall to give a well vascularized (via the inferior epigastric artery) skin pedicle. It can be harvested at laparotomy without creating additional donor site wounds and is generally reliable with few wound problems [49]. A VRAM flap may not be feasible, however, if the abdominal wall is scarred from previous laparotomies or stomas, or if a laparoscopic approach is employed. A gracilus flap is generally considered less reliable than rectus abdominus, due to its inferiorly situated vascular pedicle. A viable alternative is the gluteus maximus flap reconstruction, as described by Holm et al. in conjunction with ELAPE, which offers good outcomes (4/28 wound complications) and has the advantage over the VRAM of being a local flap [13]. However, some concerns exist over postoperative musculoskeletal function and quality of life, and further evaluation is needed [50].

Given the rate of perineal wound problems associated with primary closure, some argue that the use of a flap should be routine in APE, particularly in ELAPE. However, potential disadvantages of myocutaneous flaps are an increase in operative time, risk of flap necrosis, donor site morbidity, and the need for specialist reconstructive surgeons.

Biological mesh

The use of biological mesh is gaining popularity and is a useful alternative to the myocutaneous flap in reconstruction of the perineal defect. The advantages are no donor site morbidity, a reduced operating time, and an easily learnt technique for mesh implantation that negates the need for a plastic surgeon. Christensen et al. published a series comparing reconstruction of the perineal defect, following ELAPE, with a fasciocutaneous gluteal flap versus biological mesh and found that there was no significant difference in septic complications (11% overall) but a significantly higher perineal hernia rate in the flap group [51]. Han et al. [52] have also reported good early results with biological mesh repair of the perineal wound and it may that this could become the standard technique if future larger studies corroborate these findings.

Omentoplasty

The technique of raising a pedicled omental flap, to fill the presacral 'dead space' created by APE, has also been proposed. However, although there is some evidence of improved wound healing [53], this remains controversial as a reconstructive technique. The use of a Myocutaneous flap (VRAM) is reported to be associated with fewer perineal wound complications and a lower incidence of perineal hernia formation than in the use of omentoplasty alone [54].

Morbidity and quality of life in low anterior resection compared with ELAPE

It is a historical and commonly held belief that a permanent stoma has a negative impact on a patients quality of life (QOL), and that consequently APE should be avoided if at all possible. However, the poor functional outcomes that can be associated with low anterior resection, with approximately 60% of patients experiencing some degree of incontinence and up to a third suffering from urgency and frequency, also have adverse effects on QOL. This could particularly apply to low rectal cancer, where the eventual anastomosis is very low and many patients have neo-adjuvant therapy. Thus a literature review in 2005 [55] concluded, 'no apparent differences in quality of life are found in rectal cancer patients with a permanent stoma when compared to non- stoma patients.'

A 2007 Meta analysis [56] confirmed these initial findings, that there was no difference in the quality of life experienced following APE or low anterior resection. This has been further supported by data published from the Cleveland clinic in 2011, which used validated QOL questionnaires to follow up rectal cancer survivors and found that there was no difference between those with a permanent stoma and those without [57].

For patients undergoing TME dissection, up to a third will develop urinary or sexual dysfunction, with overall early morbidity rates of approximately 40%. Low anterior resection is associated with a substantial risk of anastomotic leak and most patients will have a disfunctioning stoma (up to 20% permanent), with loop ileostomy closure associated with a 17% morbidity [58]. Countering this, ELAPE is associated with perineal wound problems in 38% of patients [11].

Interestingly if the patients are asked to make the decision as to type of surgery, 65% are willing to defer the decision to their surgeon and of the patients who do choose, the majority would choose anterior resection rather than APE. However, at longer-term follow-up, 80% of patients who had an APE indicated they would choose it again if given the choice [59].

How et al. have recently published longitudinal QOL follow-up on a small number of patients, all with low rectal cancer, who had either low anterior resection or APE [60]. QOL was similar at one year except that a number of patients who had low anterior resection had substantial impairment of continence with sleep disturbance.

The main priority in low rectal cancer should be optimal oncological outcomes and restoration of continuity should be secondary. Optimal staging, patient preference, a second opinion, and awareness of issues with ultra-low reconstruction will help in decision-making.

Neo-adjuvant and adjuvant therapies

Although in selected cases it is necessary to downsize tumors prior to excision, it is possible to achieve excellent oncological results by precision surgery alone for low rectal cancer. If appropriate use is made of optimal imaging to select patients, many even with T3 and/or node positive disease can be cured by surgery alone [61]. A recent paper by Mathis et al. [40] reported the results in 655 patients who underwent curative surgery without radiotherapy, including 246 (37%) who had an APE, with a local recurrence rate of 5.5%. These results confirm that complete tumor excision with negative margins will cure the majority of patients and should add to the call for selective use of radiotherapy. The current 1990 NIH consensus guidelines are out-dated, unfit for purpose in the modern era, dangerous for patients and for those of us who have to look after them, and expensive for society [62].

With the improved understanding of the extended excision planes involved in ELAPE, and the ability of modern imaging to accurately predict margin involvement, it should be possible to reduce the current level of radiotherapy use for low rectal cancer and therefore reduce the significant associated morbidity.

Summary

Although indications for APE have fallen in the last half of the 20th century, APE is still essential for many patients with low rectal cancer. The historical poor results in those who had APE have focused attention on technique. ELAPE represents an exciting development in improving outcomes for advanced low rectal cancer. As always, case selection, technical expertise, and on-going evaluation are required.

CASE STUDY

ELAPE case history

Male 10/5/47 – Presented Jan 2008

- DRE – Anterior rectal tumor 3 cm from anal verge, tender and suspicion of tethering to sphincter
- MRI – low rectal anterior tumor extending to internal sphincter – possible T2 and may be right obturator node involved
- Histology – moderately differentiated adenocarcinoma
- CRT – (45-Gy in 25 fractions) with Capecitabine
- Residual ulcer/biopsy positive

Sept 08 – ELAPE

- Open abdominal/prone perineal and omentolpasty
- Adenocarcinoma/internal sphincter involved ypT2NO

Oct 08 – Buttock/perineal pain++, ?Neuropathy – gradually settled

Jan 10 – Large perineal hernia
Feb 2010 – MRI and CT – What to do now?

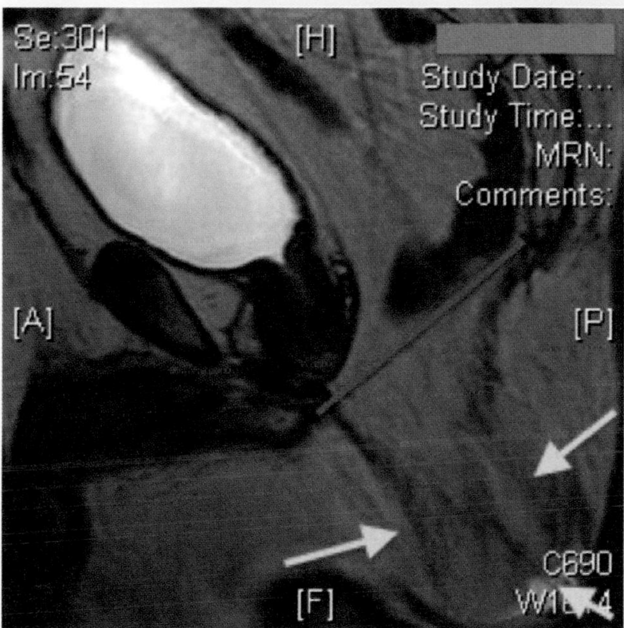

MRI: Sagittal section through pelvis showing pelvic floor (red line) and prolapsing hernia sac (yellow arrows)

TIPS AND TRICKS

- Decide on the surgical excision plane preoperatively.
- Care must be taken with the lateral dissection of the pelvic floor, near the sacrotuberal ligament, to avoid the main pudendal nerve and artery.
- The prone position and coccygectomy enhance visualization for anteriorly placed tumors in a narrow pelvis.

MUTIPLE-CHOICE QUESTIONS

1 Conventional Abdominoperineal Excision:

A. Gives better oncological outcomes than low anterior resection.

B. Is associated with the formation of a 'surgical waist' leading to higher rates of involved CRM and intraoperative perforation.

C. Has been increasing in popularity since the advent of the 'TME' plane for rectal surgery.
D. Was first described 10 years ago.
E. Is the treatment of choice for all low rectal cancers.

2 Extralevator Abdominperineal Excision is associated with:
A. Perineal hernia rate of 60%.
B. An increasing need for neo-adjuvant radiotherapy.
C. The use of the intersphincteric plane of dissection.
D. Similar impact on a patient's quality of life to low anterior resection.
E. An increase in local recurrence rates.

3 Good outcomes in Extralevator Abdominoperineal Excision are dependent upon:
A. Patient positioning.
B. Sequence of surgery, perineal versus abdominal component.
C. The use of precise surgical planes to incorporate a portion of the pelvic floor within the specimen.
D. The use of Laparoscopic or Open approaches to excision.
E. Intra-operative decision-making of the preferred surgical plane.

References

1 Heald RJ, Husband EM, Ryall RD. The mesorectum in rectal cancer surgery – the clue to pelvic recurrence? *Br J Surg* 1982; 69: 613–16.
2 Heald RJ, Moran BJ, Ryall RD, et al. Rectal cancer; the Basingstoke experience of total mesorectal excision, 1978–1997. *Arch Surg* 1998; 133: 894–9.
3 Miles EJ. A method of performing abdomino-perineal excision for carcinoma of the rectum and terminal portion of the pelvic colon. *The Lancet,* 19 Dec 1908; 1812–13.
4 Heald RJ, Smedh RK, Kald A, Sexton R, Moran BJ. Abdominoperineal excision of the rectum – an endangered operation. Norman Nigro Lectureship. *Dis Colon Rectum* 1997 Jul; 40(7): 747–51.
5 Marr R, Birbeck K, Garvican J, et al. The modern abdominoperineal excision: the next challenge after total mesorectal excision. *Ann Surg* 2005; 242: 74–82.
6 Marijnen CA, Nagtegaal ID, Kapiteijn E, Kranenbarg EK, Noordijk EM, van Krieken JH, et al. Radiotherapy does not compensate for positive resection margins in rectal cancer patients: report of a multicenter randomized trial. *Int J Radiat Oncol Biol Phys* 2003; 55: 1311–20.
7 MERCURY Study Group. Diagnostic accuracy of preoperative magnetic resonance imaging in predicting curative resection of rectal cancer: prospective observational study. *BMJ* 2006; 333: 779–82.
8 Jayne DG, Thorpe HC, Copeland J, Quirke P, Brown JM, Guillou PJ. Five-year follow-up of the Medical Research Council CLASICC trial of laparoscopically assisted versus open surgery for colorectal cancer. *Br J Surg* 2010; 97(11): 1638–45.
9 Guillou PJ, Quirke P, Thorpe H, Walker J, Jayne DG, Smith AM, et al. Short-term endpoints of conventional versus laparoscopic-assisted surgery in patients with colorectal cancer (MRC CLASICC trial): multicentre, randomised controlled trial. *Lancet* 2005; 365: 1718–26.

10 Nagtegaa ID, Van de Velde CJ, Marijnen CA, Van Krieken JH, Quirke P. Low rectal cancer: a call for a change of approach in abdominoperineal resection. *J Clin Oncol* 2005 Dec; 23: 9257–64.

11 West NP, Anderin C, Smith KJ, Holm T, Quirke P. Multicentre experience with extralevator abdominoperineal excision for low rectal cancer. *Br J Surg* 2010 Apr; 97(4): 588–99.

12 Moore TJ, Moran BJ. Precision surgery, precision terminology: the origins and meaning of ELAPE. *Colorectal Disease* Oct 2012; 14(10): 1173–4.

13 Holm T, Ljung A, Häggmark T, Jurell G, Lagergren J. Extended abdominoperineal resection with gluteus maximus flap reconstruction of the pelvic floor for rectal cancer. *Br J Surg* 2007; 94: 232–8.

14 Bebenek M, Pudelko M, Cisarz K, Balcerzak A, Tupikowski W, Wojciechowski L, et al. Therapeutic results in low-rectal cancer patients combined with abdominosacral resection are similar to those obtained by means of anterior resection in mid- and upper-rectal cancer cases. *Eur J Surg Oncol* 2007; 33: 320–3.

15 N, McFadden N, McNamara DA, Guiguet M, Tiret E, Parc R. Oncologic results following abdominoperineal resection for adenocarcinoma of the low rectum. *Dis Colon Rectum* 2003; 46: 867–74.

16 Lisfranc J. Mémoire sur l'éxcision de la partie inférieure du rectum devenue carcinomateuse. *Mém Ac R Chir* 1833; 3: 291–02.

17 Lange MM, Rutten HJ, Van de Velde CJH. One hundred years of curative surgery for rectal cancer: 1908–2008. *Eur J Surg Oncol* May 2009; 35(5): 456–63.

18 Goligher J. *Surgery of the Anus, Rectum and Colon*. London: Baillière Tindall, 1984: 590–779.

19 Nestorovic M, et al. One hundred years of Miles' operation – What has changed? *Acta Medica Medianae* 2008; 47: 43–6.

20 Miles WE. *Cancer of the rectum*. London: Lettsomiam lectures, 1923.

21 Lloyd-Davies OV. Lithotomy-Trendelenburg position for resection of rectum and pelvic colon. *Lancet* 1939; 2: 74–6.

22 Moynihan BGA. The surgical treatment of cancer of the sigmoid flexure and rectum. *Surg Gynecol Obstet* 1908; 463.

23 Dixon CF. Anterior resection for malignant lesions of the upper part of the rectum and lower part of the sigmoid. *Annals of Surgery* 1948; 128(3): 425–42.

24 Balfour DC. VIII. A method of anastomosis between sigmoid and rectum. *Ann Surg* 1910; 51: 239–41.

25 Pollett WG, Nicholls RJ. The relationship between the extent of distal clearance and survival and local recurrence rates after curative anterior resection for carcinoma of the rectum. *Ann Surg* 1983; 198: 159–63.

26 Heald RJ. Rectal cancer: the surgical options. *Eur J Cancer* 1995; 31A: 1189–92.

27 Mella J, Biffin A, Radcliffe AG, Stamatakis JD, Steele RJ: Population-based audit of colorectal cancer management in two UK health regions. Colorectal Cancer Working Group, Royal College of Surgeons of England Clinical Epidemiology and Audit Unit. *Br J Surg* 1997; 84(12): 1731–6.

28 Last R, McMinn RMH (eds). *Last's Anatomy, Regional and Applied*, 8th edn. Edinburgh: Churchill Livingstone, 1990.

29 Gray H, Williams PL, Bannister LH (eds). *Gray's Anatomy: the Anatomical Basis of Medicine and Surgery*, 38th edn. New York: Churchill Livingstone, 1995.

30 Goligher J, Duthie HL, Nixon HH (eds). *Surgery of the Anus, Rectum and Colon*, 5th edn. London: Baillière Tindall, 1984.

31 *www.lorec.nhs.uk*

32 Shihab OC, How P, West N, George C, Patel U, Quirke P, et al. Can a novel MRI staging system for low rectal cancer aid surgical planning? *Dis Colon Rectum* 2011; 54: 1260–4.

33 Brown G, Davies S, Williams GT et al. Effectiveness of preoperative staging in rectal cancer: digital rectal examination, endoluminal ultrasound or magnetic resonance imaging? *Br J Cancer* 2004; 91(1): 23–9.

34 Brown G, Kirkham A, Williams GT, Bourne M, Radcliffe AG, Sayman J, et al. High-resolution MRI of the anatomy important in total mesorectal excision of the rectum. *AJR Am J Roentgenol* 2004; 182: 431–9.

35 Bartram CI, Brown G. Endorectal ultrasound and magnetic resonance imaging in rectal cancer staging. *Gastroenterol Clin North Am* 2002; 31: 827–39.

36 Salerno G, Chandler I, Wotherspoon A, Thomas K, Moran B, Brown G. Sites of surgical waisting in the abdominoperineal specimen. *Br J Surg* 2008; 95: 1147–54.

37 Stelzner S, Holm T, Moran B, Heald R, Witzigmann H et al. Deep pelvic Anatomy Revisited for a Description of Crucial Steps in Extralevator Abdominoperineal Excision for Rectal Cancer. *Dis Colon Rectum* 2011 Aug; 54(8): 947–57.

38 de Campos-Lobato LF, Stocchi L, Dietz DW, Lavery IC, Fazio VW, Kalady MF. Prone or lithotomy positioning during an abdominoperineal resection for rectal cancer results in comparable oncologic outcomes. *Dis Colon Rectum* 2011; 54: 939–46.

39 Matijnse IS, Dudink RL, West NP, Wasowicz D, Nieuwenhuijzen GA, et al. Focus on extralevator perineal dissection in supine position for low rectal cancer has led to better quality of surgery and oncological outcome. *Ann Surg Oncol* 2012; 19: 786–93.

40 Mathis KL, Larson DW, Dozois EJ, Cima RR, Huebner M, Haddock MG. Outcomes following surgery without radiotherapy for rectal cancer. *Br J Surg* 2012; 99: 137–43.

41 Clinical Outcomes of Surgical Therapy Study Group. A comparison of laparoscopically assisted and open colectomy for colon cancer. *N Engl J Med* 2004; 350: 2050–9.

42 Veldkamp R, Kuhry E, Hop WC, Jeekel J, Kazemier G, Bonjer HJ, et al. Laparoscopic surgery versus open surgery for colon cancer: short-term outcomes of a randomised trial. *Lancet Oncol* 2005; 6: 477–84.

43 Aziz O, Constantinides V, Tekkis PP, Athanasiou T, Purkayastha S, Paraskeva P et al. Laparoscopic versus open surgery for rectal cancer: a meta-analysis. *Ann Surg Oncol* 2006; 13: 413–24.

44 Ng SS, Leung KL, Lee JF, Yiu RY, Li JC, Teoh AY, et al. Laparoscopic-assisted versus open abdominoperineal resection for low rectal cancer: A prospective randomized trial. *Ann Surg Oncol* 2008; 15(9): 2418–25.

45 Quah HM, Jayne DG, Eu KW, Seow-Choen F. Bladder and sexual dysfunction following laparoscopically assisted and conventional open mesorectal resection for cancer. *Br J Surg* 2002; 89: 1551–6.

46 Vaughan-Shaw PG, King AT, Cheung T et al. Early experience with laparoscopic extralevator abdominoperineal excision within an enhanced recovery setting: analysis of short-term outcomes and quality of life. *Ann R Coll Surg Engl* 2011; 93(6), 451–9.

47 Bullard KM, Trudel JL, Baxter NN, Rothenberger DA. Primary perineal wound closure after preoperative radiotherapy and abdominoperineal resection has a high incidence of wound failure. *Dis Colon Rectum* 2005; 48: 438–43.

48 Christian CK, Kwaan MR, Betensky RA, Breen EM, Zinner MJ, Bleday R. Risk factors for perineal wound complications following abdominoperineal resection. *Dis Colon Rectum* 2005; 48: 43–8.

49 Chessin DB, Hartley J, Cohen AM, Mazumdar M, Cordeiro P, Disa J, et al. Rectus flap reconstruction decreases perineal wound complications after pelvic chemoradiation and surgery: a cohort study. *Ann Surg Oncol* 2005; 12: 104–10.

50 Haapamåki MH, Pihlgren V, Lundberg O, Sandzén B, Rutegård J. Physical performance and quality of life after extended abdominoperineal excision of rectum and reconstruction of the pelvic floor with gluteus maximus flap. *Dis Colon Rectum* 2011; 54: 101–6.

51 Christensen HK, Nerstrom P, Tei T, Laurberg S. Perineal repair after extralevator abdominoperineal excision for low rectal cancer. *Dis Colon Rectum* 2011; 54: 711–17.

52 Han JG, Wang ZJ, Gao SG, Xu HM, Yang ZH, Jin ML. Pelvic floor reconstruction using human acellular dermal matrix after cylindrical abdominoperineal resection. *Dis Colon Rectum* 2010; 53: 219–23.

53 Nilsson PJ. Omentoplasty in abdominoperineal resection: a review of the literature using a systematic approach. *Dis Colon Rectum* 2006; 49: 1354–61.

54 Lefevre JH, MD, Parc Y, Kernéis S, Shields C, Touboul E, Chaouat M, Tiret E. Abdomino-perineal resection for anal cancer: impact of a vertical rectus abdominis myocutaneus flap on survival, recurrence, morbidity, and wound healing. *Ann Surg* 2009; 250: 707–11.

55 Pachler J, Wille-Jørgensen P. Quality of life after rectal re-section for cancer, with or without permanent colostomy. *Cochrane Database Syst Rev* 2005; CD004323.

56 Cornish JA, Tilney HS, Heriot AG, Lavery IC, Fazio VW, Tekkis PP. A meta-analysis of quality of life for abdominoperineal excision of rectum versus anterior resection for rectal cancer. *Ann Surg Oncol* 2007; 14: 2056–68.

57 de Campos-Lobato LF, Alves-Ferreira PC, Lavery IC, Kiran RP. Abdominoperineal resection does not decrease quality of life in patients with low rectal cancer. *Clinics* 2011; 66(6): 1035–40.

58 Perez RO, Habr-Gama A, Seid VE, Proscurshim I, Sousa AH Jr, Kiss DR. Loop ileostomy morbidity: timing of closure matters. *Dis Colon Rectum* 2006; 49: 1539–45.

59 Zolciak A, Bujko K, Kepka L, Oledzki J, Rutkowski A, Nowacki MP. Abdominoperineal resection or anterior resection for rectal cancer: patient preferences before and after treatment. *Colorectal Dis* 2006; 8: 575–80.

60 How P, Stelzner S, Branagan G, Bundy K, Chandrakumaran K, Heald RJ, Moran B. comparative quality of life in patients following abdominoperineal excision and low anterior resection for low rectal cancer. *Dis Colon Rectum* 2012; 55: 400–6.

61 Taylor FG, Quirke P, Heald RJ, Moran B, Blomqvist L, Swift I, et al. Preoperative high-resolution magnetic resonance imaging can identify good prognosis stage I, II, and III rectal cancer best managed by surgery alone: a prospective, multicenter, European study. *Ann Surg* 2011 Apr; 253(4): 711–9.

62 NIH consensus conference. Adjuvant therapy for patients with colon and rectal cancer. *JAMA* 1990 Sep 19; 264(11): 1444–50.

ANSWERS TO MULTIPLE-CHOICE QUESTIONS

1 B
2 D
3 C

CHAPTER 7

Neoadjuvant therapy without surgery for early stage rectal cancer?

Thomas D. Pinkney & Simon P. Bach
University Hospital Birmingham, UK

KEY POINTS

- Bowel cancer screening will change how rectal cancer presents, as a high proportion of early-stage tumors are identified.
- Due to lead-time bias, small tumors detected by screening may not show the same propensity for biological indolence compared to equivalent staged, symptomatic lesions.
- Early diagnosis provides an opportunity to develop minimally invasive strategies that preserve the rectum, avoiding the considerable morbidity and mortality associated with traditional radical surgery, to enhance the patient's quality of life.
- Local excision with transanal endoscopic microsurgery (TEMS) cures the majority of early-stage rectal cancer, but oncological efficacy does not match that of radical surgery for unselected cases.
- Low rectal cancer may be a special case, where lateral tumor spread in high-risk cases means that conventional total mesorectal excision (TME) surgery alone is not the most rational strategy.
- Combining pre-operative radiotherapy with transanal endoscopic microsurgery (TEMS) is appealing as:
  1. radiotherapy may effectively treat microscopic nodal metastases within the mesorectum or pelvic sidewall;
  2. tumor downsizing should facilitate TEMS with clear margins;
  3. tumor downstaging is measured objectively rather than relying upon clinical evaluation of response; and
  4. histopathological non-responders may be converted to radical surgery.
- Pathological complete response (pCR), i.e. the absence of viable tumor cells within the resected specimen, may obviate the requirement for local excision in some circumstances. While pCR is vital for organ conservation in the context of locally advanced

Colorectal Cancer: Diagnosis and Clinical Management, First Edition. Edited by John H. Scholefield and Cathy Eng.

disease, it is unlikely to be a prerequisite for successful treatment in the majority of early stage lesions when combined with TEMS. Hence, employing toxic treatment schedules in order to optimize pCR may not be a rational approach to the treatment of early stage rectal cancer.

- Contact radiotherapy has been suggested as a potential treatment for early rectal cancers, but data are limited and use of such 'topical' treatment in isolation does not encompass lymph nodes of the mesorectum or pelvic sidewall that can harbor foci of occult tumor spread.

Introduction

Symptomatic rectal cancer presents as a broad spectrum of disease with a bias towards advanced stage at presentation and less than 10% early-stage (T1–2) tumors. Bowel cancer screening identifies a much higher proportion of early-stage tumors; in the order of 50% Dukes A when faecal occult blood testing is used as a screening tool, rising to 62% for one-off flexible sigmoidoscopy [1;2]. Radical TME evolved to treat locally advanced, symptomatic tumors, but can also offer high rates of cure for early-stage rectal cancer with only 3–6% of patients subsequently relapsing [3;4]. Nevertheless there are concerns that this major surgery, with its attendant morbidity and mortality risks, may not be the optimal treatment for early tumors. Local treatment, with radical therapy salvage in the event of recurrence, could be safer and functionally far superior without substantially compromising cancer survival.

The principal disadvantage of radical TME surgery for treatment of early-stage rectal cancer is that for the majority of cases it is akin to using 'a sledgehammer to crack a nut'. This is especially true for low rectal cancer. In addition, the fact that rectal cancer predominantly affects the elderly provides a further incentive to explore less hazardous treatment options. Six-month mortality following radical curative surgery for rectal cancer is 4.6% for patients aged 65–74 years and 13.4% for patients aged 75–84 years, according to the Netherlands registry and randomized controlled trial (RCT) data which has been collated since 1990 [5]. The same study found that mortality may reach 30% at 6 months in those aged over 85 years. TME surgery for rectal cancer is associated with significant morbidity in the form of sexual and urinary dysfunction, surgical site infection, wound herniation, and anastomotic leak. The Dutch TME trial reported clinical bowel leaks in 16% of non-irradiated subjects [6] and despite the advent of nerve sparing techniques, pelvic dissection may cause autonomic nerve damage leading to urinary (25–34%) and sexual dysfunction [7;8]. Over 50% of patients experience some form of faecal incontinence following TME, and 30–40% suffer daily symptoms of urgency, incomplete emptying, and stool frequency [8;9]. Three prospective cohort studies have examined health related quality of life scores following rectal cancer surgery [10–12]. Each demonstrated persistently poor social role, body image, and defaecation scores. Permanent colostomy is required in 10–30% of cases.

A second potential problem with radical TME surgery lies in its use low in the rectum. It is a widely held view that radical TME surgery is the optimal oncological approach for early-stage, low rectal tumors. This may not be true. We know from the Japanese literature, and more recently the UK MERCURY trial, that overt pelvic sidewall involvement is a feature of 15% of low rectal cancer [13–15]. We might argue that for low risk T1-2 tumors lying close to the anus, local excision with TEMS is optimal. Meanwhile T1-2 at higher risk of dissemination may be inadequately treated by radical TME alone if the pelvic sidewalls are not also treated. Indeed it may not be fanciful to suggest that a combination of radiotherapy and local excision should be strongly considered within clinical trials as part of the treatment algorithm for these cancers. Several studies are ongoing in this area; the UK randomized controlled TREC study compares radical surgery with short-course preoperative radiotherapy (SCPRT) plus delayed TEMS, and also France's GRECCAR II, the Dutch CARTS trial, and the recently completed ACOSOG Z6041 study [16–19].

While we hope that these studies will provide the robust evidence required to treat early rectal cancer effectively, it is worth exploring current evidence regarding use of the modalities at our disposal; chemo-radiotherapy (CRT), SCPRT, contact radiotherapy, and excision biopsy with TEMS. It is also interesting to explore what we understand about response to radiotherapy and indeed the phenomenon of complete pathological response.

Conventional neoadjuvant chemoradiotherapy (CRT) and the apparent complete response

Long-course chemoradiotherapy followed by an 8–12 week gap to TME surgery is currently the standard of care for locally advanced rectal cancer with a threatened circumferential resection margin. The 8–12 week break is generally sufficient time for tumor regression to occur, but can also lead to a small chance of progression in non-responders. This timescale has largely been arrived at through trial and error, without high-quality RCT data (see section below on 'Timing of tumor assessment after neoadjuvant therapy'). Higher grades of tumor regression after neoadjuvant CRT are associated with improved survival [20]. A proportion of tumors will seem to completely resolve so that they disappear from the rectal lumen after treatment leaving only a fibrous scar – the 'apparent complete response'.

Up until now, standard practise in most centers has been to proceed with planned radical resection in cases where complete response is suspected. This is viewed as a safe option, due to difficulties establishing that complete response has occurred without recourse to supporting histopathological analysis [21], anxiety that subsequent salvage surgery may not be curative, and a general lack of outcome data to support the non-operative approach. Nonetheless, due to the morbidity and mortality associated with performing radical surgery, clinicians are interested to learn if a non-operative approach can be safely adopted in apparent complete responders. Enthusiasm stems from a series of intriguing publications by Angelita Habr-Gama of the University of Sao Paulo, Brazil. This research reported long-term outcomes in a cohort of patients with radiological and clinical evidence of complete response after neoadjuvant CRT for resectable locally advanced rectal cancer. The findings represented a landmark shift in the way rectal cancer treatment is viewed.

The Brazilian experience

Habr-Gama et al. initially reported an 11-year experience of utilizing their policy of strict observation and deferred surgery in a subgroup of patients who exhibited a complete or near-complete clinical response [22]. In their series, 265 patients with potentially resectable and non-metastatic distal rectal cancers (0–7 cm height from the anal verge) underwent standard neoadjuvant CRT using 5040 cGy and concurrent 5-fluorouracil 425 mg/m^2/day and leucovorin 20 mg/m^2/day. Pre-treatment staging investigation consisted of digital rectal examination (DRE), proctoscopy, colonoscopy, abdominal and pelvic computed tomography, chest X-ray, and serum carcinoembryonic antigen (CEA) measurement. Some patients also underwent endorectal ultrasound assessment.

The baseline (pre-treatment) staging of this group were as follows: 4.5% T2, 86.5% T3, and 9% T4 disease. In addition, 27% of their cohort exhibited nodal involvement at baseline. Following neoadjuvant CRT, patients were re-evaluated by a colorectal surgeon using the same modalities as in the pre-treatment phase. Biopsies were obtained during proctoscopy. At this stage colonoscopy was also performed for those patients with an initially obstructing tumor that had precluded full endoscopic examination previously. Patients with no residual abnormality detectable on these combined clinical, endoscopic, and radiological parameters were considered to have a complete clinical response. This group entered a strict protocol-driven pathway of observation rather than undergoing immediate surgical resection. They were followed monthly with physical and digital rectal examination, proctoscopy with biopsy where feasible, and serum CEA assay. They underwent chest X-ray and Computed tomography (CT) scan of the abdomen and pelvis every 6 months. If they had sustained complete tumor regression at 1 year, patients were considered 'complete responders' and subsequently underwent the same follow-up in years 2 and 3 at a frequency of every 2 and 6 months respectively. The group with an incomplete clinical response underwent immediate surgery with either an anterior resection or abdomino-perineal resection (APR), both utilizing a TME excision.

This series reported a 27% complete clinical response rate and these 71 patients followed the observation pathway as outlined above. Conversely, 22 other patients (8.3%) were deemed to have an incomplete response and underwent resection, but were found to have no residual tumor cells on histopathological examination of the specimen (a pCR). A comparison of the 5-year survival rates showed the rate in the complete clinical responders (100% 5-year survival) versus the pCR group (88%) was significantly higher ($p = 0.01$). There were three systemic recurrences in each group and two endorectal recurrences in the observation group. No patient in the observation group experienced extraluminal pelvic recurrence. At overall median follow-up of 57 months, the 5-year disease-free survival was similar at 92% versus 83% ($p = 0.09$).

A subsequent paper from the same unit explored patterns of failure of this conservative treatment strategy for an updated cohort of 361 patients with a median follow-up of 60 months [23]. The overall rate of clinical complete response was similar at 28%. Once again, 7% of patients judged as incomplete responders had radical resections showing a pCR. A failure rate was reported of 13% in the non-operative patients with 5% endorectal, 7% systemic, and 1% combined recurrence. Of note is that these local recurrences occurred late, with a mean time to recurrence of at least 4 years. All endorectal recurrences underwent successful salvage surgery and the overall 5-year survival rate for these patients was 93%. No extraluminal pelvic recurrences were seen.

This adds fuel to the suggestion that initial surgical resection may not be necessary in complete responders, as it appears that the small proportion of patients for whom the non-operative regime fails can be successfully recovered with highly reasonable success rates.

There are some notable caveats when considering the Brazilian data. First, considering the composition of this cohort, by relying upon pelvic CT and in some cases endorectal ultrasound to differentiate T2 from T3 disease, it is possible that a higher proportion of early stage tumors were included than had been appreciated. Inclusion of patients with T2 disease would favorably affect outcomes and also lead to difficulties in replicating response rates for patients staged using magnetic resonance imaging (MRI). Second, the timescales of treatment failure are not yet well established and it remains possible that some may not have been identified within the 5-year follow-up period. As such, some believe that the long-term failure rates may be underestimated, although this remains conjecture.

Other evidence on the efficacy of non-operative treatments after apparent clinical complete response

The Brazilian findings have been corroborated by numerous other single center series supporting the feasibility of a non-operative approach after apparent clinical complete response [24;25]. It has been noted, however, that there is little consistency between studies in what exactly constitutes a complete response, and the subsequent non-operative observational follow-up strategy, which makes comparing outcomes difficult. Glynne-Jones et al. recently performed a systematic review on the topic, in which original data were extracted and tabulated and study quality evaluated [26]. A total of 9 series, containing 650 patients were identified and included. Again, significant heterogeneity was found with the selection of patients, imaging modalities, staging method, cytotoxic drugs used in CRT, and the radiotherapy regime, as well as the methods of identifying complete response patients and follow-up frequency and duration. These differences between studies precluded any meaningful meta-analysis of results. The main conclusion of the research was that the majority of studies reporting a 'watch and wait' approach had major limitations due to their mainly small and retrospective nature, with short and insufficiently rigorous follow-up. Functional and quality-of-life outcomes were noticeably lacking for these patients, being reported only by one group. The authors highlighted the need for better quality prospective evidence on the risks versus benefits of a non-operative approach in patients who appear to have completely responded to neoadjuvant therapy, and cautioned against the current evidence being inappropriately extrapolated to an unselected group of rectal cancer patients. It is hoped that the currently recruiting 'deferral of surgery' multicenter UK trial will provide this high-quality prospective evidence that is desperately needed [27].

The difference between apparent complete response and pathological complete response

It is important at this stage to ensure that the reader appreciates the difference between these two related but inherently different types of response to neoadjuvant therapy. pCR can be defined as the absence of any residual cancer cells within the resected surgical specimen – as such it can only be diagnosed after formal surgical resection of the tumor site and its surroundings. pCR rates cannot therefore be quoted for patients who have undergone purely observational treatment – these cases, such as those reported by Habr-Gama above, report apparent complete response (aCR) rate evidenced by appearance on imaging investigations, direct macroscopic visualization of the tumor area, and sometimes biopsy samples. This is also referred to as 'clinical complete response' by some authors.

The difference is an important one, as it is accepted that a pre-operative aCR does not always correlate with a pCR after the operation. A study by Hiotis et al. from Memorial Sloan-Kettering found that despite 19% of patients showing aCR in their retrospective series of 488 patients undergoing neoadjuvant therapy, only 10% were subsequently found to have pCR [21]. The pCR rate amongst apparent complete responders was only 25%, and whilst being a significant predictive factor for pCR, the majority (75%) actually had persistent foci of tumor present on histological examination. The authors suggested, when this paper was published in 2002, that patients displaying aCR should routinely undergo radical surgical resection. This is unlikely to be the final word on the subject, as this paper is weakened by its retrospective design combined with a short standard delay between completion of radiotherapy and surgery of only six weeks. Proponents of the watch and wait policy would argue that this is insufficient, as tumor regression may continue beyond this point. Histopathological evaluation at 12 weeks may have produced completely different results.

Long-term outcomes after pathological complete response

Individual studies have generally reported a trend towards an improved long-term prognosis in patients who underwent resectional surgery and were found to have exhibited a pCR on examination of their resected specimen. These findings were often not statistically significant, due to the generally small number of patients in this situation in each series. If definite outcome benefit was shown in a study, it could still sometimes be difficult to draw general conclusions due to the heterogeneity of tumors included, different chemoradiotherapy regimens, and the variable outcome measures including censoring in survival analyses due to abridged follow-up. A review by Maas et al. attempted to address this by pooling together the individual patient-level data from several studies to generate a large sample size, thereby allowing multivariable analysis [28]. Authors of all studies reporting long-term outcome data for patients whose resected specimens showed a pCR were contacted and raw data were requested. A total of 14 (of 17) authors participated and the subsequent data pool available consisted of individual patient-level data for 3105 patients, of whom 484 had a pCR. The crude 5-year disease-free survival was 83.3% (95% CI 78.8–87.0) in pCR patients compared to 65.6% (63.6–68.0) for those without a pCR. This was highly significant and confirmed by the adjusted hazard ratio for PCR for failure of 0.54 (0.40–0.73), indicating that patients with pCR had a significantly increased probability of disease-free survival. The authors concluded that pCR might be a marker of a prognostically favorable tumor biological profile, which may have less propensity for local recurrence and distant metastases and a better long-term survival profile than for patients with less or no response to neoadjuvant therapy.

Factors affecting response to neo-adjuvant therapy

At least five factors may affect response (or the appearance of response) to neo-adjuvant therapy; initial tumor stage, type of neoadjuvant therapy, timing of tumor assessment, the assessment method, and thoroughness of pathological examination.

Initial tumor stage

Available evidence suggests that response rates are inversely associated with stage at presentation. Small, localized T1/2 tumors appear to have a much better chance of complete response following neoadjuvant therapy than larger, bulkier T3 or T4 tumors. In the 385 patients within the CAO/ARO/AIO-94 trial who received preoperative CRT, pCR occurred in 25% of T2 tumors, 10% of T3 tumors, and 0% of T4 tumors [29]. The ACOSOG Z6041 study ($n = 77$) used CAPOX to derive 51% pCR/Tis in selected T2 tumors [19].

The baseline characteristics of patients' tumors pre-treatment must therefore be appreciated before reading too much into reported rates of pCR (or aCR) – and at present many series and pooled analyses in the literature suffer from a heterogenous or even undefined pre-therapy staging.

Type of neo-adjuvant therapy given

A randomized trial from Toronto assessed the dose response of rectal tumors and treated 134 patients with T3/4 cancers neoadjuvantly with either 40 Gy in 20 fractions, 46 Gy in 23 fractions, or 50 Gy in 25 fractions [30]. With rising dose there was significant improvement in 2-year local recurrence-free survivals of 72%, 90%, and 89%, respectively ($p = 0.02$). Pathological complete response was found in 15%, 23%, and 33% of patients ($p = 0.07$).

In addition to radiotherapy dose, fractionation, delivery method (see contact radiotherapy below), addition of chemotherapy, choice of drug(s), and drug scheduling may also affect response. The EORTC 22921 trial confirmed the importance of adding chemotherapy to neoadjuvant radiotherapy most conclusively [31]. This trial used a 2 × 2 factorial design with 1011 patients with T3 or resectable T4 tumors being randomized to either:

- preoperative radiotherapy alone;
- preoperative chemoradiotherapy (CRT);
- preoperative radiotherapy with 4 cycles of adjuvant chemotherapy; or
- preoperative CRT with an additional 4 cycles of adjuvant chemotherapy.

In all arms the chemotherapy was 5-FU and folinic acid and radiotherapy was 45 Gy in 25 fractions. A pCR was found in 13.7% of patients who had some form of chemotherapy, but only 5.3% in those receiving radiotherapy alone. The 5-year cumulative incidence rates for local recurrences were 8.7%, 9.6%, and 7.6% in the groups that received chemotherapy preoperatively, postoperatively, or both, respectively, and 17.1% in the group that did not receive chemotherapy (P = 0.002). Despite this clear local control advantage, of note is that 5-year overall survival was not improved by the addition of chemotherapy.

Chemotherapy regimens based upon 5FU utilize the local radio-sensitizing effects of the treatment without any appreciable impact upon metastatic microscopic disease. This has led to clinicians assessing more aggressive chemotherapy regimes to try and both improve resectability of cases with an involved CRM (ARISTOTLE trial [32]) and increase pCR rates (ACOSOG Z6041 [19]). While the rationale seems clear cut in locally advanced disease, if escalation of treatment enables resection with clear margins, simply improving pCR rates may not confer substantial benefit and specifically may lead to unacceptable side effects. This was demonstrated by early closure of the ACOSOG study.

Timing of tumor assessment after neoadjuvant therapy

As previously mentioned, the length of the deliberate time lag between ending neoadjuvant therapy and performing radical surgery has been highlighted as an important factor in rectal cancer treatment. The tumor needs to be given time to achieve maximal post-treatment shrinkage but this is offset against the risk of unnecessary delay in those patients whose disease fails to respond to neoadjuvant therapy. In terms of the pCR, a direct correlation will exist between the optimum time lag for this tumor response and the highest rates of pCR found on histological examination. Parallels can also be drawn in aCR identification, in terms of establishing the best time for reassessment of preoperative tumors to assess response to treatment.

Only one randomized trial has been completed to date exploring this timing factor; the Lyon 90-01 trial, which randomized 201 patients with T2 or T3 rectal tumors to either an interval of 2 weeks or 6–8 weeks between therapy completion and surgical resection [33]. A pCR was found in 10.3% of patients with the shorter interval as compared to a rate of 26% in those with the longer interval ($p = 0.005$). The radiotherapy regimen was not typical and patients did not receive simultaneous chemotherapy, so the results may not directly correlate with current standard practise. This said, the consensus of opinion is that an interval of 2 weeks is definitely too short after neoadjuvant therapy and most believe that a minimum of 6 or 8 weeks is appropriate to realize maximum benefit.

An ongoing current UK trial aims to provide further high-quality evidence about the optimum time interval – the National Cancer Research Institute (NCRN) '6 week vs. 12 week' trial (NCT01037049) will recruit 218 patients and assess if greater rectal cancer downstaging and regression occurs when surgery is delayed to 12 weeks after completion of CRT compared to 6 weeks [33]. Results are awaited.

The current UK guidance, issued by the colorectal clinical subgroup of the NCRI suggests that whilst earlier assessment may indicate whether a tumor is showing signs of response, the presence or absence of an apparent complete response is best judged 12 weeks after the completion of neoadjuvant chemoradiotherapy [34].

Assessment tool(s) used to assess response

The older studies first describing aCR, and treating these patients conservatively, used only digital examination, mucosal visualization with proctoscopy, CT scanning, and occasionally endorectal ultrasound to assess response to neoadjuvant therapy. Over the past decade, the role of MRI in the staging rectal cancer has been established and it stands to reason that the added sensitivity afforded by this modality would be of use in diagnosing aCR. This has been studied prospectively by the MERCURY study group in the UK, where 408 patients from 12 units in 4 different European countries underwent pelvic MRI prior to surgical resection of their rectal cancer [15]. Patients were recruited with all stages of cancer and pooled results found a sensitivity of 94% and a specificity of 92% for predicting negative circumferential margins after surgery. More importantly, the study showed that when radiologists undergo specific training and the radiological technique is standardized, results are reproducible between centers. This has far-reaching consequences for the planning of who should receive neoadjuvant therapy and for the standardization of assessments of outcome. However, as yet the predictive power of MRI scanning to correctly identify those who have had a complete response is not yet established. Positron-emission tomography (PET) may in the future be an important modality for the assessment of response, but its efficacy is still being tested. An Italian group did show that proportionate decreases in the uptake of 18-fluorodeoxyglucose (FDG) on PET scanning before and after neoadjuvant therapy correlated with the rates of pathological complete response [35]. A follow-on prospective trial from the same group, however, failed to establish useful predictive indicators from the modality on multivariate analysis [36].

The UK guidelines from the NCRI group [34] recommend the following methodology for defining an apparent complete response:

- Clinical examination under anaesthetic with palpation of the tumor site and visualization of the area with biopsy of the residual scar; and
- MRI scan of the pelvis, which shows no evidence of tumor mass as compared to the pre-treatment images, or alternatively a small amount of residual abnormal tissue which in the opinion of the multidisciplinary team (MDT) is likely to represent scar tissue only.

Thoroughness of pathological examination

The examination of the rectal specimen can be more difficult after neoadjuvant therapy, owing the resultant fibrosis and finding microscopic foci of residual tumor has been likened to 'finding the needle in a haystack'; being dependent on exactly where the slides have been taken from the tumor area and on how thoroughly they are assessed. Until recently there has been a lack of standardization of the definition of pCR and a degree of operator-dependence may be a realistic concern. The CORE II trial [37] has now led to development of a pathological consensus, which may be taken up internationally in the future in an attempt to standardize reporting of outcomes results:

1. Take 5 blocks from site of tumor; if no residual tumor:
2. Embed whole of suspicious area; if no residual tumor:
3. Take 3 levels through each block; if no residual tumor:
4. Accept diagnosis of pathological complete response.

Practical issues in the non-operative management after apparent complete response (aCR)

For many years surgical resection has been the mainstay of management of rectal cancer. As such, not performing an operation in a patient who displays aCR is still a novel step.

What to tell the patient after aCR

Because the long-term sequelae of non-operative management are not yet established, a full and frank discussion of treatment options available to the patient, including advantages and disadvantages of each course of action, is vital. This must also be fully documented with potential failure rates quoted clearly recorded. The patient and their family must be fully participatory in the decision as to whether to undergo conventional treatment and continue with resectional surgery, or to opt to defer surgery until/if there is evidence of residual or recurrent cancer in the rectum. If they elect to undergo observation alone, they must also understand that they are committing to a necessarily intense follow-up regimen, which will require numerous investigations and hospital visits.

Clinical follow-up strategy after aCR

Each of the studies exploring non-operative management of aCR patients utilizes a slightly different follow-up strategy. They all agree that the reassessment of the tumor must be structured, frequent, and rigorous to ensure that patients who do regress or recur are identified and salvaged as quickly as possible.

In the Habr-Gama studies, the observation (non-operative) group underwent monthly digital rectal examination, proctoscopy with biopsy if indicated, and serum CEA assay. They also had chest X-ray and CT scanning of the abdomen and pelvis every 6 months. If they remained clear at 1 year, the same physical examinations were undertaken in year 2 every 2 months and in year 3 every 6 months.

The current recommended policy in the UK is that patients should undergo 3-monthly examination under anaesthetic (EUA) with endoscopic vizualization and biopsy of the area, and also 3-monthly MRI scanning of the pelvis for the first year [34]. These patients should also have pre-programmed 3-monthly MDT meeting review and discussion of these results. After 12 months of negative follow-up, they should attend outpatient clinic every 3 months for the next 2 years for clinical examination, with a formal EUA and biopsy if any abnormality is seen or felt. MRI scanning is recommended at 12, 18, and 24 months. No recommendations are currently given for follow-up beyond this point.

Local resection of early rectal cancer

Local excision of rectal cancer has always existed alongside radical surgery. In the 1980s, Basil Morson reported that local excision was as effective as radical surgery for the treatment of Dukes A rectal cancer [38]. At that time excision was by Parks peranal approach or alternative sphincter splitting techniques. The peranal approach has its limitations as the surgeon only has restricted access to the lower rectum. In 2000 the Minnesota group produced a retrospective cohort study outlining high rates of treatment failure following peranal excision of T1 and T2 tumors [39]. Soon thereafter several other US institutions followed suit.

In general local recurrence rates were 20% for pT1 tumors and approaching 40% for pT2. These series all predated patient selection with pelvic MRI for evaluation of locoregional lymph node status. There were a number of associated publications suggesting that the results of salvage surgery for relapse after local excision were poor, although it seemed that these patients were not subject to intense surveillance schedules, perhaps due to frailty. Realizing that the technique of peranal excision was suboptimal, Gerhard Buess developed an elegant system for transanal excision of rectal tumors in the mid-1980s [40;41]. This became known as transanal endoscopic microsurgery (TEMS). His system was ahead of its time, providing magnified binocular vision of the rectum with regulated intraluminal pressure. This allowed surgeons to perform a variety of transanal operations, including full thickness excision of the rectal wall and associated perirectal fat to deliver rectal tumors with precise and clear margins. The efficacy of this optimized TEMS technique was examined in a UK national dataset of 487 patients undergoing TEMS at 21 centers [42]. This demonstrated 5-year local disease-free survival rate of 81.4% for T1 tumors and 70.7% for T2 tumors. Depth of invasion, maximal tumor diameter, presence of intramural lymphovascular invasion, advanced age, and poor differentiation were independently associated with local recurrence.

Patients staged with pT1 sm1 G1/2 LyV0 tumors less than 3 cm had recurrence rates below 5% (the mortality rate for radical resection in the UK). The majority of patients had tumors with intermediate risk of recurrence (10–25%). There are currently no means to precisely identify which cases will recur later following R0 local excision. Patients must decide whether they accept the possibility of under treatment in order to gain good function or rather prefer the strategy of over treatment and potentially poor function. In the future we hope that biomarkers will help refine these decisions [43]. The salvage rates for patients under surveillance will also be critically important. If surveillance detects recurrence at a suitably early stage then escalation to radical surgery may be reserved for the minority who would actually benefit from this approach.

An alternative strategy is to try and combat the factors responsible for local recurrence after TEMS. Tumor implantation at surgery or microscopic metastasis in locoregional lymphatics are both implicated in this process. External beam radiotherapy is known to half recurrence rates when applied in conjunction with radical surgery and has the potential to neutralize microscopic tumor deposits lying outside of the local excision field, shrink the tumor itself to facilitate resection with clear margins, and reduce risk of implantation at surgery.

Neoadjuvant radiotherapy and excision biopsy with TEMS for early rectal cancer

Combining pre-operative radiotherapy with TEM surgery is appealing as:

- radiotherapy may effectively treat microscopic metastases present in mesorectal and pelvic sidewall lymph nodes;
- tumor downsizing should facilitate local excision with clear margins;
- tumor downstaging is measured objectively, rather than relying upon clinical examination; and
- histopathological non-responders may be converted to radical surgery.

There is currently very little evidence to guide the use of downstaging radiotherapy and local excision as a curative treatment for early rectal tumors. Two small prospective studies have been conducted, the first comparing radical versus local excision following downstaging CRT [44], the second evaluated efficacy of long and short course neoadjuvant radiotherapy schedules prior to delayed local excision [45].

Another study from Lezoche et al. randomized 40 consecutive patients with T2N0 G1-2 rectal cancer to neoadjuvant CRT followed by either laparoscopic TME surgery or local excision using TEM after a 6–8 week interval [46]. Patients were preoperatively staged using a combination of macrobiopsy, ERUS, and MRI. The pCR rate following CRT was 35% (14 patients). A further 25% (10 patients) were staged as ypT1. With a median follow-up of 56 months (range 44–67 months), one from each group recurred (both ypT2). Salvage surgery was successful in the patient treated initially by organ preservation.

In the study of Bujko et al., 47 patients, with mainly T1 and T2 tumors (some early T3 allowed), received either neoadjuvant SCPRT or CRT prior to delayed local excision [45]. Radiotherapy was usually followed by TEMS after a planned interval of 6 weeks (range 4–15 weeks), although other local excision techniques were allowed. Tumors were less than 4 cm in diameter, staged by digital rectal examination and MRI or ERUS/ pelvic CT. Three patients did not progress to local excision. The pCR rates were 35% (11/31) following SCPRT and 54% (7/13) after CRT. Histopathology indicated pCR or completely excised ypT1 tumor in 66% (29 patients). These patients were all then observed. The remainder (n = 15) were candidates for conversion to radical surgery, of whom 7 were unfit or refused and one had a repeat local excision. APE was performed in 7 patients. Residual tumor was found within the bowel wall of 6 and 1 patient with ypT3 had mesorectal lymph node metastases. With median follow-up of 14 months (range 0–41 months) local recurrence was detected in 3/44 operated patients (2 × CRT, 1 × SCPRT), all of whom underwent successful salvage surgery.

A meta-analysis of 7 studies of CRT and local excision to treat 237 cT2-T3 rectal tumors, reported pCR rates of 22% with no local recurrences seen in this group [47]. A further 19% of tumors were staged ypT1, 36% ypT2, and 14% ypT3 with local recurrence rates of 2%, 7%, and 12%, respectively.

Recently the ACOSOG Z6031 study, a non-randomized phase II design, evaluated an enhanced chemoradiotherapy regime (Capox), combined with local excision for ERUS defined uT2 disease [19]. The aim was to optimize pCR, but unfortunately this protocol had unacceptable toxicity that led to closure of the study. Data from 77 patients were reported, with pCR rates of 44%.

SCPRT has lower acute toxicity compared to long-course in a direct comparison of the two treatments [48]. Similar differences were reported in non-comparative studies [6;49]. SCPRT can lead to high rates of pCR if surgery is delayed in both early and advanced disease [50–52]. Further improvements in surveillance following local treatment will potentially optimize successful radical therapy salvage for patients who do recur.

The role of local resection in patients exhibiting a complete response

Some have argued that a reasonable alternative to meticulous observation of a rectal cancer site, which has shown an apparent complete response, would be to remove the whole treatment site with local resection (TEMS) techniques. This has the advantage of allowing full histological assessment to confirm a *pathological* complete response, and removing the tumor bed which might logically reduce the chance of local recurrence. There is limited large-scale evidence to support this strategy, but it has been analysed retrospectively by Kundel et al., who compared outcomes in a group of patients displaying a complete response to treatment (diagnosed as a pCR after resection) who either underwent local excision (n = 14) or radical surgery (n = 23) [53]. At a median follow-up of 48 months, 4 patients in the radical surgery group had a recurrence and none in the local group did; one patient died in the former group and none in the other. Disease-free survival, pelvic recurrence-free survival, and overall survival rates were similar in both groups. Another finding in this series was that overall nodal metastases were rare in patients with pCR, with only one patient (3%) displaying this feature on examination. Several other groups have reported similar small series on local excision after pCR. Eleven such series were pooled and together compiled 100 patients showing an overall local recurrence rate of 7% and distal failure rate of 8%.

Contact radiotherapy alone in early rectal cancer

Contact radiotherapy as a curative treatment for early rectal cancer was first described in France in 1946, but gained much wider exposure through the work of Papillon when he reported his 36 years of experience with the technique in 1990 [54;55]. Currently around 1200 patients have been treated worldwide with contact radiotherapy [56].

The treatment involves the direct delivery of radiation endoluminally to the tumor using a hand-held unit. The primary advantage is the ability to deliver high radiation doses to the tumor under direct visualization with minimal toxicity to the surrounding normal tissues. The radiation dose administered falls of quickly with increasing depth from the source. The Papillon technique delivers a dose rate of 20 Gy per minute with 100% of this dose delivered at the surface, 50% at 5 mm depth, and only 20% at 10 mm. There is negligible scatter from the tube itself.

The treatment is typically given over 5 weeks, with 35 Gy delivered on day 1, 30 Gy on day 7, 20–25 Gy on day 21, and 10–20 Gy on day 35. A total of 80–110 Gy is therefore given in 4 to 5 fractions [57]. This compares with the standard external-beam dose of 45–50 Gy for rectal cancer, given over 25–28 fractions over around 5 weeks.

Gerard et al. reported a summary of the international results from contact radiotherapy in 2003 for T1 or T2 cancers, and showed a 50–70% overall survival with 80–90% local control [58]. Contact radiotherapy is only offered at one center in the UK at present. This unit (Clatterbridge, Wirral) reported their treatment policy and outcomes for the 242 patients treated with their multimodality approach (of which 124 underwent contact radiotherapy) up to that point in 2007 [56]. The outcomes were excellent, with 93% local control at 3 years, but the patients undergoing contact radiotherapy alone were not reported separately in this series.

Patients undergoing conservative treatment alone must be followed up closely over the first 2–3 years when the risk of recurrence is the highest. At Clatterbridge they are seen every 2–3 months, with digital rectal examination and visualization of the tumor area with sigmoidoscopy and a low threshold for biopsy if any suspicion of residual disease or recurrence.

Of note is that there are currently no UK guidelines for treatment with radiotherapy alone – the Association of Coloproctology of Great Britain and Ireland (ACPGBI) recommends local treatment for T1 tumors of less than 3 cm in diameter, but this local treatment here refers to local surgical excision [59]. There remains a paucity of randomized controlled trial evidence around the efficacy of contact radiotherapy as a stand-alone treatment for rectal cancer. As such it is not yet accepted as an alternative option to the 'gold standard' of surgical resection. Until further evidence is available from large-scale collaborations – which need to be international owing to the relatively small numbers of suitable patients and centers offering the treatment – the true role of contact radiotherapy in isolation is unclear.

Combining EBRT and contact radiotherapy

The concept that contact radiotherapy could be used to boost the radiotherapy dose delivered to the tumor and also treat the peri-rectal tissues whilst ameliorating complication rates relating to higher external beam radiotherapy (EBRT) doses damaging normal surrounding tissues is attractive. It draws upon the body of evidence showing that the radiosensitivity of rectal cancer is often highly dose-dependent and represents a potential further use for contact radiotherapy.

Gerard described his policy of giving initial contact radiotherapy of 60–80 Gy, followed by a course of EBRT giving a further 39 Gy in 13 fractions using a small distribution volume to irradiate both the primary tumor and any local lymph nodes [60]. A total of 116 patients with T1/T2 tumors were treated with a local control rate of 88% and an 83% 5-year survival.

The Lyon R96-02 trial was a randomized trial in which EBRT alone was compared with EBRT plus a contact boost of 60–80 Gy [61]. The same EBRT dose of 39 Gy in 13 fractions was given in both arms. Over a 5-year period, a total of 88 patients with T2 or T3 rectal tumors (lower than 6 cm from the anal verge and of less than two-thirds of the circumference) were randomized and improved rates of complete pathological response were seen in the contact therapy arm (23% vs. 15%; $p = 0.027$) along with a significant increase in sphincter preservation surgery (76% vs. 44%; $p = 0.04$). No increase in surgical complications was seen and anorectal function analysis was similar in both arms. Of note is that no concurrent radiosensitizing chemotherapy was given in this trial, which would be standard practise today and would be expected to improve pelvic control rates further. There have been no trials comparing combined EBRT/contact radiotherapy with no operation at all versus standard EBRT and surgical resection.

Future trials in contact radiotherapy

One of the main barriers to wider application and research into contact radiotherapy has been the obsolescence of the Philips RT50 machine, which is no longer commercially available. However, a new contact 50 KV machine (Papillon 50©, Ariane Medical Systems, Nottinghamshire, UK) has recently been introduced. This machine will reproduce the characteristics of the Philips unit with the added advantages of full computerization and a fiberoptic camera within the head of the applicator to allow real-time visualization of the tumor to improve treatment accuracy. This has facilitated the CONTEM (Contact and Transanal Endoscope Microsurgery) trials, which are currently in set-up [62]. The three linked trials are as follows:

1 CONTEM 1 will evaluate contact radiotherapy alone for T1–T2 N0 rectal cancers following margin-positive local excision;
2 CONTEM 2 will assess contact radiotherapy followed by EBRT plus capecitabine and oxaliplatin in patients with larger T1-2 N0 disease followed by local excision 6 weeks later; and
3 CONTEM 3 will assess contact radiotherapy plus EBRT in elderly patients with inoperable T2-3 N0-1 disease.

In the CONTEM 1 and CONTEM 2 trials, a total of 150 patients will be enrolled to demonstrate an estimated risk of local recurrence of less than 8%.

The future of non-operative treatment after neoadjuvant therapy in rectal cancer

In anal cancer, a traditionally highly destructive surgical treatment has been nearly fully subsumed over the past few decades by an organ preservation approach, which utilizes chemoradiotherapy as the mainstay of treatment. Whilst the majority of advanced rectal cancers are likely to still warrant exenterative surgery for the foreseeable future, it is interesting to contemplate if smaller, lower, or more radiosensitive rectal tumors may follow the same pathway in the future.

At present the vast majority of the evidence advocating a non-operative approach in rectal cancer is of low quality, generally retrospective in nature, and from single center case series or at best non-randomized trials. Most include patients with a range of tumor stages, different chemoradiotherapy regimens, variable diagnostic methodologies, and eclectic follow-up schedules. As such the true results can be difficult to unpick. A further concern is that because the idea is relatively new, long-term outcomes data is highly limited – it could be that all patients with apparent complete response do experience recurrence of local disease or development of distant disease, just at a later time than in the normal rectal cancer populations.

Increasing implementation of novel radiosensitizing systemic agents in neoadjuvant setting may mean that response rates (including complete response) will increase in the future. The advances in imaging, such as improved MRI images or interpretation techniques, and/or the use of FDG-PET, means that there is also the potential for more patients with complete response to be identified with a greater level of certainty. Similarly microarray gene expression may be proved to be a valuable tool in the prediction of complete responders.

Prospective and rigidly controlled data is urgently needed to best advise patients and clinicians about the safest treatment course. Consensus is required on the ideal definition, diagnostic tools, and timing of assessment for identifying complete response in a reproducible and scientific manner. Until this point, we believe that the proven efficacy of TEMS to completely remove early rectal tumors for a minimal morbidity profile outweighs the potential benefits of the non-operative approach which, at present, we do not know enough about. If a patient does undergo neoadjuvant therapy and be found to have an apparent complete response, there is probably good enough evidence to justify local resection of the tumor site with TEMS to minimize future risks.

TIPS AND TRICKS/KEY PITFALLS

- The majority of evidence on non-operative management of patients exhibiting apparent complete response comes from small and retrospective studies; as such their findings should be interpreted with a degree of caution.
- Pathological complete response (pCR) can only be diagnosed after surgical resection of the entire tumor area – until this point the diagnosis can only be an apparent (or clinical) complete response.

- The timing of tumor assessment after neoadjuvant therapy will significantly affect apparent complete response rates, as will the initial tumor stage and type of neoadjuvant therapy given.
- Primary TEMS resection of early low rectal tumors may provide a more reliable alternative to neoadjuvant CRT and non-operative treatment for responders in terms of long-term disease-free survival.

CASE STUDY AND MULTIPLE CHOICE QUESTIONS

A 64-year-old man is diagnosed with a low rectal cancer 5 cm above the dentate line. Initial radiological staging suggests a T2 tumor and he undergoes long-course neoadjuvant chemoradiotherapy (CRT) with a view to downstaging the tumor prior to radical resection with an ultra-low anterior resection.

On his post-treatment MRI scan performed 8 weeks after completion of CRT, there is no obvious remaining tumor tissue visible.

1 Regarding the current diagnosis in this patient: (select one correct answer)

A. He can now be said to exhibit a pathological complete response (pCR)

B. He can now be said to exhibit an apparent complete response (aCR)

C. A computed tomography (CT) scan must be performed before any conclusion can be made about a complete response

D. An examination under anaesthetic with palpation of the tumor site, visualization of the area, and biopsy of the tumor scar must be performed before he can be deemed as showing apparent complete response (aCR)

2 Assuming a diagnosis of apparent complete response (aCR) is subsequently made, which of the following statements are true regarding suitable subsequent management? (multiple answers may be correct)

A. Transanal endoscopic microsurgery (TEMS) resection of the scar tissue may offer lower surgical morbidity, with no known detriment in long-term survival compared to continuing with traditional resectional surgery of the rectum

B. Contact radiotherapy to the scar area has been proven to improve long term survival

C. If he continues with the predetermined management plan and undergoes ultra-low anterior resection, there is at least a 30–40% chance that he will experience daily symptoms of stool frequency, urgency, and incomplete emptying

D. An advantage of continuing with radical surgery would be that any pelvic sidewall disease would be effectively dealt with at the operation

3 The patient decides to undergo a non-operative treatment policy for his apparent complete response. All of the following are correct, *except*:

A. He should undergo 6-monthly examination under anaesthetic (EUA) with endoscopic visualization and biopsy of the area and also 3-monthly MRI scanning of the pelvis for the first year

B. The failure rate of this non-operative treatment policy is around 10–20% at 5 years

C. If the tumor recurs and he subsequently undergoes salvage resectional surgery, it is likely that the long-term outcome will not be inferior to if he had undergone primary resection

D. If the tumor is going to recur, evidence suggests that this will happen within the first 24–48 months

References

1 UK Flexible Sigmoidoscopy Screening Trial Investigators. Single flexible sigmoidoscopy screening to prevent colorectal cancer: baseline findings of a UK multicentre randomised trial. *Lancet* 2002; 359(9314): 1291–300.

2 UK Colorectal Cancer Screening Pilot Group. Results of the first round of a demonstration pilot of screening for colorectal cancer in the United Kingdom. *BMJ* 2004; 329(7458): 133.

3 Endreseth BH, Myrvold HE, Romundstad P, Hestvik UE, Bjerkeset T, Wibe A. Transanal excision vs. major surgery for T1 rectal cancer. *Dis Colon Rectum* 2005; 48(7): 1380–8.

4 Peeters KC, Marijnen CA, Nagtegaal ID, et al. The TME trial after a median follow-up of 6 years: increased local control but no survival benefit in irradiated patients with resectable rectal carcinoma. *Ann Surg* 2007; 246(5): 693–701.

5 Rutten HJ, den Dulk M, Lemmens VE, van de Velde CJ, Marijnen CA. Controversies of total mesorectal excision for rectal cancer in elderly patients. *Lancet Oncol* 2008; 9(5): 494–501.

6 Marijnen CAM, Kapiteijn E, van de Velde CJH, et al. Cooperative Investigators of the Dutch Colorectal Cancer Group. Acute side effects and complications after short-term preoperative radiotherapy combined with total mesorectal excision in primary rectal cancer: report of a multicenter randomized trial. *J Clin Oncol* 2002; 20(3): 817–25.

7 Hendren SK, O'Connor BI, Liu M, et al. Prevalence of male and female sexual dysfunction is high following surgery for rectal cancer. *Ann Surg* 2005; 242(2): 212–23.

8 Wallner C, Lange MM, Bonsing BA, et al. Causes of fecal and urinary incontinence after total mesorectal excision for rectal cancer based on cadaveric surgery: A study from the cooperative clinical investigators of the Dutch Total Mesorectal Excision trial. *J Clin Oncol* 2008; 26(27): 4466–72.

9 Temple LK, Bacik J, Savatta SG, et al. The development of a validated instrument to evaluate bowel function after sphincter preserving surgery for rectal cancer. *Dis Colon Rectum* 2005; 48(7): 1353–65.

10 Engel J, Kerr J, Schlesinger-Raab A, Eckel R, Sauer H, Holzel D. Quality of life in rectal cancer patients: a four-year prospective study. *Ann Surg* 2003; 238(2): 203–13.

11 Grumann MM, Noack EM, Hoffmann IA, Schlag PM. Comparison of quality of life in patients undergoing abdominoperineal extirpation or anterior resection for rectal cancer. *Ann Surg* 2001; 233(2): 149–56.

12 Wilson TR, Alexander DJ. Clinical and non-clinical factors influencing postoperative health-related quality of life in patients with colorectal cancer. *Br J Surg* 2008; 95(11): 1408–15.

13 Kobayashi H, Ueno H, Hashiguchi Y, Mochizuki H. Distribution of lymph node metastasis is a prognostic index in patients with stage III colon cancer. *Surgery* 2006; 139(4): 516–22.

14 Kobayashi H, Mochizuki H, Kato T, et al. Outcomes of surgery alone for lower rectal cancer with and without pelvic sidewall dissection. *Dis Colon Rectum* 2009; 52(4): 567–76.

15 MERCURY Study Group. Relevance of Magnetic Resonance Imaging-detected pelvic sidewall lymph node involvement in rectal cancer. *Br J Surg* 2011; 98(12): 1798–804.

16 *http://www.controlled-trials.com/isrctn14422743*

17 *http://clinicaltrials.gov/ct2/show/NCT00427375*

18 Bökkerink GMJ, de Graaf EJR, Punt CJA, et al. Study Protocol – The CARTS study: Chemoradiation therapy for rectal cancer in the distal rectum followed by organ-sparing transanal endoscopic microsurgery. *BMC Surg* 2011; 11: 34.

19 Garcia-Aguilar J, Shi Q, Thomas CR, et al. A Phase II Trial of neoadjuvant chemoradiation and local excision for T2N0 rectal cancer: preliminary results of the ACOSOG Z6041 trial. *Ann Surg Oncol* 2012; 9(2): 384–91.

20 Janjan NA, Crane C, Feig BW, et al. Improved overall survival among responders to preoperative chemoradiation for locally advanced rectal cancer. *Am J Clin Onc* 2001; 24(2): 107–12.

21 Hiotis SP, Weber SM, Cohen AM, et al. Assessing the predictive value of clinical complete response to neoadjuvant therapy for rectal cancer: an analysis of 488 patients. *J Am Coll Surg* 2002; 194: 131–36.

22 Habr-Gama AP, Perez RO, Nadalin W. Operative versus non-operative treatment for stage 0 distal rectal cancer following chemoradiation therapy. *Ann Surg* 2004; 240: 711–8.

23 Habr-Gama A. Assessment and management of the complete clinical response of rectal cancer to chemoradiotherapy. *Colorectal Dis* 2006; 8(supp.l 3): 21–4.

24 Dalton R, Velineni R, Osborne M, et al. A single-centre experience of chemoradiotherapy for rectal cancer: is there potential for non-operative management? *Colorectal Dis* 2012; 14: 567–71.

25 Maas M, Beets-Tan RG, Lambregts DM, et al. Wait and see policy for clinical complete responders after chemoradiation for rectal cancer. *J Clin Oncol* 2011; 29: 4633–40.

26 Glynne-Jones R, Hughes R. Critical appraisal of the 'wait and see' approach in rectal cancer for clinical complete responders after chemoradiation. *Br J Surg* 2012; 99: 897–909.

27 [Online]. *http://public.ukcrn.org.uk/Search/StudyDetail.aspx?StudyID=8565*

28 Maas M, Nelemans PJ, Valentini V, et al. Long-term outcome in patients with a pathological complete response after chemoradiation for rectal cancer. *Lancet Oncol* 2010; 11: 835–44.

29 Rodel C, Martus P, Papadoupolos T, et al. Prognostic significance of tumor regression after preoperative chemoradiotherapy for rectal cancer. *J Clin Oncol* 2005; 23: 8688–96.

30 Wiltshire KL, Ward IG, Swallow C, et al. Preoperative radiation with concurrent chemotherapy for resectable rectal cancer: effect of dose escalation on pathologic complete response, local recurrence-free survival, disease-free survival, and overall survival. *Int J Radiat Oncol Biol Phys* 2006; 64(3): 709–16.

31 Bosset JF, Collette L, Calais G, et al. Chemotherapy with preoperative radiotherapy in rectal cancer. *N Engl J Med* 2006; 355: 1114–23.

32 [Online]: *http://www.controlled-trials.com/ISRCTN09351447/*

33 [Online]: *http://clinicaltrials.gov/ct2/show/NCT01037049*

34 Gollins S, Renehan A, Saunders M, Scott N, Susnerwala S, Sun Myint A. Rectal Cancer – apparent complete response (aCR). Colorectal Clinical Subgroup, National Cancer Research Institute. Available from: *http://www.gmccn.nhs.uk/hp/portal_repository/files/RectalCancerApparentCompleteResponseafterChemoradiotherapy.pdf*
35 Di Fabio F, Pinto C, Fanti S, et al. Correlation between FDG-PET and pathologic response in patients with rectal cancer treated with neoadjuvant chemo-radiotherapy: First results of the Bologna Project. *Proc Am Soc Clin Oncol* 2005; 23: (abstr 3623).
36 Martoni AA, Di Fabio F, Pinto C, et al. Prospective study on the FDG-PET/CT predictive and prognostic values in patients treated with neoadjuvant chemoradiation therapy and radical surgery for locally advanced rectal cancer. *Ann Oncol* 2011; 22(3): 650–6.
37 Rutten H, Sebag-Montefiore D, Glynne-Jones R, et al. Capecitabine, oxaliplatin, radiotherapy, and excision (CORE) in patients with MRI-defined locally advanced rectal adenocarcinoma: Results of an international multicenter phase II study. *Proc Am Soc Clin Oncol* 2006; 24: (abstr 3528).
38 Whiteway J, Nicholls RJ, Morson BC. The role of surgical local excision in the treatment of rectal cancer. *Br J Surg* 1985 Sep; 72(9): 694–7.
39 Garcia-Aguilar J, Mellgren A, Sirivongs P, et al. Local excision of rectal cancer without adjuvant therapy – a word of caution. *Ann Surg* 2000; 231(3): 345–51.
40 Buess G, Hutterer F, Theiss J, Bobel M, Isselhard W, Pichlmaier H. A system for a transanal endoscopic rectum operation. *Chirurg* 1984; 55: 677–80.
41 Buess G, Theiss R, Hutterer F, et al. Transanal endoscopic surgery of the rectum – testing a new method in animal experiments. *Leber Magen Darm* 1983; 13: 73–7.
42 Bach SP, Hill J, Monson JR, et al. A predictive model for local recurrence after transanal endoscopic microsurgery for rectal cancer. *Br J Surg* 2009; 96(3): 280–90.
43 Leong KJ, Wei W, Tannahill LA, et al. Methylation profiling of rectal cancer identifies novel markers of early-stage disease. *Br J Surg* 2011; 98: 724–34.
44 Lezoche E, Guerrieri M, Paganini AM, et al. Long-term results in patients with T2-3 N0 distal rectal cancer undergoing radiotherapy before transanal endoscopic microsurgery. *Br J Surg* 2005; 92(12): 1546–52.
45 Bujko K, Richter P, Kolodziejczyk M, et al. Preoperative radiotherapy and local excision of rectal cancer with immediate radical re-operation for poor responders. *Radiother Oncol* 2009; 92(2): 195–201.
46 Lezoche E, Guerrieri M, Paganini AM, et al. Transanal endoscopic versus total mesorectal laparoscopic resections of T2-N0 low rectal cancers after neoadjuvant treatment: a prospective randomized trial with a 3-years minimum follow-up period. *Surg Endosc* 2005; 19(6): 751–6.
47 Borschitz T, Wachtlin D, Möhler M, et al. Neoadjuvant chemoradiation and local excision for T2-3 rectal cancer. *Ann Surg Oncol* 2008; 15(3): 712–20.
48 Bujko K, Nowacki MP, Nasierowska-Guttmejer A, Michalski W, Bebenek M, Kryj M. Long-term results of a randomized trial comparing preoperative short-course radiotherapy with preoperative conventionally fractionated chemoradiation for rectal cancer. *Br J Surg* 2006; 93(10): 1215–23.
49 Sauer R, Becker H, Hohenberger W, et al. Preoperative versus postoperative chemoradiotherapy for rectal cancer. *N Engl J Med* 2004; 351: 1731–40.
50 Pettersson D, Cedermark B, Holm T, Radu C, Påhlman L, Glimelius B, et al. Interim analysis of the Stockholm III trial of preoperative radiotherapy regimens for rectal cancer. *Br J Surg* 2010; 97(4): 580–7.

51 Bujko K, Richter P, Kolodziejczyk M, et al. Preoperative radiotherapy and local excision of rectal cancer with immediate radical re-operation for poor responders. *Radiother Oncol* 2009; 16; 92(2): 195–201.

52 Graf W, Dahlberg M, Osman MM, Holmberg L, Påhlman L, Glimelius B. Short-term preoperative radiotherapy results in down-staging of rectal cancer: a study of 1316 patients. *Radiother Oncol* 1997; 43(2): 133–7.

53 Kundel Y, Brenner R, Purim O, et al. Is local excision after complete pathological response to neoadjuvant chemoradiation for rectal cancer an acceptable treatment option? *Dis Colon Rectum* 2010; 53: 1624–31.

54 Lamarque PL, Gross CG. La radiotherapie de contact des cancer du rectum. *J Radiol Electrol* 1946; 27: 333–346.

55 Papillon J. Present status of radiation therapy in the conservative management of rectal cancer. *Radiother Oncol* 1990; 17: 275–83.

56 Sun Myint A, Grievey RJ, McDonaldz AC, et al. Combined modality treatment of early rectal cancer – the UK experience. *Clinical Oncology* 2007; 19: 674–81.

57 Higgins KA, Willett CG, Czito BG. Non-operative management of rectal cancer: current perspectives. *Clin Colo Cancer* 2010; 9(2): 83–8.

58 Gerard J, Ayzac L, Coquard R, et al. Endocavitary irradiation for early rectal carcinomas T1(T2). A series of 101 patients treated with the Papillon's technique. *Int J Radiat Oncol Biol Phys* 1996; 4: 775–83.

59 The Association of Coloproctology of Great Britain and Ireland. *Guidelines for the Management of Colorectal Cancer*, 3rd edn (2007). Available at: *http://www.acpgbi.org.uk/assets/documents/COLO_guides.pdf*

60 Gerard J, Romestaing P, Chapet O. Radiotherapy alone in the curative treatment of rectal carcinoma. *Lancet Oncol* 2003; 4: 158–66.

61 Gerard JP, Chapet O, Nemoz C. Improved sphincter preservation in low rectal cancer with high-dose preoperative radiotherapy: the Lyon R96-02 randomized trial. *J Clin Oncol* 2004; 22: 2404–9.

62 Lindegaard J, Gerard JP, Sun Myint A, Myerson R, Thomsen H, Laurberg S. Whither papillon? Future directions for contact radiotherapy in rectal cancer. *Clin Oncol* 2007; 19(9): 738–41.

ANSWERS TO MULTIPLE-CHOICE QUESTIONS

1 D
2 A, C
3 D

CHAPTER 8

Minimally invasive surgery for rectal cancer and robotics

David Jayne & Gregory Taylor
St James's University Hospital, Leeds, UK

KEY POINTS

- Laparoscopic rectal cancer surgery is gaining in popularity due to the documented short-term benefits as compared to open surgery.
- Short-term benefits include less postoperative pain, earlier recovery, shorter hospital stay, fewer wound complications, quicker return to normal function, and improved cosmesis.
- The long-term oncological outcomes of laparoscopic rectal cancer surgery, as documented in large randomized controlled trials, are comparable to open surgery.
- Robotic-assisted surgery offers several technological advantages over laparoscopic surgery, including a stable camera platform, 3-dimensional operative field, and articulating instruments.
- Whether the technological advances inherent in the robotic system translate into clinical benefits remains to be clarified.
- Preliminary evidence suggests that robotic-assistance may provide benefit in terms of reduced conversion rate to open surgery and perhaps lower circumferential resection margin positivity.
- Controversy continues as to the cost-effectiveness of robotic-assisted surgery.
- A rigorous random comparison of robotic versus laparoscopic surgery for rectal cancer is required.

Introduction

Laparoscopic techniques were introduced into general surgical practise in the 1980s and the benefits for patients' with benign disease were quickly realized in terms of shorter hospital stay, quicker recovery and return to normal

Colorectal Cancer: Diagnosis and Clinical Management, First Edition. Edited by John H. Scholefield and Cathy Eng.

function, and improved cosmesis. The application of laparoscopic techniques into colorectal practise soon followed, at first for benign disease and then for malignancy. However, the challenge in colorectal disease, as compared to other general surgical applications, was substantial. The laparoscopic colorectal surgeon was required to undertake the same multi-quadrant operations as open surgery, but with limited tactile feedback, poorly designed instruments, and under 2-dimensional operating vision. Concerns were also expressed regarding laparoscopic cancer surgery and the adequacy of oncological safety, with the reporting of unusual port-site recurrences. The guidance from national bodies at that time was therefore reserved, with the National Institute for Clinical Excellence (NICE) in the UK advising: 'For colorectal cancer, open rather than laparoscopic resection should be the preferred surgical procedure', and 'Laparoscopic surgery should only be undertaken for colorectal cancer as part of a randomized controlled clinical trial' [1].

In response, several large, multicenter, randomized controlled trials were set up to evaluate the safety and efficacy of laparoscopic colorectal cancer surgery. The first to report was the Clinical Outcomes of Surgical Therapy (COST) study group, who published the results of a US multicenter randomized controlled trial (RCT), comparing laparoscopic and open surgery for colon cancer in 2004 [2]. In their study of 872 patients recruited from 48 centers and followed up for a median of 4.4 years, they showed benefits for laparoscopic-assisted surgery, including less analgesic requirement and shorter hospital stay, with similar morbidity, mortality, and re-admission rates. There was no difference in survival outcomes, with local recurrence rates of 16% and 18% and overall 3-year survival rates of 86% and 85% for the laparoscopic-assisted and open groups respectively. Importantly, disease recurrence in surgical wounds was 1% for both the laparoscopic-assisted and open groups, indicating that abdominal wound metastasis was not peculiar to the laparoscopic approach.

The first randomized control trial to address the issue of rectal cancer was the UK MRC-CLASICC (Conventional vs. Laparoscopic-Assisted Surgery for Colorectal Cancer) trial [3]. Between 1996 and 2002, a total of 794 patients from 32 surgeons across the UK were recruited, of which 381 had rectal cancer. The early results from CLASICC were reported in 2005 and showed no significant difference in the short-term end-points, which included morbidity, mortality, and pathological surrogate markers for oncological outcome. The surgery, as judged by central pathological review of resection specimens, was generally of high quality in both laparoscopic-assisted and open arms, with similar longitudinal resection margins and lymph node yields.

However, two important concerns were raised. In patients undergoing laparoscopic-assisted anterior resection, there was a higher rate of circumferential resection margin (CRM) involvement (CRM positivity: 12% lap vs. 6% open, 95% CI: −2.1%, 14.4%, p = 0.19), although this was not statistically significant. In addition, there was a high conversion rate of 34% for laparoscopic-assisted rectal cancer surgery. This was a reflection of both a learning curve effect, as demonstrated by a fall in conversion rates throughout the study period, but also the increased technical difficulty associated with laparoscopic rectal cancer surgery. The main reasons for conversion were excessive tumor fixity or uncertainty of tumor clearance (41% of conversions), obesity (26%), anatomical uncertainty (21%), and inaccessibility of tumor (20%). Importantly, conversion appeared to have a negative influence on early postoperative morbidity and mortality, with significantly worse outcomes seen in those patients who were converted. Three factors were subsequently found to be independent predictors for conversion to open surgery; namely body mass index, male sex, and extent of tumor spread from the muscularis mucosa [4]. Thus, the obese male patient with a locally advanced rectal cancer is much less likely to complete a laparoscopic operation.

In addition to concerns regarding the oncological aspects of laparoscopic rectal cancer surgery, there were also issues relating to functional outcomes, in particular the preservation of bladder and sexual function [5]. Although this is a recognized complication following open surgery, with reported rates of bladder and sexual dysfunction between 0%–15% and 10%–5% respectively, the incidence of sexual dysfunction following laparoscopic surgery in male patients in particular seems to be increased (overall sexual function: difference lap vs. open −11.18; 95% CI: −10.94, −0.74; p = 0.063).

In 2006, NICE updated its guidance for laparoscopic colorectal cancer surgery stating: 'Laparoscopic (including laparoscopically assisted) resection is recommended as an alternative to open resection for individuals with colorectal cancer in whom both laparoscopic and open surgery are considered suitable' [6]. This statement was qualified by the caveat that: 'Laparoscopic colorectal surgery should be performed only by surgeons who have completed appropriate training in the technique and who perform this procedure often enough to maintain competence'. The NICE statement failed to distinguish between laparoscopic surgery for colon and rectal cancer and was generally taken as a 'green light' for widespread implementation. Subsequently, a UK Department of Health initiative, LAPCO, was launched in 2006 to promote the training and encourage uptake of the laparoscopic approach for colorectal cancer [7].

The current status of laparoscopic rectal cancer surgery

There has been a slow but progressive uptake of laparoscopic colorectal cancer surgery over the past 5 years. In 2011, the penetration rate in the UK was approximately 30% (8), which is still far below the ceiling for uptake, but more than most other European countries and the USA. This is undoubtedly a reflection of the long learning curve associated with laparoscopic surgery. Current estimates of the learning curve vary greatly, depending on the case-mix studied and the criteria used to assess proficiency, but are most often reported in the region of 50–60 cases for anterior resection [9;10].

The evidence base for laparoscopic colon cancer is now well established, and that for laparoscopic rectal cancer surgery is quite compelling. Over 50 studies have reported outcomes following laparoscopic rectal cancer surgery, a selection of which are shown in Table 8.1 comparing laparoscopic and open surgery. The conversion rates range from 0% to 33%, with few studies reporting rates greater than 20%. The majority of studies have reported no difference in morbidity following laparoscopic surgery. The duration of surgery is consistently longer with the laparoscopic approach, but with no obvious differences in short-term survival measures.

Two meta-analyses specifically addressing laparoscopic rectal cancer surgery have attempted to collate the available evidence. In 2006, Aziz et al. reported a meta-analysis, including 20 studies and 2071 patients with 44% undergoing laparoscopic and 56% open surgery for rectal cancer [11]. Significant benefits in favor of the laparoscopic approach were found for time to stoma function, first bowel movement, feeding solids, and length of hospital stay. Additional benefit was found for those undergoing laparoscopic abdominoperineal resection in terms of decreased postoperative analgesic requirement and less wound infections. No difference was found between the laparoscopic and open groups in extent of oncological clearance. In 2008, Anderson et al. reported a meta-analysis focusing on the oncological outcomes following laparoscopic rectal cancer resection [12]. Over 3000 patients from 24 studies were compared for differences in oncological outcome between laparoscopic and open surgery. At 3 years, no significant difference was seen between the two treatment groups: radial margin positivity was 5% (lap) versus 8% (open); overall survival was 76% (lap) versus 69% (open); and local recurrence was 7% (lap) versus 8% (open). The authors concluded that there was no oncological difference between laparoscopic and open resections for primary rectal cancer. This conclusion accords with the long-term results from

Table 8.1 Selected series comparing laparoscopic and open rectal cancer surgery.

Study author	Year	n		Procedure (%)		Conversion rate (%)	5-year survival (%)		Morbidity (%)		Duration of surgery (mins)		Lymph nodes removed		Hospital stay (days)		Local recurrence (%)		Follow-up (months)
		Lap	Open	LAR	APR		Lap	Open	Lap	Open	Lap	Open	Lap	Open	Lap	Open	Lap	Open	
Leung	2004	203	200	100	0	23.2	75.3	78.3	19.7	22.5	190*	144*	11.1	12.1	8.2*	8.7*	-	-	49.2
Wu	2004	18	18	61	39	0	-	-	5.6*	27.8*	189*	146*	7.8	8.2	-	-	-	-	-
Zhou	2004	82	89	100	0	-	-	-	6.1*	12.4*	120*	106*	-	-	8.1*	13.3*	-	-	-
Anthube	2003	101	334	77	23	11	-	-	11	25	218	218	12*	22*	14	20	-	-	-
Feliciotti	2003	81	43	74	26	12.3	62.5	60.6	-	-	-	-	10.3	9.8	-	20.8	20.8	-	43.8
Hartley	2001	21	22	71	29	33	-	-	28.5	18	180*	125*	6	7	13.5	15	5	4.5	38
Hu	2001	20	25	100	0	0	-	-	0	8	227*	146*	-	-	18.3	18	-	-	8
Pasupathy	2001	11	22	100	0	-	-	-	18	9	97.5	90	-	-	6.5	6	-	-	12
Vithiananthan	2001	27	17	100	0	-	-	-	26*	28*	-	-	12	11	6.1*	11.1*	-	-	-
Leung	2000	25	34	0	100	8	-	-	48	62	215*	166*	10	12	16*	25.5*	-	-	28.3
Fleshmann	1999	42	152	100	0	21	54	60	76	50	234	209	9.7	7.9	7.4*	11.9*	21.4	-	55
Schwander	1999	32	32	59.3	40.7	0	-	-	31.3	31.3	281*	209*	13	13	15.3*	21.9*	3.1	0	32
Goh	1997	20	20	100	100	0	-		-	-	90	73	20	19	5	5.5	-	-	38
Ramos	1997	18	18	0	100	10	-	-	44	66	229	208	11.1	7.8	7.4*	12.9*	6	17	20
Seow-Choen	1997	16	11	0	100	-	-	-	-	-	-	-	10	10	6.5*	8*	0	0	12 vs 33
Darzi	1995	12	16	0	100	0	-	-	33	56	195	104	9.5	6	11	17.5	-	-	-
Tate	1993	11	14	100	0	-	-	-	45	29	205*	123*	10	13	12.3	14.3	-	-	-

Data not reported marked with '-'. Values marked with '*' were reported as being statistically significant ($p \leq 0.05$). Lap: laparoscopic; LAR: laparoscopic anterior resection; APR: abdominoperineal resection the CLASICC trial [13]. Initial concerns regarding the higher rate of circumferential margin involvement following laparoscopic anterior resection failed to translate into a difference in local recurrence, overall survival, or disease-free survival.

The most recent evidence to emerge on laparoscopic rectal cancer surgery is from the COLOR II study. This multicenter study, involving 30 centers across the world and recruiting 1103 rectal cancer patients between 2004 to 2010, has recently presented its initial results at the European Society of Surgical Oncology (ESSO) conference in Stockholm in 2011 (unpublished). Patients undergoing laparoscopic rectal cancer resection had less blood loss but longer operations than those undergoing open surgery. Conversion to open operation was still observed in 16.4% of cases. There was no difference in the circumferential or longitudinal resection margins or the number of retrieved lymph nodes. However, laparoscopic surgery had the advantage of earlier recovery of bowel function, less analgesic requirement, and shorter hospital stay.

Two other trials of laparoscopic rectal cancer surgery are currently in progress: a US trial of laparoscopic-assisted versus open resection for rectal cancer (Clinical Trials.gov Identifier: NCT00726622) and the Australasian A La Cart trial (*www.australiancancertrials.gov.au*). The results of these trials are eagerly awaited.

TIPS AND TRICKS AND KEY PITFALLS

Laparoscopic rectal cancer surgery

- Patient selection is the key to a successful laparoscopic rectal cancer operation. Patients most likely to be converted to open operation include males, the obese, and those with advanced cancers.
- The patient should be correctly positioned on the operating table in a modified Lloyd-Davies position and adequately supported on a bean-bag to allow for extremes of table tilt.
- A combination of 5 mm and 10 mm ports should be placed to allow adequate retraction and triangulation, and a 12 mm port in the right iliac fossa to enable use of a laparoscopic stapler.
- The operation begins with laparoscopic assessment of the abdomen and the tumor site. For ease of identification, it is preferable to mark the distal tumor margin preoperatively by colonoscopic tattooing. The patient is placed in a steep head-down position with right-sided tilt, and the small bowel is deflected out of the pelvis and to the patient's right, away from the root of the inferior mesenteric vessels and duodenojejunal flexure. If necessary, the uterus can be retracted ventrally, out of the rectal operating field, by either stapling of the round ligaments to the anterior abdominal wall or by a trans-abdominal supra-pubic suture passed through the uterine fundus.

- The dissection should follow a pre-determined sequence. This usually involves:
  i) medial-to-lateral dissection with high division of the inferior mesenteric vessels;
  ii) retroperitoneal dissection of the left colon;
  iii) release of the lateral peritoneal attachments and taken-down of the splenic flexure;
  iv) rectal mobilization in the TME planes with autonomic nerve visualization and preservation;
  v) division of the distal rectum with a laparoscopic stapler;
  vi) specimen retrieval and insertion of stapler head through a Pfannenstiel incision with wound protection; and
  vii) intra-corporeal colo-rectal anastomosis.
- The autonomic nerves are at risk during:
  i) high vessel division as they run along the anterior surface of the aorta;
  ii) the pelvic brim as the sympathetic nerves form the two pelvic nerve bundles;
  iii) the lateral pelvic side walls where the sympathetic nerves intermingle with the parasympathetic afferents to form the pelvic plexi; and
  iv) the antero-lateral aspect of the rectum at the peritoneal reflection where they pass to the external genitalia and bladder.

  Particular care should be taken at all these points of dissection with prudent use of diathermy.
- The left ureter is at risk during:
  i) division of the inferior mesenteric vessels – the left ureter should be visualized and deflected posteriorly prior to vessel division; and
  ii) the pelvic brim, where it crosses the left iliac vessels and has a tendency to be tented upwards during the retroperitoneal dissection.
- The splenic flexure may or may not need to be taken down, depending on the redundancy of the sigmoid colon and the level of the colo-rectal anastomosis; much of the required colonic length is obtained by high ligation of the inferior mesenteric vessels. If splenic flexure mobilization is required, this may be aided by:
  i) insertion of a swab to mark the flexure during retroperitoneal dissection of the left colon;
  ii) slight head-up and right-side down tilt on the operating table; and
  iii) the operator assuming a position between the patient's legs.
- Rectal dissection in a tight pelvis may be aided by:
  i) the assistant providing retraction on the recto-sigmoid junction to lift the rectum out of the pelvis;
  ii) a sling placed around the upper rectum to facilitate assistant retraction;
  iii) an expandable retracting device placed through a supra-pubic port to facilitate anterior dissection.
- Any difficulty in accurately identifying the distal tumor margin can be resolved with the use of a rigid sigmoidoscope to provide transillumination of the transection level, which can be marked with a laparoscopic clip.
- Laparoscopic division of the distal rectum can be difficult in a tight pelvis and may be accomplished through either a right iliac fossa or supra-pubic port. Multiple stapler firings to transect the distal rectum should be avoided as it increases the risk of anastomotic failure. If necessary, stapling and transection of the distal rectum can be performed through the Pfannenstiel incision.

Robotic rectal cancer surgery

Robotic-assistance, in the form of the da Vinci™ Surgical System (Intuitive Surgical, Sunnyvale, Ca, USA), was introduced into surgical practise in the 1990s, with the potential to extend the boundaries of laparoscopic surgery. It consists of a surgical cart carrying 3 or 4 robotic arms to which the effectors (instruments) are attached, a digital integration/insufflation stack, and the surgeon's operating console. The robotic system offers several technological advantages that may overcome many of the difficulties of laparoscopic surgery. It provides the surgeon with a pseudo 3-dimensional immersive operating environment, intuitive operating without a fulcrum effect, a stable camera platform, and articulating instruments with 7-degrees freedom of motion. Originally developed for cardiac surgery, it soon found a niche in operations that demanded surgical precision within a confined operating environment. The first reported use of the da Vinci system for segmental colectomy performed for diverticular disease was reported in 2001 by Weber et al. [14]. Since then, the da Vinci has been used in many colorectal applications, including right hemicolectomy [15], rectopexy [16], and transanal surgery [17], although by far the most popular application has been in rectal cancer surgery.

The feasibility of robotics for rectal cancer resection was established by Pigazzi et al. in a series of 6 low rectal cancers [18]. A subsequent follow-up study, by the same authors, of 39 rectal cancers treated prospectively by robotic-assisted resection, reported a zero rate of conversion with a mortality of 0% and morbidity of 12.8% [19]. Table 8.2 documents the reported studies of robotic-assisted rectal cancer surgery up to 2011. The majority are small personal series with limited follow-up, but combined, they give the impression of potential benefits in terms of low rates of conversion, and more importantly, low rates of circumferential margin positivity. The only randomized trial compared 18 patients assigned to robotic-assisted resection with 18 patients assigned to standard laparoscopic resection [20]. No difference was observed in the operative times, the conversion rates (2 laparoscopic, 0 robotic), or the quality of mesorectal resection. The only difference was the length of hospital stay, which was significantly shorter following robotic-assisted laparoscopic surgery (robotic-assisted: 6.9 ± 1.3 days; standard laparoscopic: 8.7 ± 1.3 days, $p < 0.001$) and attributed to a reduction in surgical trauma. Whilst it is accepted that these studies are very preliminary and may include a degree of selection bias, they have also been performed on the learning curve for robotic surgery. In addition to original reports, there has been one systematic review of robotic-assisted rectal cancer surgery [21]. This included 7 studies and a total of 353 robotic-assisted and 401 conventional laparoscopic rectal cancer

Table 8.2 Published series of robotic-assisted rectal cancer surgery. Complication rates and lengths of hospital stay are comparable to conventional laparoscopic surgery. Conversion rates and rates of CRM involvement are lower than conventional laparoscopic surgery. Operative time is increased.

Author (year)	No.	Complication rate (%)	Conversion rate	Length of stay (days)	Operative time (mins)	CRM positivity (%)
Baik SH (2009)	56	5.4	0.0	5.7	190	7.1
Bianchi (2010)	25	16.0	0.0	6.5	240	0.0
Park (2010)	52	19.2	0.0	10.4	232	1.9
Patriti (2009)	29	30.6	0.0	11.9	202	0.0
Pigazzi (2010)	41	22.0	7.3	6.5	296	2.4
Choi GS (2010)	41	29.3	0.0	9.9	231	4.9
Pigazzi (2007)	39	12.8	2.6	4.0	285	0.0
Pigazzi, Luca (2010)	143	24.0	4.9	8.3	297	0.7
Kim SH (2009)	50	18.0	0.0	9.2	304	2.0
Prasad (2010)	51	22.0	3.9	6.5	350	0.0
Da Vinci	**527**	**20.2**	**2.5**	**7.9**	**271**	**1.9**

resections. Robotic surgery was associated with a significantly lower conversion rate, but no difference was seen in complications, circumferential margin involvement, distal resection margin, lymph node yield, or hospital stay.

The lack of good evidence to support robotic-assisted rectal cancer surgery prompted the design and implementation of the MRC/EME/NIHR ROLARR (Robotic versus Laparoscopic Rectal Cancer Resection) trial [22]. This pan-World randomized controlled trial aims to evaluate the technical and oncological safety and efficacy, and cost-effectiveness of robotic-assisted rectal cancer resection. Recruitment commenced in 2011 and short-term outcomes are eagerly awaited in 2013.

TIPS AND TRICKS AND KEY PITFALLS

Robotic rectal cancer surgery

- Patient selection is the key to a successful robotic-assisted rectal cancer operation. If the patient is suitable for laparoscopic rectal cancer resection, he/she will be suitable for a robotic-assisted operation. Male patients, the obese, and those with locally advanced cancers will be more likely to require conversion to open operation, although preliminary data suggests that this is less often the case than when similar patients undergo conventional laparoscopic procedures.
- The patient should be correctly positioned on the operating table in a modified Lloyd-Davies position and adequately supported on a bean-bag to allow for extremes of table tilt.

- Particular care is required in the positioning of ports, with consideration given to the range of dissection required within the abdomen as well as the potential for external collisions of the robotic arms. A combination of robotic and conventional laparoscopic ports will be required. A minimum distance of 'one-hand's breadth' is required to avoid external collisions of the robotic arms.
- The operation begins with laparoscopic assessment of the abdomen and the tumor site. For ease of identification, it is preferable to mark the distal tumor margin pre-operatively by colonoscopic tattooing. The patient is placed in a head-down position with right-sided tilt, and the small bowel deflected out of the pelvis and to the patient's right, away from the root of the inferior mesenteric vessels and the duodenojejunal flexure.
- The operation can either be performed as either a hybrid or totally robotic procedure. In the hybrid operation, the left colon, splenic flexure, and inferior mesenteric vessels are dissected using standard laparoscopic technique, and then the robot is docked between the patient's legs for the rectal dissection. The totally robotic operation is performed either with a single docking, or with docking/re-docking to facilitate the colonic and rectal phases of the operation. It is the author's preference to perform a re-docking manoeuvre for the majority of cases, particularly in the larger patient. In this scenario, the left colonic dissection and splenic flexure mobilization is performed with the robotic cart approaching the patient from the left side and the robotic arms docked to ports on the patient's right-side (Figure 8.1A). For the rectal dissection, the robot is de-docked and the operating table and patient rotated such that the robotic cart approaches the patient from the left knee; the robotic cart remains in the same position (Figure 8.1B). The robot is re-docked with the arms orientated for the pelvic approach. To facilitate movement of the robotic arms, a 'port-within-port' technique is used.
- Robotic-assisted rectal resection should follow the same pre-determined steps to those described above for laparoscopic anterior resection.
- Identification and preservation of the left ureter and autonomic nerves is the same as for conventional laparoscopic surgery.
- The technological advances of the robotic system enable novel techniques to be undertaken that would otherwise be very difficult in conventional laparoscopy. Natural orifice specimen extraction (NOSE) [23] has been advocated for mid- and low-rectal cancers, whereby the distal rectum is transected with the Endowrist™ robotic scissors below the distal cancer margin to enable extraction of the specimen through a wound protector placed through the anus. The specimen is resected at the perineum end and the stapler head secured in the colon with a proximal purse-string suture before being returned to the abdominal cavity. The wound retractor is removed from the anal canal and a distal purse-string suture placed with the use of the robot. A transanal double purse-string, single stapled colo-rectal anastomosis is performed. The need for an abdominal wound to retrieve the specimen is avoided, with potential benefits in terms of postoperative discomfort. Alternatively, for low rectal cancers requiring abdomino-perineal excision, division of the lateral and posterior pelvic floor can be performed from the abdominal robotic approach, facilitating an easy completion of the extra-levator excision from the perineum [24].

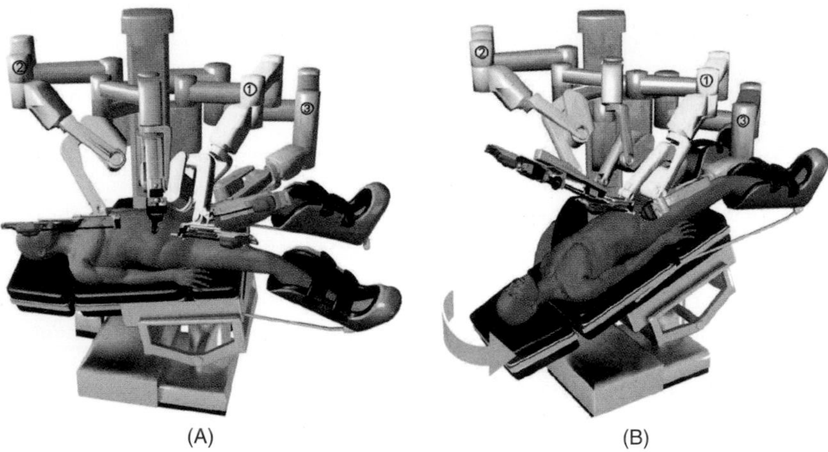

Figure 8.1 (A) Left colonic mobilization and taken-down of the splenic flexure is first undertaken with the robot approaching the patient from the left side, with slight patient head-down and right-sided tilt. (B) For the rectal dissection, the robot is de-docked and the operating table and patient rotated such that the robotic cart approaches the patient's left knee. The robot is re-docked with the arms arranged in a pelvic orientation.

CASE STUDY

A 65-year-old male presents with a 6-week history of fresh rectal bleeding and increase in bowel frequency, with a tendency to loose motions. Colonoscopy reveals a posteriorly located tumor at 8 cm from the anal verge, which on biopsy turns out to be an adenocarcinoma. A CT scan shows no evidence of metastatic disease and an MRI scan stages the cancer as a T3, N0 lesion with clear circumferential resection margins. The patient has a history of controlled hypertension, but is otherwise fit and well. He has a Body Mass Index of 35 kg/m^2 and a right iliac fossa scar from a previous appendicectomy.

MULTIPLE-CHOICE QUESTIONS

1 When counselling the above patient for anterior resection, which of the following statements are false?

- **A.** The patient is suitable for anterior resection by either laparoscopic or robotic-assisted approach.
- **B.** The patient's BMI of 35 kg/m^2 does not increase the chance of conversion to an open operation.
- **C.** The fact that the patient is male increases his risk of conversion to open operation.
- **D.** Previous appendicectomy will not increase the patient's risk of conversion to open operation.
- **E.** A robotic-assisted operation is more likely to result in conversion to open operation.

2 The proven benefits of laparoscopic as compared to open rectal cancer surgery include:
- **A.** A quicker resolution of postoperative ileus with return of bowel function.
- **B.** Improved pelvic autonomic nerve visualization with better preservation of bladder and sexual function.
- **C.** A quicker recovery with shorter hospital stay.
- **D.** Better oncological outcomes with improved disease-free and overall survival.
- **E.** Increased cost-effectiveness due to shorter operating times.

3 When undertaking a robotic-assisted rectal cancer operation, one should *always*:
- **A.** Place the patient in a steep head-down position with left-sided tilt.
- **B.** Allow 3 fingers-breaths between robotic ports to minimize external collisions of the robotic arms.
- **C.** De-dock the robot if any change in patient position is planned.
- **D.** Mobilize the splenic flexure using conventional laparoscopy.
- **E.** Allow for more operating time as compared to conventional laparoscopy.

References

1 National Centre for Clinical Excellence: Technology Appraisal Guidance No. 17: Guidance on the Use of Laparoscopic Surgery for Colorectal Cancer. December 2000. Available from: *www.nice.org.uk*

2 The Clinical Outcomes of Surgical Therapy Study Group: A comparison of laparoscopically assisted and open colectomy for colon cancer. *N Engl J Med* 2004; 350: 2050–9.

3 Guillou PJ, Quirke P, Thorpe H, Walker J, Jayne DG, Smith AMH, et al. for the MRC CLASICC trial group. Short-term end-points of conventional versus laparoscopic-assisted surgery in patients with colorectal cancer (MRC CLASICC trial): multicentre, randomised controlled trial. *Lancet* 2005; 365: 1718–26.

4 Thorpe H, Jayne DG, Guillou PJ, Quirke P, Copeland J, Brown JM for the Medical Research Council Conventional versus Laparoscopic-Assisted Surgery in Colorectal Cancer Trial Group. Patient factors influencing conversion from laparoscopically assisted to open surgery for colorectal cancer. *Br J Surg* 2008; 95: 199–205.

5 Jayne DG, Brown JM, Thorpe H, Walker J, Quirke P, Guillou PJ. Bladder and sexual function following resection for rectal cancer in a randomized clinical trial of laparoscopic versus open technique. *Br J Surg* 2005; 92: 1124–32.

6 NICE Technology Appraisal Guidance 105: Laparoscopic surgery for colorectal cancer. Aug 2006. Available from: *www.nice.org.uk/TA105*

7 LAPCO: National Training Programme in Laparoscopic Colorectal Surgery. Available from: *www.lapco.nhs.uk*

8 Morris EJ, Jordan C, Thomas JD, Cooper M, Brown JM, Thorpe H, et al. CLASICC trialists. Comparison of treatment and outcome information between a clinical trial and the National Cancer Data Repository. *Br J Surg* 2011; 98: 299–307.

9 Tekkis PP, Senagore AJ, Delaney CP, Fazio VW. Evaluation of the learning curve in laparoscopic colorectal surgery: comparison of right-sided and left-sided resections. *Ann Surg* 2005; 242: 83–91.

10 Park I, Choi G-S, Lim K-H, Kang B-M, Jun S-H. Multidimensional analysis of the learning curve for laparoscopic colorectal surgery: lessons from 1,000 cases of laparoscopic colorectal surgery. *Surg Endosc* 2009; 23: 839–46.

11 Aziz O, Constantinides V, Tekkis PP, Athanasiou T, Purkayatha S, Paraskeva P, et al. Laparoscopic versus open surgery for rectal cancer: a meta-analysis. *Ann Surg Oncol* 2006; 13: 413–24.
12 Anderson C, Uman G, Pigazzi A. Oncological outcomes of laparoscopic surgery for rectal cancer: a systematic review and meta-analysis of the literature. *J Cancer Surg* 2008; 34: 1135–42.
13 Jayne DG, Thorpe H, Copeland J, Quirke P, Brown JM, Guillou PJ. Five-year follow-up of the Medical Research Council CLASICC trial of laparoscopically assisted versus open surgery for colorectal cancer. *Br J Surg* 2010; 97: 1638–45.
14 Weber PA, Merola S, Wasielewski A, Ballantyne GH. Telerobotic-assisted laparoscopic right and sigmoid colectomies for benign disease. *Dis Colon Rect* 2001; 45: 1689–94.
15 deSouza AL, Prasad LM, Park JJ, Marecik SJ, Blumetti J, Abcarian H. Robotic assistance in right hemicolectomy: is there a role? *Dis Colon Rect* 2010; 53: 1000–6.
16 Munz Y, Moorthy K, Kudchadkar R, Hernandez JD, Martin S, Darzi A, et al. Robotic assisted rectopexy. *Am J Surg* 2004; 187: 88–92.
17 Atallah SB, Albert MR, deBeche-Adams TH, Larach SW. Robotic transanal minimally invasive surgery in a cadaveric model. *Tech Coloproct* 2011; 15: 461–4.
18 Pigazzi A, Ellenhorn JD, Ballantyne GH, Paz IB. Robotic-assisted laparoscopic low anterior resection with total mesorectal excision for rectal cancer. *Surg Endosc* 2006; 20: 1521–5.
19 Hellan M, Anderson C, Ellenhorn JD, Paz B, Pigazzi A. Short-term outcomes after robotic-assisted total mesorectal excision for rectal cancer. *Ann Surg Oncol* 2007; 14: 3168–73.
20 Baik SH, Ko YT, Kang CM, Lee WJ, Kim NK, Sohn SK, et al. Robotic tumor-specific mesorectal excision of rectal cancer: short-term outcome of a pilot randomized trial. *Surg Endosc* 2008; 22: 1601–8.
21 Memon S, Heriot AG, Murphy DG, Bressel M, Lynch AC. Robotics versus laparoscopic proctectomy for rectal cancer: a meta-analysis. *Ann Surg Oncol* July 2012; 19(7): 2095–101.
22 Collinson FJ, Jayne DG, Pigazzi A, Tsang C, Barrie JM, Edlin R, et al. An international, multicentre, prospective, randomised, controlled, unblinded, parallel-group trial of robotic-assisted versus standard laparoscopic surgery for the curative treatment of rectal cancer. *Int J Colorect Dis* 2012; 27: 233–41.
23 Prasad LM, deSouza AL, Marecik SJ, Park JJ, Abcarian H. Robotic purse-string technique in low anterior resection. *Dis Colon Rect* 2010; 53: 230–4.
24 Marecik SJ, Zawadzki M, Desouza AL, Park JJ, Abcarian H, Prasad LM. Robotic cylindrical abdominoperineal resection with transabdominal levator transection. *Dis Colon Rect* 2011; 54: 1320–5.

ANSWERS TO MULTIPLE-CHOICE QUESTIONS

1 B, E
2 A, C
3 C, E

CHAPTER 9

Surgery for anal cancer

John H. Scholefield
University Hospital, Nottingham, UK

KEY POINTS

- HPV is an aetiological factor in anal squamous cell carcinomas (SCC). Women with previous gynaecological lesions on the cervix and vulva and the immunosuppressed (transplant recipients and HIV patients) are at risk for AIN. These premalignant lesions may be rapidly progressive in immunocompromised patients. (*pen nib*)
- The management of anal squamous carcinoma has changed dramatically in the last few years. Chemradiation is the treatment of first choice for most lesions. (*scalpel*)
- Surgery may be the primary treatment modality for small perianal lesions that can be locally excised. (*pen nib*)
- Melanoma of the anus is very rare and has a dismal prognosis, radical surgery, chemotherapy, and radiotherapy are of little benefit. Local excision may provide useful palliation. (*pen nib*)

Introduction

Anal cancer is rare, accounting for approximately 4% of large bowel malignancies; however, there is some evidence that its incidence is increasing. Most anal cancers arise from the squamous epithelium of the anal margin or anal canal, although a few arise from anal glands and ducts.

The surgical literature on surgical treatment for anal cancer makes a distinction between the anal canal and perianal area, but these distinctions are not precise. This distinction between anal verge and anal canal has become less important as surgery plays a lesser role in treatment, but reports of surgical results from past decades are confused by this variation in definition.

Although anatomists see the anal canal as lying between the dentate line and the anal verge, surgically it is defined as lying between the anorectal ring

Colorectal Cancer: Diagnosis and Clinical Management, First Edition. Edited by John H. Scholefield and Cathy Eng.

and the anal verge. For pathologists, the canal has been defined as corresponding to the longitudinal extent of the internal anal sphincter. The canal above the dentate line is lined by rectal mucosa, except for a small zone immediately above the line called the transitional or junctional zone. Inferiorly, the canal is covered by stratified squamous epithelium. Further confusion relates to the definition of the anal canal and anal margin as sites for cancer. The anal margin is variously described as the visible area external to the anal verge, or as the area below the dentate line.

Over 80% of anal cancers are of squamous origin, arising from the squamous epithelium of the anal canal and perianal area; 10% are adenocarcinomas arising from the glandular mucosa of the upper anal canal, the anal glands, and ducts. A very rare and particularly malignant tumor is anal melanoma. Lymphomas and sarcomas of the anus are even less common but have increased in incidence in recent years, particularly among patients with human immunodeficiency virus (HIV) infection. There has also been a rise in the incidence of other anal epidermoid tumors among patients with HIV.

Most of what follows relates to the treatment of anal squamous cancers, which comprise the largest part of the surgical treatment of this condition.

Aetiology and pathogenesis

Anal squamous cell carcinomas are relatively uncommon tumors; there are between 300 and 400 new cases per year in England and Wales. Based on these figures, each consultant general surgeon might expect to see one anal carcinoma every 2–3 years. Anal cancers are probably under-reported, since some anal canal tumors are misclassified as rectal tumors and some perianal tumors as squamous carcinomas of skin.

The increasing incidence of HIV infection has resulted in a rise in the incidence of anal cancer, particularly in areas such as San Francisco, with a large homosexual population, seeing a dramatic increase. A recent study from Denmark has reported a doubling in the incidence of anal cancer over the last 10 years, particularly in women [1]. No other countries have reported similar increases to date, but the Cancer Registry data in Denmark are renowned for their remarkable accuracy and completeness.

Epidemiological and molecular biological data have shown an association between a sexually transmissible agent and female genital cancer [2]. Human papillomavirus (HPV) type 16 and less commonly types 18, 31, and 33 DNA have been identified in approximately 80% anal squamous cell carcinomas [3].

HPVs, which are DNA viruses, comprise more than 60 types capable of causing a wide variety of lesions on squamous epithelium. Common warts can be found on the hands and feet of children and young adults, and are caused by the relatively infectious HPV types 1 and 2. Anogenital papillomaviruses are less infective than types 1 and 2 and are exclusively sexually transmissible. The epidemiology of genital papillomavirus infection is poorly understood, largely due to the social and moral taboos surrounding sexually transmissible infections. Anogenital papillomavirus-associated lesions range from condylomas through intraepithelial neoplasia to invasive carcinoma. Although HPV is probably important in the pathogenesis of anal cancer, other carcinogens probably play a role too – there is evidence that other co-carcinogens may be metabolites from cigarette smoke, and other sexually transmissible agents such as Herpes Simplex and Chlamydia. The host response to these agents is also important in the pathogenesis of the disease – such that immunosuppressed individuals such as transplant recipients and those on systemic immunosuppressive such as steroids azothiaprine are at increased risk of anal cancer.

Once one area of the anogenital epithelium is infected, spread of papillomavirus infection throughout the rest of the anogenital area probably follows, but remains occult in the majority of individuals. Therefore the commonly held belief that anal cancer occurs only in individuals who practise anal intercourse is unfounded. This myth is often a source of great anxiety to heterosexual patients who develop anal cancer.

Premalignant lesions

Anal and genital papillomavirus-associated lesions may be identified clinically either by naked eye inspection or more usually with an operating microscope (colposcope) and the application of acetic acid to the epithelium, resulting in an 'aceto-white' lesion. Colposcopy of the anus (sometimes referred to as 'anoscopy') may suggest the degree of dysplasia and permits targeted biopsy of a lesion, but histological examination remains the diagnostic standard. Although the natural history of cervical papillomavirus infection and intraepithelial neoplasia is reasonably well understood, the same is not true for anal lesions, probably because they have been diagnosed only over the last 15–20 years. Consequently, the natural history and malignant potential of anal intraepithelial neoplasia are both uncertain.

Anogenital intraepithelial neoplasia of the cervix (CIN), vulva (VIN), vagina (VAIN), and anus (AIN) is graded from I to III, according to the number of thirds of epithelial depth that appear dysplastic on histological section. Thus in grade III the cells of the whole thickness of the epithelium appear dysplastic, being synonymous with carcinoma *in situ*.

High-grade anal intraepithelial lesions may be characterized by hyperkeratosis or changes in the pigmentation of the epithelium. Thus carcinoma *in situ* may appear white, red, or brown, the pigmentation commonly being irregular. The lesions may be flat or raised; but ulceration is suggestive of invasive disease. It is important that any suspicious area is biopsied and examined histologically. The terms 'Bowen's disease of the anus' and 'leukoplakia' are best avoided as they are confusing and convey no specific information, the malignant potential of both being uncertain.

At present, multifocal genital intraepithelial neoplasia represents a difficult clinical problem, which may be further complicated by the occurrence of synchronous or metachronous AIN [4]. The management of these patients is uncertain, as the natural history of these lesions remains poorly understood.

Histological types

Included within the category of epidermoid tumors are squamous cell, basaloid (or cloacogenic) carcinomas, and muco-epidermoid cancers. The different morphological types of anal cancer do not appear to have different prognoses. Tumors arising at the anal margin tend to be well differentiated and keratinizing, whereas those arising in the canal are more commonly poorly differentiated. Basaloid tumors arise in the transitional zone around the dentate line and form 30–50% of all anal canal tumors.

Patterns of spread

Anal canal cancer spreads locally, mainly in a cephalad direction, so that the tumor may appear to have arisen in the rectum. The tumor also spreads outwards into the anal sphincters and into the rectovaginal septum, perineal body, scrotum, or vagina in more advanced cases (Figure 9.1). Lymph node metastases occur frequently, especially in tumors of the anal canal. Spread occurs initially to the perirectal group of nodes and thereafter to inguinal, haemorrhoidal, and lateral pelvic lymph nodes. The frequency of nodal involvement is related to the size of the primary tumor together with its depth of penetration. Approximately 14% of patients will present with inguinal lymph node involvement, but this rises to approximately 30% when

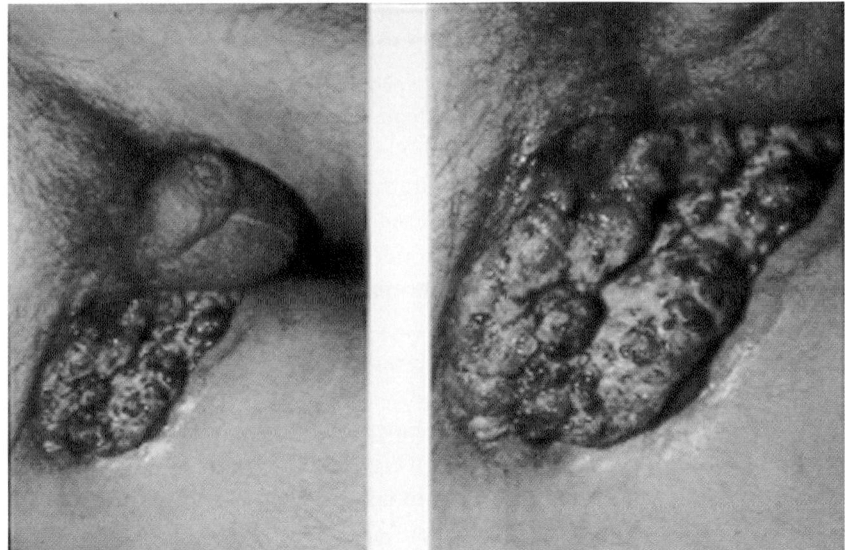

Figure 9.1 Locally advanced anal cancer involving the anal canal, perianal skin, perineal skin, and base of scrotum. Treatment with chemoradiation failed to control the disease and the patient underwent a salvage abdominoperineal excision.

the primary tumor is greater than 5 cm in diameter. Only 50% of patients with enlarged nodes at presentation will subsequently be shown to contain tumor. Synchronously involved nodes carry a particularly poor prognosis, whereas when metachronous spread develops the salvage rate is much higher.

Haematogenous spread tends to occur late and is usually associated with advanced local disease. The principal sites of metastases are the liver, lung, and bones. However, metastases have been described in the kidneys, adrenals, and brain

Clinical presentation

The predominant symptoms of epidermoid anal cancer are pain and bleeding, which are present in about 50% of cases. The presence of a mass is noted by a minority of patients, around 25%. Pruritus and discharge occur in a similar proportion. Advanced tumors may involve the sphincter mechanism, causing faecal incontinence. Invasion of the posterior vaginal wall may cause a fistula.

Cancer of the anal margin usually has the appearance of a malignant ulcer, with a raised, everted, indurated edge. Lesions within the canal may not be visible, though extensive lesions spread to the anal verge, or can extend via the ischiorectal fossa to the skin of the buttock. Digital examination of the anal canal is usually painful, and may reveal the distortion produced by the tumor. Since anal cancer tends to spread upwards, there may be involvement of the distal rectum, perhaps giving the impression that the lesion has arisen there. Involvement of the perirectal lymph nodes may be palpable on digital examination, rather more than may be apparent in disseminating rectal cancer. If the tumor has extended into the sphincter muscles, the characteristic induration of a spreading malignancy may be felt around the anal canal.

Although up to one-third of patients will have inguinal lymph nodes that are enlarged, biopsy will confirm metastatic spread in only 50% of these; the rest are due to secondary infection. Biopsy or fine needle aspiration is recommended by many to confirm involvement of the groin nodes if radical block dissection is contemplated. Distant spread is unusual in anal cancer, so hepatomegaly, though it must be looked for, is very uncommon. Frequently, other benign perianal conditions will exist in association with anal cancer, such as fistulas, condylomas, or leukoplakia.

Investigation

The most important investigation in the management of anal cancer is examination under anaesthetic, which permits optimum assessment of the tumor in terms of size, involvement of adjacent structures, and nodal involvement, and also provides the best opportunity to obtain a biopsy for histological confirmation. Sigmoidoscopic examination is probably best performed at this examination.

Clinical staging

No one system of staging for anal tumors has been adopted universally. However, that of the UICC is the most widely used. For anal canal lesions, this system has been criticised as it has required assessment of involvement of the external sphincter. To overcome this, a system has been suggested by Papillon et al. [5] as follows:

- T1 <2 cm;
- T2 2–4 cm;
- T3 >4 cm, mobile;

- T4a invading vaginal mucosa;
- T4b extension into structures other than skin, rectal, or vaginal mucosa.

In recent years, magnetic resonance imaging (MRI) has taken over from endo anal ultrasound in staging these lesions. MRI is better than endo anal ultrasound, providing information on spread beyond the anal canal.

Serum tumor markers are unhelpful as they do not provide reliable information.

Treatment

Historical

Traditionally, anal cancer has been seen as a 'surgical' disease. Anal canal tumors were treated by radical abdominoperineal excision and colostomy, whereas anal margin lesions were treated by local excision. Over the past decade, non-surgical radical treatments, such as radiotherapy with or without chemotherapy, have taken over as primary treatments of choice in most cases.

Overall, the results of surgery for anal cancer are disappointing for what is essentially a locoregional disease. For decades, radical abdominoperineal excision of the rectum and anus was the preferred method of treatment at most centers around the world.

Abdominoperineal excision for anal canal cancer differs little from the procedure used for rectal cancer, but particular care is taken to clear the space below the pelvic floor. Around 20% of cases are incurable surgically at presentation. Results published since the mid-1980s reporting series collected over the previous several decades have varied widely in their survival outcome, but on average the 5-year survival has been around 55–60%. Most post-surgical relapses occur locoregionally.

Around 75% of cancers at the anal margin have been treated in the past by local excision. The rationale for this was based on the perception that margin lesions rarely metastasise, though this has not always been confirmed by prolonged follow-up. It may be postulated that disappointing 5-year survival rates (~50–70%) might have been better if radical surgery had been applied more frequently.

Current

Chemoradiation therapy (combined modality therapy)

Combined modality therapy for anal cancer was championed by Norman Nigro, who chose to use 5-fluorouracil (5FU) and mitomycin C empirically as a preoperative regimen aimed at improving the results of radical surgery [6]. It was evident to Nigro that this regime led to dramatic tumor shrinkage: in his 1974 publication, the tumor was reported to have disappeared completely in all three patients. No tumor was found in the surgical specimen in both of the patients who underwent abdominoperineal excision; the third refused surgery. As he became more confident, Nigro no longer routinely pressed his patients to undergo radical surgery, initially confining himself to excising the site of the primary tumor after combined modality therapy. Later, he dropped even this relatively minor surgical step if the primary site looked and felt normal after treatment [7].

The most recent data on combined modality therapy from the UK Coordinating Committee on Cancer Research compared chemoradiation with radiotherapy alone in a randomized multicenter study [8]. This study randomized 585 patients, making it the largest single trial in anal cancer. This trial showed that combined modality therapy gave superior local control of disease compared with radiotherapy alone. Only 36% of patients receiving combined therapy had 'local failure' compared with 59% of those receiving radiotherapy alone. Although there was no significant overall survival advantage for either treatment regimen, the risk of death from anal cancer was significantly less in the group receiving combined modality therapy (Figure 9.2). As a result

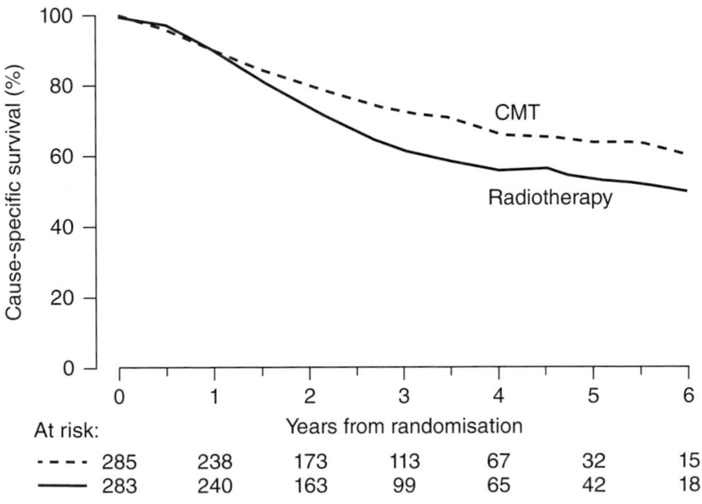

Figure 9.2 (A) Deaths from anal cancer. Number of events: radiotherapy 105, combined modality therapy (CMT) 77 (RR = 0.71, 95% CI 0.53–0.95, $P = 0.02$) [8] Figure 5, with permission. Number at risk = number alive. (B) UKCCCR Anal Cancer trial: risk of local failure (T1–2 and N0) [10]. Reproduced with permission of Elsevier.

of this trial, it seems that the standard treatment for anal squamous carcinoma should be a combination of radiotherapy and intravenous 5FU with mitomycin, which remains the gold standard [9].

Mitomycin causes much of the toxicity of chemoradiation (particularly a problem in elderly patients) and thus trials of the use of cisplatin as an alternative to mitomycin have been performed (RTOG, 2006). This trial randomized 652 patients but showed that cisplatin had no advantage over mitomycin and may be inferior. The search for the optimal regimen goes on.

Complications of chemoradiation for anal carcinoma include diarrhoea, mucositis, myelosuppression, skin erythema, and desquamation. Late complications include anal stenosis and fistula formation. HIV patients with anal epidermoid cancers are probably best treated with chemoradiation, but have increased toxicity [11].

The role of surgery today

Although surgeons no longer play the central therapeutic role, they nevertheless have important contributions to make.

Initial diagnosis

Most patients present to surgeons, who are best suited to perform examination under anaesthesia to confirm diagnosis and assess local extent.

Lesions at the anal margin

Small lesions at the anal margin may still best be treated by local excision alone, obviating the need for protracted courses of non-surgical therapy. There is some evidence that the risk of regional lymph node metastasis is not related to primary tumor size, which may explain the disappointing results sometimes reported after local excision. This conflicts with the view that tumor size is related to stage, which explains the excellent results of local excision in small tumors.

Treatment of complications and disease relapse

Surgeons retain an important role in the treatment of anal cancer after failure of primary non-surgical therapy, either early or late. Four situations may require surgery after primary non-surgical treatment: residual tumor, complications of treatment, incontinence, or fistula after tumor resolution, and subsequent tumor recurrence:

1 The appearance of the primary site is often misleading after radiotherapy. In most patients complete remission is indicated by the tumor disappearing completely. In some, however, an ulcer may remain, occasionally

looking like an unchanged primary tumor. Only generous biopsy will reveal whether the residual ulcer contains tumor or consists merely of inflammatory tissue. Histological proof of residual disease is essential before radical surgery is recommended to the patient. For patients with proven residual disease, a salvage abdominoperineal resection may be the only option. In fit patients with extensive pelvic disease extending around the vagina or bladder, pelvic exenteration may need to be considered. This type of surgery carries a high morbidity with impaired wound healing due to the radiotherapy. A primary reconstruction of the perineal area using a myocutaneous flap is strongly recommended in these cases.

2 Complications of non-surgical treatment for anal cancer do occur in a proportion of patients, including radionecrosis, fistula, and incontinence. Severe anal pain due to radio-necrosis of the anal lining may necessitate either a colostomy, in the hope that the lesion may heal after faecal diversion, or radical anorectal excision with a flap used to reconstruct the perineum.

3 Occasionally, a tumor is so locally extensive that the patient will be rendered incontinent as a consequence of primary tumor shrinkage. Although rectovaginal fistula may be amenable to repair, sphincter damage is unlikely to improve with local surgery, necessitating abdominoperineal excision of the anorectum. Abdominoperineal excision of the rectum under these circumstances is usually best undertaken in conjunction with a rectus abdominis myocutaneous flap to aid perineal wound healing.

4 In the case of recurrent disease developing after initial resolution, biopsy is mandatory prior to surgical intervention. These biopsies need to be of reasonable size, number, and depth, as the histological appearances following radiotherapy can make histopathological interpretation difficult. If high-dose radiotherapy was used for primary treatment, further non-surgical therapy for recurrence is usually contraindicated, making radical surgical removal necessary.

Inguinal metastases

Inguinal lymph nodes are enlarged in 10–25% of patients with anal cancers. Although inguinal lymph node involvement may be treated by radiotherapy, some argue in favor of surgery; however, histological confirmation is advisable before radical groin dissection, as up to 50% of cases of inguinal lymphadenopathy may be due to inflammation alone. Enlargement of groin nodes some time after primary therapy is most likely due to recurrent tumor;

radical groin dissection is indicated in this situation, with up to 50% 5-year survival.

Treatment of intraepithelial neoplasia

HPV infection of the anogenital area is very common, and it is reported that over 70% of sexually active adults have at some time had occult or overt genital HPV infection. In most individuals the infection remains occult, but in a minority the infection manifests itself as either condylomas or intraepithelial neoplasia. As with other viral infections, it is impossible to eradicate HPV infection by surgical excision; for this reason, surgical excision of condylomas is effectively performed more for relief of symptoms and cosmesis.

Similarly, the natural history of low-grade AIN (I and II) is relatively benign and therefore a policy of observation alone is adequate. This is likely to be particularly advisable when large areas of the anogenital epithelium are affected. However, for high-grade AIN (III), the advice is more circumspect, as we do not know the natural history of this condition. If the area of AIN III is small, it is probably prudent to excise it locally and then to observe the patient at regular intervals for a number of years. If the area of AIN III is too large for local excision without risk of anal stenosis, then a careful observational policy with 6-monthly review may be an option.

Aggressive surgical excision of the whole perianal skin and anal canal and resurfacing with split skin with a defunctioning colostomy has been used to treat wide areas of AIN III. This sort of surgery necessitates multiple procedures and carries significant morbidity, which for a condition of uncertain malignant potential may make the treatment worse than the disease.

The use of immunomodulators in AIN has been investigated as a potential therapeutic option. While some authors report encouraging results, these are all small studies of short duration. Photodynamic therapy using topical photosensitizers may be useful, but experience is currently very limited. All these treatments are painful and this often limits their use.

Rarer tumors

Adenocarcinoma

Adenocarcinoma in the anal canal is usually a very low rectal cancer that has spread downwards to involve the canal; however, true adenocarcinoma of the anal canal does occur, probably arising from the anal glands which arise around the dentate line and pass radially outwards into the sphincter muscles. This is a very rare tumor, quite radiosensitive, and is increasingly being treated by chemoradiation.

Malignant melanoma

Malignant melanoma is another very rare tumor, accounting for just 1% of anal canal malignant tumors. The lesion may mimic a thrombosed external pile due to its color, although amelanotic tumors also occur. Anal melanomas have a dismal prognosis, the literature suggests a median survival of around 18 months after diagnosis and only 10–20% 5 year survival. All treatment options appear to be equally unsuccessful and liver and lung metastases are common. As the chances of cure are minimal, radical surgery as primary treatment should be abandoned, but local excision may provide useful palliation [12].

TIPS AND TRICKS

1 Prophylactic antibiotics given with the chemotherapy help to reduce the risk of systemic sepsis caused by chemotherapy in elderly, or frail patients with anal SCC.
2 Local excision of small anal margin squamous carcinomas is an effective treatment with low recurrence rates, provided the margins of resection are clear of tumor.

CASE STUDY

A 67-year-old lady presented with an increasingly symptomatic anal fistula on a background of Crohn's disease for 20 years. The fistula had been present for around 10 years and treated with a long-term loose seton. In the last 6 months, the fistula had started to discharge more pus and blood. An MRI scan showed an area of high signal and a complex supra lavator abscess with a trans-sphincteric tract. The fistula was treated by further drainage on 3 occasions over the next 6 months and although some tissue was excised, none was sent for histopathological examination. Finally, at a third examination under anaesthesia, some of the discharge appeared to contain necrotic tissue which was sent for histopathological examination. This showed anal SCC, a staging CT showed that the supralevator collection had grown and was probably tumor, and there were also multiple liver and para aortic nodal metastases. Unfortunately, despite chemoradiotherapy, the patient died 2 years later of metastatic disease.

Note: A high index of suspicion is required to diagnose anal cancer, any excised tissue should be sent for histopathological examination.

MULTIPLE CHOICE QUESTIONS

1 Basaloid anal cancers are a subtype of which type of anal cancer?
  A. Adenocarcinoma
  B. Squamous cell carcinoma
  C. Melanoma
  D. Bushke-Lowenstien tumor

2 Risk factors for progression of anal intra-epithelial neoplasia include:
  A. Smoking
  B. Genital Herpes
  C. Transplant recipients
  D. Prolonged steroid therapy

3 Chemoradiotherapy for anal squamous carcinomas may be associated with the following late complications:
  A. Recto vaginal fistula
  B. Fracture of the pubic rami
  C. Recurrent rectal bleeding
  D. Lymphoedema

References

1 Frische M, Melbye M. Trends in the incidence of anal carcinoma in Denmark. *Br Med J* 1993; 306: 419–22.

2 Daling J, Weiss N, Hislop T, et al. Sexual practices, sexually transmitted diseases and the incidence of anal cancer. *N Engl J Med* 1987; 317: 973–7. Excellent epidemiological paper on anal squamous cell carcinoma.

3 Palmer JG, Scholefield JH, Shepherd N, et al. Anal cancer and human papillomaviruses. *Dis Colon Rectum* 1989; 32: 1016–22. Very relevant paper reporting the association between anal cancer and papillomaviruses.

4 Scholefield J, Hickson W, Smith J, et al. Anal intraepithelial neoplasia: part of a multifocal disease process. *Lancet* 1992; 340: 1271–3.

5 Papillon J, Mayer M, Mountberon J, et al. A new approach to the management of epidermoid carcinoma of the anal canal. *Cancer* 1987; 51: 1830–7.

6 Nigro N, Vaitkevicius V, Considine B Jr, et al. Combined therapy for cancer of the anal canal. A preliminary report. *Dis Colon Rectum* 1974; 27: 354–6. A classic paper – first experience of using chemoradiation in anal cancer.

7 Nigro N. An evaluation of combined therapy for squamous cell cancer in the anal canal. *Dis Colon Rectum* 1984; 27: 763–6.

8 UKCCCR Anal Cancer Trial Working Party. Epidermoid anal cancer: results from the UKCCCR randomised trial of radiotherapy alone versus radiotherapy, 5-fluorouracil, and mitomycin. *Lancet* 1996; 348: 1049–54. A large well-run randomized trial that changed the management of this cancer in the UK.

9 Cummings B, Keane T, O'Sullivan B, et al. Mitomycin in anal canal carcinoma. *Oncology* 1993; 50(suppl 1): 63–9.

10 Northover J, Meadows A, Ryan C, Gray R, on behalf of UKCCCR Anal Cancer Trial Working Party. *The Lancet,* 1996; 349: 206, UKCCCR.

11 Uronis HE, Bendell JC. Anal cancer – an overview. *Oncologist* 2007; 12: 524–34.

12 Ross M, Pezzi C, Pezzi T, et al. Patterns of failure in anorectal melanoma. A guide to surgical therapy. *Arch Surg* 1990; 125: 313–16.

ANSWERS TO MULTIPLE-CHOICE QUESTIONS

1 B
2 A, B, C, D
3 A, B, C, D

PART 4
Oncology

CHAPTER 10

Controversies in adjuvant chemotherapy

Stephen Staal, Karen Daily & Carmen Allegra
Hematology/Oncology, Medicine, University of Florida, Gainseville, FL 32601, USA

KEY POINTS

- Stage III colorectal cancer survival rates can be improved with cytotoxic chemotherapy with 5-Flurouracil (FU)/Leucovorin (LEU) or Capecitabine (CAP) and oxaliplatin (OX); irinotecan (IR), and addition of bevacuzimab (BEV) and cetuximab (CTX) were failures in the adjuvant setting.
- Patients over the age of 70 require careful drug selection; benefit from addition of OX to FU or CAP is questionable and toxicity is increased.
- Stage II patients overall have only a 4% benefit from adjuvant therapy and should be selected for treatment based on clinical and pathological prognostic features.
- The 15% of colon cancers with DNA Mismatch Repair Defects/Microsatellite Instability (MSI) have an improved prognosis. MSI Stage II patients should probably not be treated; our interpretation of the data is that Stage III patients can potentially benefit from both FU/LEU and FU/LEU/OX.
- Tumor gene expression signature testing is commercially available to aid in determining prognosis, but its inability to predict benefits from chemotherapy limits its clinical applicability.
- Molecular profiling of tumors and rational therapies targeting predictive subtypes will ultimately replace the all-inclusive trial.
- Enhanced understanding of the relationship between host factors and the tumor, particularly immune parameters, will provide new therapeutic opportunities.

CASE STUDIES

Stage II – A young woman in the setting of ulcerative colitis

A 32-year-old woman with a 10-year history of well controlled ulcerative colitis was found to have high grade dysplasia on biopsy of a high rectal/sigmoid abnormality during a routine surveillance endoscopy. Endoscopic ultrasound staged the lesion as uT2N0. CT

Colorectal Cancer: Diagnosis and Clinical Management, First Edition. Edited by John H. Scholefield and Cathy Eng.

of the chest, abdomen, and pelvis showed no additional disease and the patient proceeded to colectomy with permanent ostomy. Pathology revealed a T3N0 adenocarcinoma with 16 lymph nodes examined, microsatellite stable (MSS), KRAS, and BRAF genes both non-mutated. Oncotype testing was performed to clarify the benefit of adjuvant chemotherapy; the patient was ambivalent after considering risks and benefits. When the Recurrence Score returned in the high risk category at 55, she decided to proceed with adjuvant chemotherapy and was treated with CAP.

Stage III – An elderly woman with partial obstruction

A 72-year-old woman was admitted to the hospital after presenting to the emergency room with constipation. A partially obstructing sigmoid colon adenocarcinoma was stented to facilitate discharge and preoperative evaluation. Her medical history included osteoporosis and rehabilitation for a recent hip fracture. Definitive surgery was deferred for a course of parenteral nutrition to improve her nutrition and she required evaluation and management for a persistent sinus tachycardia. She eventually underwent a scheduled laparoscopic anterior resection of a 13 cm moderately differentiated adenocarcinoma. The tumor was ulcerated and necrotic with perineural invasion. It extended through the muscularis propria into the pericolonic adipose tissue and involved 1 of 33 lymph nodes (pT3N1a). Tumor markers included MSS and KRAS mutated. The patient was treated with 6 months of FU/LEU.

TIPS AND TRICKS / KEY PITFALLS

- Primary prognostic factors are histology (signet ring/mucinous worse), depth of tumor penetration and invasion (T stage, obstruction, local perforation), extent of nodal involvement (N stage) and number of nodes harvested, grade (high vs. low). Microsatellite status (MSI better than MSS), but to date no other acquired genetic features, has correlated with prognosis. This will certainly change as tumor genome analysis becomes a common feature of ongoing clinical trials.
- Data supports a similar benefit of adjuvant FU/LEU for the half of all colon cancer patients over the age of 70 as for younger patients. Individual prognostic factors, comorbidities (and their impact on survival), and a general geriatric assessment should govern the use of chemotherapy. The addition of OX to FU or CAP is of questionable benefit in the elderly, but can be considered in the high risk, fit patient.
- Tumor gene expression testing can provide additional prognostic information and may be of use in both Stage II and III colon cancer patients, where further individual assessment of recurrence risk will affect the decision for treatment or not. Gene expression data has, disappointingly, not been predictive of benefit from chemotherapy.

Adjuvant therapy proves effective

Prior to 1990, despite several decades of effort, convincing evidence for benefits of adjuvant chemotherapy for colorectal cancer was lacking. Initial efforts involved perioperative use of short courses of both intraluminal and systemic chemotherapy (thiotepa, flurodeoxyuridine, and FU), with the intention of limiting spread of cancer cells occurring at the time of surgery. As early as 1971, a report comparing controls to a 5-day course of FU given 14 days after surgery showed no benefit. With the realization that recurrence was more related to occult metastatic disease present at the time of surgery than spread by the surgeon, and that a prolonged treatment course was necessary to eradicate disease, more rational controlled trials using FU for up to 18 months were conducted but again failed to show benefit. Trials with combinations (FU and the alkylataing agent 1-(2chlorethyl-3-4 mehtylcyclohexyl)-1-nitrosourea(Me-ccnu)) proved no more efficacious, and for a while the focus, based on animal data, switched to boosting the immune system. In the absence of specific immunotherapy, clinical trials employed non-specific stimulants such as Bacillus Calmette Guerin (BCG), *Corynebacterium parvum*, and an antihelminthic with immunostimulatory properties, levamisole (LV). Trials of immune stimulants, both alone and in combination with chemotherapy, were designed in the late 1970s in the continuing search for an effective approach, although the lack of information regarding the combination of immune and cytotoxic therapy was recognized as a concern [1].

A review article published in 1988 on adjuvant therapy of colorectal cancer by Buyse et al. was subtitled: 'Why We Still Don't Know'. The authors attempted a meta-analysis of 27 controlled trials reported at that time examining radiation, chemotherapy, and immunotherapy in the adjuvant setting. They concluded that although retrospective subsets showed the best benefits – a 17% reduction in death and overall 3.4% higher survival at 5 years – in those receiving at least a year of 5-FU, there was no convincing evidence of benefit from the lumped chemotherapy trials (6791 patients, 3384 deaths) [2]. Further data was not long in coming.

In early 1990, Moertel et al. reported on 1296 patients randomized for observation, LV for 3 days every 2 weeks for 1 year, or LV plus FU given for 5 consecutive days monthly for 12 cycles [3]. The results were striking, with a highly significant 33% reduction in death rate and 41% reduction in rate of recurrence in node positive, Stage C disease. The absolute improvement in survival was about 10%. LV, an antihelminthic drug, had been chosen for its immunostimulatory properties [4] based on a preliminary trial [5]; alone it showed no benefit with a survival curve matching observation. Other trials had confirmed the lack of efficacy of single agent LV and the authors admitted some welcome surprise that this study had proven so positive and struggled to explain the role, if any, of LV. Tests for synergy between LV and FU at physiological doses were negative *in vitro* [6], although high doses did demonstrate an effect possibly mediated by inhibition of tyrosine phosphatases

[7] – a mechanism which would impact on many cellular functions. This combination may be particularly immunogenic or there is a cryptic *in vivo* pharmacodynamic synergy leading to more effective tumor cell kill by FU. A trial of high dose versus standard dose LV in combination with FU was reported 16 years after the initial report [8]; there was no additional benefit to increasing the LV dose. However, interest rapidly faded in LV, as LEU-modulated FU regimens and combination cytotoxics entered the adjuvant arena.

In the early 1980s, attempts to improve the efficacy of FU cytotoxicity led to the discovery that increased intracellular reduced folates improved the binding of FU metabolites to their ultimate target, thymidylate synthase. Clinical trials in metastatic disease showed a 2–3-fold increased response rate with a combination of FU and LEU [9]. NSABP C-04 compared FU/LEU to FU/LV and FU/LV/LEU [10]. There was a significant 5% improvement in disease-free survival (DFS) and a marginal improvement in overall survival (OS), favoring FU/LEU versus 5FU/LV with no additional benefit to FU/LEU/LV. Similar results were seen in Intergroup 0089, which examined 2 different doses of LEU in combination with FU given for either 6 or 12 months [11]. A third arm added LV to the low dose LEU arm and the control arm was FU/LV. At 10 years of follow-up, there was no significant DFS or OS difference amongst the four arms. Based on these and other studies [12], LEU modulated FU became the standard adjuvant approach. The various schedules of FU administration remained an area of interest, but ultimately no significant difference in survival between daily times 5 monthly, weekly, continuous infusion [13] (although treatment could be abbreviated to 12 weeks with results equal to 24 weeks of bolus [14]) or fortnightly bolus with 48-hour infusion (FU2/LEU) could be demonstrated [15]; the last, as the least toxic and with an improved response rate, was adopted in further combination trials in Europe. QUASAR, a 5000 patient community based trial enrolling Stage II and III patients, was reported in 2000, showing no benefit from additional LV added to two different FU/LEU regimens [16]. CAP, an oral fluoropyrimidine, was equivalent to intravenous FU/LEU in a trial randomizing close to 2000 patients [17]. It had a favorable adverse event profile and offered a convenient alternative to infusional FU/LEU programs.

The combination OX/FU/LEU proved effective in FU/LEU-refractory metastatic patients [18]. In 2004, the MOSAIC trial reported a comparison of FU/LEU to OX/FU/LEU(FOLFOX), demonstrating a significant 6% (DFS and 4% OS benefit for Stage III patients on FOLFOX [19;20]; OS for the Stage II patients was the same in both arms. Addition of OX added to the weekly FU/LEU schedule (FLOX) was examined in NSABP C-07, reported in 2007 [21], and updated in 2011 [22] – subset analysis showed no benefit to OX addition in patients over the age of 70 (the median age at diagnosis). Although the overall trial did not show an OS benefit to addition of oxaliplatin, this was statistically significant in the under-70 sub-set. The benefit of adding OX is clear, the DFS benefit is statistically significant in the largest trials, and OS is improved (a conclusion supported by SEER data), but given the increased toxicity and diminished benefits in the elderly, age and comorbidities should figure in the treatment decision. Trials comparing OX added to CAP(XELOX) demonstrated incremental benefits similar to FLOX and FOLFOX when compared to FU/LEU [23], providing a third option. Although there are no head-to-head comparisons of these regimens, the outcomes are similar; they differ with respect to toxicity profile (more GI toxicity with FLOX) and convenience of administration.

FOLFOX and FLOX proved effective, providing about one-third again the benefit to survival as 5FU/LV. The same was not true for irinotecan (IR), a drug equally effective against metastatic disease as OX. Three trials examining addition of IR to a FU/LEU regimen with a total of close to 4000 patients were unanimously negative. With the approval of BEV, an anti-vascular growth factor (VEGF) antibody, and CTX, an anti-epidermal growth factor (EGFR) antibody, in metastatic colon cancer, these drugs were quickly moved into the adjuvant setting with great expectations.

First-generation biologics: Bevacuzimab and Cetuximab ineffective

NSABP C-08 compared FOLFOX6 for 6 months with or without BEV, for 12 months in Stage II and III colon cancer patients. The study failed to meet its goal of improved DFS at 3 years [24]. Interestingly, results at 15 months favored the BEV arm, leading to the speculation that BEV may transiently suppress cancer cells or render them less detectable, or its cessation may figure in the observed rebound of the tumor. The AVANT trial [25], adding 48 weeks of BEV to XELOX or FOLFOX4, showed similar results. A subset analysis failed to demonstrate any group by age, sex, ethnicity, or nodal status that benefited from BEV addition. The strength of the data to date has led to the abandonment of trials of BEV in the adjuvant setting, unless biomarkers or subsets that predict benefit can be identified.

An antibody targeting an EGFR receptor, Her2, has validated the concept of targeting growth factors in the adjuvant breast cancer setting; similar expectations for CTX in colon cancer were not realized. Despite the identification of mutated KRAS as a predictor of no benefit from CTX, in metastatic

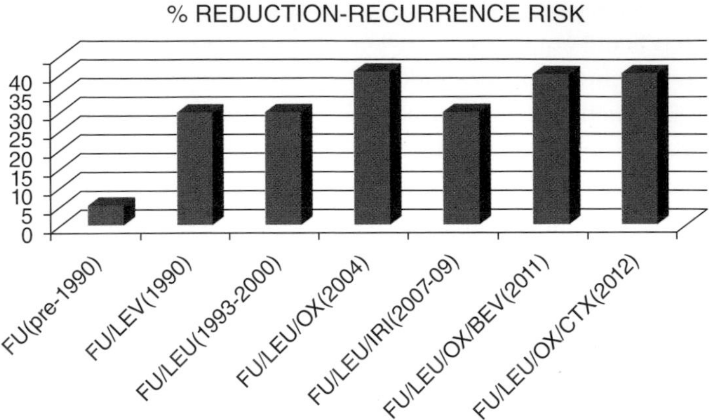

Figure 10.1 Adjuvant chemotherapy benefits (author's interpretation of published studies).

disease [26], which allows elimination of non-responders, there is no evidence that EGFR is a driver for colorectal cancer in the same way that Her2 amplification drives breast cancer. Two trials were initiated in 2004/5 to examine the addition of CTX to mFOLFOX-6, N0147 [27], or FOLFOX-4, PETACC8 [28]. With the subsequent knowledge that only patients with non-mutated KRAS or BRAF benefited from CTX in the metastatic setting, entry was restricted to this genotype. Consistent with the increased toxicity of CTX, only half the patients over the age of 70 were able to complete chemotherapy plus CTX versus close to 80% in this age group on chemotherapy alone – there was also a trend to worse outcomes in this age group.

As illustrated in Figure 10.1, the largest reduction in risk of recurrence was achieved with the initial trials of modulated FU with a second, lesser, gain achieved with the addition of OX. The last 10 years have seen no significant progress in the benefits of adjuvant therapy for colorectal cancer, although we have a better understanding of selection criteria and a bank of tumors correlated with clinical outcomes for assessment of new knowledge to identify more effective therapies.

Patient age, pathological features, and biomarkers for treatment selection

The median age for patients with colorectal cancer is 70 and the ability of a major portion of this population to tolerate and benefit from chemotherapy has long been a concern. In 2001, a pooled analysis of over 3000 patients over

70 from 7 randomized phase III FU-based trials was reported. Toxicity in this age group was similar to younger patients, except for an increased risk of leucopenia [29]. A similar benefit from therapy was seen regardless of age. Age was also examined as a factor in benefit in the MOSAIC [20] and NSABP C-07 [22] trials. Approximately one-third of the patients in MOSAIC were over the age of 65 and demonstrated equivalent OS with or without OX. It seems unlikely that the biology of colon cancer is dramatically different in the older patient; fewer elderly patients enrolled in trials, competing causes of death due to co-morbidities, and abbreviated or delayed treatments due to toxicity seem more likely causes for the inferior outcome [30]. The data from FU trials and SEER data would favor not excluding the elderly from the most effective therapy; however, individual assessment and patient involvement is necessary. Adjuvant! (*adjuvantonline.com*) is a useful online tool using pathological criteria for graphic depiction of individualized recurrence risk and benefit of therapy; it has been clinically validated [31] and incorporates age and comorbidities which can be helpful in deliberations with the elderly. Included Help files, which review the various regimens and their toxicities in tabular form, can also aid with individualization of treatment choice.

The benefit of adjuvant chemotherapy in Stage II disease was difficult to document due to the overall good prognosis of this stage, requiring large numbers to achieve statistically significant outcomes. A trial enrolling over 3000 Stage II patients in Britain between 1994 and 2003 and reporting in 2007 estimated a 3.6% survival benefit with FU/LV therapy; all-cause mortality and DFS were both statistically significant, and benefit over the age of 70 was not seen. A pooled analysis (IMPACT B2) of over 1000 Stage II patients drawn from 5 randomized trials failed to show a significant benefit to therapy [32]; an update and extension of this data showed a 17% RFS and 15% OS benefit compared with 40% and 35% respectively for Stage III disease [33].

Combined analysis of the first 4 NSABP adjuvant colon trials totaling 2255 Stage II patients showed a consistent benefit similar to that for Stage III patients [34]; a more recent update of NSABP data again showed a similar reduction in DFS and OS between Stage II and III patients [35], and the authors argued in favor of their data as being better controlled with strict entry criteria versus other populations. The addition of OX in the MOSAIC and NSABP C-07 trials did not affect OS in Stage II, although there was a trend for DFS benefit. SEER data analysis has failed to demonstrate a benefit for chemotherapy in Stage II, despite poor prognostic features [36], suggesting little impact of chemotherapy in Stage II disease in the general community. The current National Comprehensive Cancer Network (*www.nccn.org*) guidelines recommend clinical trial, observation, or FU based chemotherapy for low risk Stage II; an OX-FU regimen is recommended for those Stage II patients with high risk features (T4, bowel obstruction, local perforation, questionable margins, less than 12 nodes harvested, or lymphovascular invasion), who have a recurrence risk similar to Stage III patients.

The hope of personalized therapy is that detailed biological analysis of the individual patient's tumor will offer a precise assessment of prognosis and, most important, predict benefit from the available therapies. Over the last two decades, a variety of biological features of colorectal cancer has been correlated with prognosis and, where the clinical data allows, benefit from treatment (Table 10.1).

One of the earliest studies examined levels of thymidylate synthase (TS) expression; the 70% of patients with high levels had a worse prognosis but benefited from chemotherapy [38]. Analysis of a larger data set confirmed the prognostic impact of higher level TS expression but could find no interaction with adjuvant chemotherapy [38]. The difference in TS expression can also be examined at the genetic level; polymorphisms in the vicinity of the TS gene promoter correlate with levels of TS protein and have been used to intensify therapy in high expressors [39–41], although this approach requires prospective evaluation in a larger patient population.

Loss of heterozygosity (LOH) of chromosome 18q was one of the earliest acquired genetic defects described in colon cancer [42]. Subsequent studies have yielded conflicting data on the prognostic significance of this marker. A systematic review pointed out the problems of varying assays utilized and designs of the clinical studies examined [43]. Ultimately, there was no definitive prognostic impact found, although a trend towards worse outcome with LOH18q was noted.

Table 10.1 Molecular features of colorectal cancer that may have prognostic and/or predictive significance for recommending therapy. For commonly altered path proteins, see [37]. Only MSI and KRAS status are incorporated into a standard algorithm.

Molecular feature	Frequency	Prognostic significance	Predictive significance
Thymidylate Synthase	~30% low	Low is better	FU?
18qLOH	~70%	?	5FU ≥ better
Hypermutated (MSI)	16%	favorable (HR 0.47)	?
TP53 altered	47–67%	unclear	No definitive evidence
WNT path	92–97%	–	?
MAPK path	59–80%	–	–
PI3K-AKT path	50–53%	–	–
TGF-β path deficient	27–87%	–	–
CIMP high	16% (assoc. with MSI)	assoc. with MSI	assoc. with MSI

There are several known gene alterations in colon cancer with therapeutic implications. Mutation of the KRAS gene occurs early in the carcinogenic cascade and has been found in 40% of patients – additional mutations accrue during the course of tumor development. In a study of 2300 patients enrolled in NSABP C-07 and C-08 (FU/LEU ± OX; FOLFOX ± BEV resp.), none of the mutations examined impacted prognosis – KRAS-35.3%, BRAF-14.3%, P13K-12.4%, NRAS-2.9%, and MET-3.7% prevalent were all interrogated and affected neither outcome or benefit form OX [44]. BRAF mutations did predict for worse outcomes at relapse, explaining the previously reported effect on survival in CALGB 89803 (Stage III FU/LEU vs IRI/FU/LEU [45]). TP53 mutations were identified in 274/607 (45%) of assayable tumors from this same trial.

Mutations can occur in different regions of the TP53 gene; these can be divided into those involving DNA binding (ZB) or non-binding (NZB) regions. Only amongst women in this study [46] was there a significant correlation with DFS and OS (5-year OS HR 0.90, 0.72, and 0.59 resp.). Although limited by subset numbers, the data suggests that ZB mutated women benefit from IRI/FU/LEU, whereas NZB mutated patients do better with FU/LEU. This analysis points out the potential complexities of interactions between host, interventions, and detailed molecular alterations – identifying and mapping all the relevant factors will be challenging.

DNA mismatch repair (MMR) enzyme mutations were initially identified as the cause of Lynch syndrome, which accounts for 3% of colon cancer. About 15% of colon cancers are mismatch repair deficient, mostly due to acquired epigenetic silencing of these genes [47;48]. This results in MSI, which can be detected along with MMR protein deficiency to identify such patients. MSI colon cancers are characteristically proximal, poorly differentiated, and with a marked lymphocytic infiltrate [49;50]. Unlike Lynch syndrome patients, the sporadic MSI patients are commonly older, female, and smokers. MSI tumors have a normal DNA content, in contrast to the marked chromosome alterations seen in the majority of colorectal cancer [51;52]. That MSI tumors have a better prognosis is a consistent finding, but the benefits of FU/LEU therapy remain controversial [52;53]. Although the retrospective clinical studies are somewhat inconsistent, a recent large retrospective study suggests that sporadic cases may be particularly resistant to FU; presumptive germline-mutated patients seemed to retain sensitivity to FU [54], but the data is limited by the small numbers. Stage III presumptive germline patients had a significant benefit from FU based therapy. The NCCN recommends testing for MSI status for Stage II patients where FU alone would be contemplated, which seems reasonable given the improved prognosis. Re-examination of the overall negative IRI/FU/

LV adjuvant trial (CALGB 89803) looking at the MSI subset showed an improved outcome in this group in comparison to FU/LV alone [55]; analysis of the PETACC3 trial showed no benefit [56]. Analysis of the MOSAIC trial showed similar improvement in MSI and MSS patients with the addition of OX to FU [57]; the NSABP data set favored benefit with addition of OX in MSS, but not MSI patients [58]. The NCCN recommends testing for MSI status for Stage II patients, since the well established improved prognosis would minimize the absolute benefit of adjuvant chemotherapy. There have been too few patients and events in these retrospective studies, as well as varying assay approaches, to definitively settle the predictive value of MMR status for either FU/LEU or FU/LEU/OX.

High throughput genomic scanning technology is providing an increasingly complex portrait of colon cancer molecular alterations. Readily accessible tissue, in both the premalignant and advanced stages, has allowed an outline of tumor molecular pathogenesis. Studies initiated over two decades ago defined the common role of upregulation of the β-catenin pathway, primarily via mutation of the APC gene, the loss of heterozygosity, and gene deletion (DCC) occurring on the long arm of chromosome 18 (18qLOH), as well as the additional contributions of the frequently mutated KRAS, PI3K, and TP53 genes (reviewed in [59]).

Identification of mutations present in large numbers of colon cancers confirmed these known drivers of malignancy, as well as adding many more additional candidates and confirming the complexity and heterogeneity of genetic changes amongst colorectal tumors [60;61]. A more global analysis has recently reported on the mutations, DNA methylation patterns, DNA copy number and rearrangements, and messenger RNA and microRNA expression levels of 276 colorectal tumors [37]. The variety of molecular events could be sorted into known cellular networks, which pointed to a particular effect on MYC, a transcription factor which has been implicated in many of the biological alterations found in cancer cells [62]. The DNA methylation studies confirmed a subset of CRCs that were heavily methylated (CIMP for CpG island methylator phenotype); the role of epigenetics in CRC pathogenesis is more difficult to define than the hard-wired DNA changes, but there is a clear, poorly understood, link between MSI and CIMP high. A preliminary attempt at clinical correlation sorted molecular alterations with classical pathological criteria of tumor aggression, pointing towards the next generation of clinical trials, which will necessarily need to include such extensive marker panels to better refine prognosis.

The relevance of specific molecular changes was illustrated by recent data on the benefits of aspirin in the prevention of colon cancer recurrence [63].

Genotyping of tumors has shown this benefit to occur only in colon cancers driven by mutated P13K [64;65], where the effect was dramatic, although this has been disputed in a recent conference presentation [66]. Regardless, it points to new opportunities to match therapies to individual tumor genotypes in the future.

Gene expression profiling of tumors has been available for over a decade; commercially available tests are an option in the decision tree for chemotherapy or not for some breast cancer patients based on retrospective studies [67]; significant numbers of patients thought to be low or high risk by clinical criteria are reclassified discordantly by genomic criteria. Both companies currently offering commercial tests for breast cancer, Agendia (*www.agendia.com*) and Genomic Health (*oncotypedx.com*), now have tests available to stratify colorectal cancer patients into high and low risk categories.

The PARSC trial utilizes the Coloprint assay prospectively with the ultimate goal of comparing the initially hidden molecular prognosis with current best clinical practise and outcomes of both treated and untreated patients [68]. Genomic Health has developed the Recurrence Score (RS), a 12-gene signature for Stage II prognosis; simultaneously they attempted development of a FU therapy score in the hope of predicting chemosensitivity. The validation trial for the assay was performed on the QUASAR tumor specimens; there was a positive correlation between the gene signature and recurrence, although the risk spread was only 7–8%. Disappointingly, the gene signature for FU based sensitivity showed no correlation with FU benefit; with a constant proportional benefit of treatment, the difference in outcome would likely be in the 1–2% range. In an analysis of specimens from CALGB 9581, a trial of ineffective immunotherapy in Stage II patients with T4 tumors excluded, only RS and MMR status were prognostic – lymphovascular invasion, grade, and number of nodes examined were not useful [69]. Gene profiling for breast cancer has been adopted in part because it can predict benefits from chemotherapy (although results from prospective trials will not be available for several years); modest improvements in predicting prognosis alone may be useful for those Stage II colon cancer patients unsure of the decision for chemotherapy or not.

Immunotherapy – back to the future?

Frustration with the failure of active drugs for metastatic disease (IRI, BEV, and CTX) to improve the adjuvant cure rate is reminiscent of the early adjuvant trials, where a similar frustration and lack of effective chemotherapeutic agents led to the inclusion of non-specific immunotherapies, such as BCG and LEV, in treatment arms. NSABP C01 was a 3-arm trial of MOF, BCG, and no therapy; although early data showed a benefit for BCG, subsequent analysis showed no advantage for DFS, although there was a survival advantage to BCG in this elderly population due to a reduction in other causes of mortality [70]. An autologous tumor cell vaccine was tested over the course of more than 20 years. Technically arduous with reagents likely of varying quality at different institutions, initial reports of benefit were met with skepticism [71;72], although a report 10 years later suggested benefit from this approach in Stage II patients [73]. Humoral, vaccine, and cellular therapies have all been aimed at CRC [74] without convincing evidence of efficacy.

Interest in the balance between colon cancer and the immune system has been rekindled with advances in immunology, allowing a more precise evaluation of local tumor-immune interactions and opportunities for rationally designed therapy. During the last decade, French researchers have focused on analyzing immune infiltrates associated with colon cancer and demonstrated the correlation between improved prognosis and the presence of effector memory T cells [75–77]; in their hands the immunoscore bests the TNM system for predicting outcome. An international consortium is working to refine and standardize this technology to allow its dissemination to the pathology community. This group has recently published a more comprehensive 'immunome' analysis of colon cancer [78], mimicking in scope and ambition the tumor genome project.

Just as molecular analysis has informed our cytoxic therapy, new knowledge and results in the field of cancer immunotherapy offers the hope that immune manipulation will ultimately prove effective. The increased understanding of immune suppression by tumor cells [79;80], the interplay between chemotherapy and the immune system [81], and the availability of new reagents and cellular constructs to engineer an immune attack against tumor cells [82], provides a rational approach to anticancer immunotherapy not available to the early investigators. MSI tumors would be a particularly attractive target, since their hypermutable phenotype is likely to generate a large number of unique antigens, and lymphocyte infiltration is a prominent histologic feature.

Rectal cancer

The recently published comprehensive molecular analysis of CRC included 69 rectal cancers amongst the 277 tumors [37]. Their molecular characteristics were identical to those of tumors from elsewhere in the colon, with the exception of the MSI and hypermethylated tumors most commonly found in the proximal colon. This confirms the clinical impression that the only distinguishing feature of rectal cancer is its anatomical location deep in the pelvis; the rectum is arbitrarily defined as within 12 cm from the anal verge, but anatomically it begins at the peritoneal reflection. Tumors arising in this location are more likely to recur locally in the pelvis, metastasize to the sacrum and vertebral bodies, and spread distantly to the lungs via venous drainage that bypasses the liver [83]. Adjuvant radiation therapy (RT) has an established role for limiting the risk of local recurrence, but has not consistently demonstrated a survival advantage; chemotherapy improved survival given either alone or in combination with RT [84;85]. Neoadjuvant proved superior to adjuvant RT in preventing local recurrence with less morbidity [86–88]; neoadjuvant chemoradiotherapy (nCRT) similarly won out over a similar adjuvant program [89], although it raises the dilemma of patient selection and risk of overtreatment, since patients are selected on clinical rather than pathological criteria. The benefit of radiation is modest, but with careful surgical technique utilizing a sleeve, or total mesorectal excision, local recurrences are reduced by about 5%. Not surprisingly, response to nCRT correlates with survival as well as benefit from additional systemic therapy.

Additional drugs [90] have been added to either FU/RT or CAP/RT in an attempt to improve the pathological complete response (pCR) rate and long-term survival of rectal cancer patients. Three large trials of several thousand patients total have reported on the addition of OX – despite increased toxicity there was limited or no additional benefit to pCR or long-term outcome to date [91–93]. Addition of CTX to CAP produced an inferior outcome [94].

As discussed in a recent review [95], the complexity of rectal cancer management requires close collaboration between surgeons, radiation therapists, and medical oncologists, to ensure the best functional and survival outcomes for the patient.

Designing the next generation of adjuvant trials

There is a need for rapid assessment of new therapies, as the genomic and immunologic revolution will continue to provide us with an abundance of candidates. The failure of most candidate drugs to reach market and the depressing litany of large negative trials has led to new 'adaptive' models [96;97] for drug testing, to select only the most active agents and rapidly move them to the clinic. The lesson from the first several decades of colon cancer adjuvant therapy is 'never give up'. Despite the frustration of the last decade, we now have available new tools and knowledge that all but guarantee dramatic advances in the future, we require only the organization and wisdom to achieve the next therapeutic breakthroughs to benefit our patients.

MULTIPLE-CHOICE QUESTIONS

1 Poor prognostic factors for Stage II colon cancer include which of the following?
- **A.** Bowel obstruction at presentation
- **B.** Perforation at the site of the tumor
- **C.** Lymphovascular invasion
- **D.** MSI (mismatch repair deficient)
- **E.** High grade

2 Which of the following statements are true?
- **A.** Patients over the age of 70 have the same consistent statistical benefit from FU/LEU/OX chemotherapy as younger patients.
- **B.** The only study showing a statistically significant benefit for chemotherapy for Stage II patients is QUASAR1.
- **C.** BEV and CTX, active biological agents in the metastatic setting, improve outcome in the adjuvant setting.
- **D.** The median age for patients with colon cancer is 62.
- **E.** Infusional FU provides a statistically significant survival benefit over bolus FU and oral CAP in the adjuvant setting.

References

1 Nystrom JS, Bateman JR, Weiner J. Adjuvant treatment of colorectal cancer. *Western J Med* 1977 Feb; 126: 95–101.

2 Buyse M, Zeleniuch-Jacquotte A, Chalmers TC. Adjuvant therapy of colorectal cancer. Why we still don't know. *JAMA* 1988 Jun 24; 259(24): 3571–8.

3 Moertel CG, Fleming TR, Macdonald JS, Haller DG, Laurie JA, Goodman PJ, et al. Levamisole and fluorouracil for adjuvant therapy of resected colon carcinoma. *N Engl J Med* 1990 Feb 8; 322(6): 352–8.

4 Janik J, Kopp WC, Smith JW 2nd, Longo DL, Alvord WG, Sharfman WH, et al. Dose-related immunologic effects of levamisole in patients with cancer. *J Clin Oncol* 1993 Jan; 11(1): 125–35.

5 Laurie JA, Moertel CG, Fleming TR, Wieand HS, Leigh JE, Rubin J, et al. Surgical adjuvant therapy of large-bowel carcinoma: an evaluation of levamisole and the combination of levamisole and fluorouracil. The North Central Cancer Treatment Group and the Mayo Clinic. *J Clin Oncol* 1989 Oct; 7(10): 1447–56.

6 Grem JL, Allegra CJ. Toxicity of levamisole and 5-fluorouracil in human colon carcinoma cells. *J Natl Cancer Inst* 1989 Sep 20; 81(18): 1413–7.

7 Kovach JS, Svingen PA, Schaid DJ. Levamisole potentiation of fluorouracil antiproliferative activity mimicked by orthovanadate, an inhibitor of tyrosine phosphatase. *J Natl Cancer Inst* 1992 Apr 1; 84(7): 515–9.

8 O'Connell MJ, Sargent DJ, Windschitl HE, Shepherd L, Mahoney MR, Krook JE, et al. Randomized clinical trial of high-dose levamisole combined with 5-fluorouracil and leucovorin as surgical adjuvant therapy for high-risk colon cancer. *Clin Colorectal Cancer* 2006 Jul; 6(2): 133–9.

9 Poon MA, O'Connell MJ, Moertel CG, Wieand HS, Cullinan SA, Everson LK, et al. Biochemical modulation of fluorouracil: evidence of significant improvement of survival and quality of life in patients with advanced colorectal carcinoma. *J Clin Oncol* 1989 Oct; 7(10): 1407–18.

10 Wolmark N, Rockette H, Mamounas E, Jones J, Wieand S, Wickerham DL, et al. Clinical trial to assess the relative efficacy of fluorouracil and leucovorin, fluorouracil and levamisole and fluorouracil, leucovorin and levamisole in patients with Dukes' B and C carcinoma of the colon: results from National Surgical Adjuvant Breast and Bowel Project C-04. *J Clin Oncol* 1999 Nov 1; 17(11): 3553–9.

11 Haller DG, Catalano PJ, Macdonald JS, O'Rourke MA, Frontiera MS, Jackson DV, et al. Phase III study of fluorouracil, leucovorin, and levamisole in high-risk stage II and III colon cancer: final report of Intergroup 0089. *J Clin Oncol* 2005 Dec 1; 23(34): 8671–8.

12 Multicentre Pooled Analysis of Colon Cancer Trials (IMPACT) investigators. Efficacy of adjuvant fluorouracil and folinic acid in colon cancer. *International Lancet* 1995 Apr 15; 345(8955): 939–44.

13 Poplin EA, Benedetti JK, Estes NC, Haller DG, Mayer RJ, Goldberg RM, et al. Phase III Southwest Oncology Group 9415/Intergroup 0153 randomized trial of fluorouracil, leucovorin, and levamisole versus fluorouracil continuous infusion and levamisole for adjuvant treatment of stage III and high-risk stage II colon cancer. *J Clin Oncol* 2005 Mar 20; 23(9): 1819–25.

14 Chau I, Norman AR, Cunningham D, Tait D, Ross PJ, Iveson T, et al. A randomised comparison between 6 months of bolus fluorouracil/leucovorin and 12 weeks of protracted venous infusion fluorouracil as adjuvant treatment in colorectal cancer. *Ann Oncol* 2005 Apr 1; 16(4): 549–57.

15 de Gramont A, Bosset JF, Milan C, Rougier P, Bouché O, Etienne PL, et al. Randomized trial comparing monthly low-dose leucovorin and fluorouracil bolus with bimonthly high-dose leucovorin and fluorouracil bolus plus continuous infusion for advanced colorectal cancer: a French intergroup study. *J Clin Oncol* 1997 Feb; 15(2): 808–15.

16 QUASAR Collaborative Group. Comparison of fluorouracil with additional levamisole, higher-dose folinic acid, or both, as adjuvant chemotherapy for colorectal cancer: a randomised trial. *Lancet* 2000 May 6; 355(9215): 1588–96.

17 Twelves C, Wong A, Nowacki MP, Abt M, Burris H 3rd, Carrato A, et al. Capecitabine as adjuvant treatment for stage III colon cancer. *N Engl J Med* 2005 Jun 30; 352(26): 2696–704.

18 André T, Bensmaine MA, Louvet C, François E, Lucas V, Desseigne F, et al. Multicenter phase II study of bimonthly high-dose leucovorin, fluorouracil infusion, and oxaliplatin for metastatic colorectal cancer resistant to the same leucovorin and fluorouracil regimen. *J Clin Oncol* 1999 Nov; 17(11): 3560–8.

19 André T, Boni C, Mounedji-Boudiaf L, Navarro M, Tabernero J, Hickish T, et al. Oxaliplatin, fluorouracil, and leucovorin as adjuvant treatment for colon cancer. *N Engl J Med* 2004 Jun 3; 350(23): 2343–51.

20 André T, Boni C, Navarro M, Tabernero J, Hickish T, Topham C, et al. Improved overall survival with oxaliplatin, fluorouracil, and leucovorin as adjuvant treatment in stage II or III colon cancer in the MOSAIC trial. *J Clin Oncol* 2009 Jul 1; 27(19): 3109–16.

21 Kuebler JP, Wieand HS, O'Connell MJ, Smith RE, Colangelo LH, Yothers G, et al. Oxaliplatin combined with weekly bolus fluorouracil and leucovorin as surgical adjuvant chemotherapy for stage II and III colon cancer: results from NSABP C-07. *J Clin Oncol* 2007 Jun 1; 25(16): 2198–204.

22 Yothers G, O'Connell MJ, Allegra CJ, Kuebler JP, Colangelo LH, Petrelli NJ, et al. Oxaliplatin as adjuvant therapy for colon cancer: updated results of NSABP C-07 trial, including survival and subset analyses. *J Clin Oncol* 2011 Oct 1; 29(28): 3768–74.

23 Haller DG, Tabernero J, Maroun J, de Braud F, Price T, Van Cutsem E, et al. Capecitabine plus oxaliplatin compared with fluorouracil and folinic acid as adjuvant therapy for stage III colon cancer. *J Clin Oncol* 2011 Apr 10; 29(11): 1465–71.

24 Allegra CI, Yothers G, O'Connell MJ, Dharif S, Petrelli NJ, Colangelo LH, et al. Phase III trial assessing bevacizumab in stages II and III carcinoma of the colon: results of NSABP protocol C-08. *J Clin Oncol* 2011 Jan 1; 29(1): 11–6.

25 De Gramont A, Van Cutsem E, Schmoll H-J, Tabemero J, Clarke S, Moore MJ, et al. Bevacizumab plus oxaliplatin-based chemotherapy as adjuvant treatment for colon cancer (AVANT): a phase 3 randomised controlled trial. *Lancet Oncol* 2012 Dec 13; 13(12): 1225–33.

26 Allegra CJ, Jessup JM, Somerfield MR, Hamilton SR, Hammond EH, Hayes DF, et al. American Society of Clinical Oncology provisional clinical opinion: testing for KRAS gene mutations in patients with metastic colorectal carcinoma to predict response to anti-epidermal growth factor receptor monoclonal antibody therapy. *J Clin Oncol* 2009 April 20; 27(12): 2091–6.

27 Alberts SR, Sargent DJ, Nair S, Mahoney MR, Mooney M, Thibodeau SN, et al. Effect of oxaliplatin, fluorouracil, and leucovorin with or without cetuximab on survival among patients with resected Stage II colon cancer – a randomized trial. *JAMA* 2012 Apr 4; 307(13): 1383–93.

28 Taieb J, Tabernero J, Mini E, Subtil F, Folprecht G, Laethem J-LV, et al. Subgroup analyses results of the PETACC8 phase III trial comparing adjuvant FOLFOX4 with or without cetuximab (CTX) in resected stage III colon cancer (CC). *J Clin Oncol* [Internet] 2013 (cited 2013 Oct 25); 31(supply. abstr. 3525). Available from: *http://meetinglibrary.asco.org/content/110568-132*

29 Sargent DJ, Goldberg RM, Jacobson SD, Macdonald JS, Labianca R, Haller DG, et al. A pooled analysis of adjuvant chemotherapy for resected colon cancer in elderly patients. *N Engl J Med* 2001 Oct 11; 345(15): 1091–7.

30 Ades S. Adjuvant chemotherapy for colon cancer in the elderly: moving from evidence to practice. *Oncology* 2009; Feb; 23(2): 162–7.

31 Gill S, Loprinzi C, Kennecke H, Grothey A, Nelson G, Woods R, et al. Prognostic web-based models for stage II and III colon cancer: A population and clinical trials-based validation of numeracy and adjuvant! online. *Cancer* 2011 Sep 15; 117(18): 4155–65.

32 International Multicentre Pooled Analysis of B2 Colon Cancer Trials (IMPACT B2) Investigators. Efficacy of adjuvant fluorouracil and folinic acid in B2 colon cancer. *J Clin Oncol* 1999 May; 17(5): 1356–63.

33 Gill S, Loprinzi CL, Sargent DJ, Thomé SD, Alberts SR, Haller DG, et al. Pooled analysis of fluorouracil-based adjuvant therapy for stage II and III colon cancer: who benefits and by how much? *J Clin Oncol* 2004 May 15; 22(10): 1797–806.

34 Mamounas E, Wieand S, Wolmark N, Bear HD, Atkins JN, Song K, et al. Comparative efficacy of adjuvant chemotherapy in patients with Dukes' B versus Dukes' C colon cancer: results from four National Surgical Adjuvant Breast and Bowel Project Adjuvant Studies (C-01, C-02, C-03, and C-04). *J Clin Oncol* 1999 May 1; 17(5): 1349.

35 Wilkinson NW, Yothers G, Lopa S, Costantino JP, Petrelli NJ, Wolmark N. Long-term survival results of surgery alone versus surgery plus 5-fluorouracil and leucovorin for stage II and stage III colon cancer: pooled analysis of NSABP C-01 through C-05. A baseline from which to compare modern adjuvant trials. *Ann Surg Oncol* 2010 Apr; 17(4): 959–66.

36 O'Connor ES, Greenblatt DY, LoConte NK, Gangnon RE, Liou J-I, Heise CP, et al. Adjuvant chemotherapy for stage II colon cancer with poor prognostic features. *J Clin Oncol* 2011 Sep 1; 29(25): 3381–8.

37 The Cancer Genome Atlas Network. Comprehensive molecular characterization of human colon and rectal cancer. *Nature* 2012 Jul 19; 487(7407): 330–7.

38 Allegra CJ, Paik S, Colangelo LH, Parr AL, Kirsch I, Kim G, et al. Prognostic value of thymidylate synthase, Ki-67, and p53 in patients with Dukes' B and C colon cancer: A National Cancer Institute-National Surgical Adjuvant Breast and Bower Project collaborative study. *J Clin Oncol* 2003 Jan 15; 21(2): 241–51.

39 Horie N, Aiba H, Oguro K, Hojo H, Takeishi K. Functional analysis and DNA polymorphism of the tandemly repeated sequences in the 5′-terminal regulatory region o the human gene for thymidylate synthase. *Cell Struct Funct* 1995 Jun: 20(3): 191–7.

40 Pullarkat ST, Stoehlmacher J, Ghaderi V, Xiong YP, Ingles SA, Sherrod A, et al. Thymidylate synthase gene polymorphism determines response and toxicity of 5-FU chemotherapy. *Pharmacogenomics J* 2001; 1(1): 65–70.

41 Tan BR, Thomas F, Myerson RJ, Zehnbauer B, Trinkaus K, Malyapa RS, et al. Thymidylate synthase genotype-directed neoadjuvant chemoradiation for patients with rectal adenocarcinoma. *J Clin Oncol* 2011 Mar 1; 29(7): 875–83.

42 Fearon ER, Cho KR, Nigro JM, Kern SE, Simons JW, Ruppert JM, et al. Identification of a chromosome 18q gene that is altered in colorectal cancer. *Science* 1990 Jan 5; 247(4938): 49–56.

43 Popat S, Houlston RS. A systematic review and meta-analysis of the relationship between chromosome 18q genotype, DCC status and colorectal cancer prognosis. *Eur J Cancer* 2005 Sept; 41(14): 2060–70.

44 Gavin PG, Colangelo LH, Fumagalli D, Tanaka N, Remillard MY, Yothers G, et al. Mutation profiling and microsatellite instability in stage II and III colon cancer: an assessment of their prognostic and oxaliplatin predictive value. *Clin Cancer Res* 2012 Dec 1; 18(23): 6531–41.

45 Ogino S, Shima K, Meyerhardt JA, McCleary NJ, Ng I, Hollis D, et al. Predictive and prognostic roles of BRAF mutation in stage III colon cancer: results from intergroup trial CALGB 89803. *Clin Cancer Res* 2012 Feb 1; 18(3): 890–900.

46 Warren RS, Atreya CE, Niedzwiecki D, Weinberg VK, Donner DB, Mayer RJ, et al. Association of TP53 mutational status and gender with survival after adjuvant treatment for stage III colon cancer: results of CALGB 89803. *Clin Cancer Res* 2013 Oct 15; 19(20): 5777–87.

47 Aaltonen LA, Peltonmäki P, Leach FS, Sistonen P, Pylkkänen L, Mecklin JP, et al. Clues to the pathogenesis of familial colorectal cancer. *Science* 1993 May 7; 260(5109): 812–6.

48 Thibodeau SN, Bren G, Schaid D. Microsatellite instability in cancer of the proximal colon. *Science* 1993 May 7; 260(5109): 816–9.

49 Kim H, Jen J, Vogelstein B, Hamilton SR. Clinical and pathological characteristics of sporadic colorectal carcinomas with DNA replication errors in microsatellite sequences. *Am J Pathol* 1994 Jul; 145(1): 148–56.

50 Lothe RA, Peltomäki P, Meling GI, Aaltonen LA, Nyström-Lahti M, Pylkkänen L, et al. Genomic instability in colorectal cancer: relationship to clinicopathological variables and family history. *Cancer Res* 1993 Dec 15; 53(24): 5849–52.

51 Ribic CM, Sargent DJ, Moore MJ, Thibodeau SN, French AJ, Goldberg RM, et al. Tumor microsatellite-instability status as a predictor of benefit from fluorouracil-based adjuvant chemotherapy for colon cancer. *N Engl J Med* 2003 Jul 17; 349(3): 247–57.

52 Kim GP, Colangelo LH, Wieand HS, Paik S, Kirsch IR, Wolmark N, et al. Prognostic and predictive roles of high-degree microsatellite instability in colon cancer: a National Cancer Institute-National Surgical Adjuvant Breast and Bowel Project Collaborative Study. *J Clin Oncol* 2007 Mar 1; 25(7): 767–72.

53 Sinicrope FA. DNA mismatch repair and adjuvant chemotherapy in sporadic colon cancer. *Nat Rev Clin Oncol* 2010 Mar; 7(3): 174–7.

54 Sinicrope FA, Foster NR, Thibodeau SN, Marsoni S, Monges G, Labianca R, et al. DNA mismatch repair status and colon cancer recurrence and survival in clinical trials of 5-fluorouracil-based adjuvant therapy. *J Natl Cancer Inst* 2011 Jun 8; 103(11): 863–75.

55 Bertagnolli MM, Niedzwiecki D, Compton CC, Hahn HP, Hall M, Damas B, et al. Microsatellite instability predicts improved response to adjuvant therapy with irinotecan, fluorouracil, and leucovorin in stage III colon cancer: Cancer and Leukemia Group B Protocol 89803. *J Clin Oncol* 2009 Apr 10; 27(11): 1814–21.

56 Roth AD, Delorenzi M, Tejpar S, Yan P, Klingbiel D, Fiocca R, et al. Integrated analysis of molecular and clinical prognostic factors in stage II/III colon cancer. *J Nat Cancer Inst* 2012 Nov 7; 104(21): 1635–46.

57 Flejou J-F, André T, Chibaudel B, Scriva A, Hickish T, Tabernero J, et al. Effect of adding oxaliplatin to adjuvant 5-fluorouracil/laucovorin (5FU/LV) in patients with defective mismatch repair (dMMR) colon cancer stage II and III included in the MOSAIC study. *J Clin Oncol* (Internet) 2013 [cited 2013 Nov 1); 31 (suppl; abstr 3524). Available from: *http:// meetinglibrary.asco.org/content/112291-132*

58 Gavin PG, Paik S, Yothers G, Pogue-Geile KL. Colon cancer mutation: prognosis/ prediction-response. *Clin Cancer Res* 2013 Mar 1; 19(5): 1301.

59 Fearon ER. Molecular genetics of colorectal cancer. *Ann Rev Path: Mech Dis* 2011; 6(1): 479–507.

60 Wood LD, Parsons DW, Jones S, Lin J, Sjöblom T, Leary RJ, et al. The genomic landscapes of human breast and colorectal cancers. *Science* 2007 Nov 16; 318(5853): 1108–13.

61 Sjöblom T, Jones S, Wood LD, Parsons DW, Lin J, Barber TD, et al. The consensus coding sequences of human breast and colorectal cancers. *Science* 2006 Oct 13; 314(5797): 269–74.

62 Dang CV. MYC on the path to cancer. *Cell* 2012 Mar 30; 149(1): 22–35.

63 Bastiaannett E, Sampieri K, Dekkers OM, de Craen AJM, van Herk-Sukel MPP, Lemmens V, et al. Use of aspirin postdiagnosis improves survival of colon cancer patients. *Br J Cancer* 2012 Aug 24; 106(9): 1564–70.

64 Domingo E, Church DN, Sieber O, Ramamoorthy R, Yanagisawa Y, Johnstone E, et al. Evaluation of PIK3CA mutation as a predictor of benefit from nonsteroidal anti-inflammatory drug therapy in colorectal cancer. *J Clin Oncol* 2013 Dec 1; 31(34): 4297–305.

65 Liao X, Lochhead P, Nishihara R, Morikawa T, Kuchiba A, Yamauchi M, et al. Aspirin use, tumor PIK3CA mutation, and colorectal-cancer survival. *New Eng J Med* 2012; 367(17): 1596–606.

66 ECC 2013 Press Release: New research shows how aspirin may act on blood platelets to improve survival in colon cancer patients (Internet). Available from: *http://www.esmo.org/Conferences/European-Cancer-Congress-2013/News/ECC-2013-Press-Release-New-Research-shows-how-Aspirin-may-act-on-Blood-Platelets-to-Improve-Survival-in-Colon-Cancer-Patients*

67 Paik S. Is gene array testing to be considered routine now? *Breast* 2011 Oct; 20 Suppl. 3: S87–91.

68 Salazar R, Rosenberg R, Lutke Holzik M, et al. The PARSC trial: a prospective study for the assessment of recurrence risk in stage II colon cancer (CC) patients using ColoPrint. *J Clin Oncol* (Meeting Abstracts) 2011; 29(suppl. 4: abstr. 602).

69 Venook AP, Niedzwiecki D, Lopatin M, Ye X, Lee M, Friedman PN, et al. Biologic determinants of tumor recurrence in Stage II colon cancer: validation study of the 12-gene recurrence score in Cancer and Leukemia Group B (CALGB) 9581. *J Clin Oncol* 2013 May 10; 31(14): 1775–81.

70 Smith RE, Colangelo L, Wieand HS, Begovic M, Wolmark N. Randomized trial of adjuvant therapy in colon carcinoma: 10-year results of NSABP Protocol C-01. *J Natl Cancer Inst* 2004 Aug 4; 96(15): 1128–32.

71 Hoover HC Jr, Brandhorst JS, Peters LC, Surdyke MG, Takeshita Y, Madariaga J, et al. Adjuvant active specific immunotherapy for human colorectal cancer: 6.5-year median follow-up of a phase III prospectively randomized trial. *J Clin Oncol* 1993 Mar; 11(3): 390–9.

72 Moertel CG. Vaccine adjuvant therapy for colorectal cancer: 'very dramatic' or ho-hum? *J Clin Oncol* 1993 Mar; 11(3): 385–6.

73 Hanna MG Jr, Hoover HC Jr, Vermorken JB, Harris JE, Pinedo HM. Adjuvant active specific immunotherapy of stage II and stage III colon cancer with an autologous tumor cell vaccine: first randomized phase III trials show promise. *Vaccine* 2001 Mar 21; 19(17–19): 2576–82.

74 Foon KA, Yannelli J, Bhattacharya-Chatterjee M. Colorectal cancer as a model for immunotherapy. *Clin Cancer Res* 1999 Feb 1; 5(2): 225–36.

75 Pagès F, Berger A, Camus M, Sanchez-Cabo F, Costes A, Molidor R, et al. Effector memory T cells, early metastasis, and survival in colorectal cancer. *N Eng J Med* 2005 Dec 22; 353(25): 2654–66.

76 Galon J, Costes A, Sanchez-Cabo F, Kirilovsky A, Mlecnik B, Lagorce-Pagès, et al. Type, density, and location of immune cells within human colorectal tumors predict clinical outcome. *Science* 2006 Sep 29; 313(5795): 1960–4.

77 Mlecnik B, Tosolini M, Kirilovsky A, Berger A, Bindea G, Meatchi T, et al. Histopathologic-based prognostic factors of colorectal cancers are associated with the state of the local immune reaction. *J Clin Oncol* 2011 Feb 20; 29(6): 610–8.

78 Bindea G, Mlecnik B, Tosolini M, Kirilovsky A, Waldner M, Obenauf AC, et al. Spatiotemporal dynamics of intratumoral immune cells reveal the immune landscape in human cancer. *Immunity* 2013 Oct 17; 39(4): 782–95.

79 Pardoll DM. The blockade of immune checkpoints in cancer immunotherapy. *Nat Rev Cancer* 2012 Apr; 12(4): 252–64.

80 Lesterhuis WJ, Haanen JBAG, Punt CJA. Cancer immunotherapy – revisited. *Nat Rev Drug Discov* 2011; 10(8): 591–600.

81 Zitvogel L, Kepp O, Kroemer G. Immune parameters affecting the efficacy of chemotherapeutic regimens. *Nat Rev Clin Oncol* 2011 Mar; 8(3): 151–60.

82 Rosenberg SA. Raising the bar: the curative potential of human cancer immunotherapy. *Sci Transl Med* 2012 Mar 28; 4(127): 127ps8.

83 Niederhuber JE. Colon and rectum cancer. Patterns of spread and implications for workup. *Cancer* 1993 Jun 15; 71(12 Suppl.): 4187–92.

84 Fisher B, Wolmark N, Rockette H, Redmond C, Deutsch M, Wickerham DL, et al. Postoperative adjuvant chemotherapy or radiation therapy for rectal cancer: results from NSABP protocol R-01. *J Natl Cancer Inst* 1988 Mar 2; 80(1): 21–9.

85 Wolmark N, Wieand HS, Hyams DM, Colangelo L, Dimitrov NV, Romond EH, et al. Randomized trial of postoperative adjuvant chemotherapy with or without radiotherapy for carcinoma of the rectum: National Surgical Adjuvant Breast and Bowel Project Protocol R-02. *J Natl Cancer Inst* 2000 Mar 1; 92(5): 388–96.

86 Frykholm GJ, Glimelius B, Påhlman L. Preoperative or postoperative irradiation in adenocarcinoma of the rectum: final treatment results of a randomized trial and an evaluation of late secondary effects. *Dis Colon Rectum* 1993 Jun; 36(6): 564–72.

87 Cammà C, Giunta M, Fiorica F, Pagliaro L, Craxì A, Cottone M. Preoperative radiotherapy for resectable rectal cancer: A meta-analysis. *JAMA* 2000 Aug 23; 284(8): 1008–15.

88 Kapiteijn E, Marijnen CA, Nagtegaal ID, Putter H, Steup WH, Wiggers T, et al. Preoperative radiotherapy combined with total mesorectal excision for resectable rectal cancer. *N Engl J Med* 2001 Aug 30; 345(9): 638–46.

89 Sauer R, Becker H, Hohenberger W, Rödel C, Wittekind C, Fietkau R, et al. Preoperative versus postoperative chemoradiotherapy for rectal cancer. *N Engl J Med* 2004 Oct 21; 351(17): 1731–40.

90 Sanghera P, Wong DWY, McConkey CC, Geh JI, Hartley A. Chemoradiotherapy for rectal cancer: an updated analysis of factors affecting pathological response. *Clin Oncol (R Coll Radiol)* 2008 Mar; 20(2): 176–83.

91 Rödel C, Liersch T, Becker H, Fietkau R, Hohenberger W, Hothorn T, et al. Preoperative chemoradiotherapy and postoperative chemotherapy with fluorouracil and oxaliplatin versus fluorouracil alone in locally advanced rectal cancer: initial results of the German CAO/ARO/AIO-04 randomised phase 3 trial. *Lancet Oncol* 2012 Jul; 13(7): 679–87.

92 Gérard J-P, Azria D, Gourgou-Bourgade S, Martel-Laffay I, Hennequin C, Etienne P-L, et al. Clinical outcome of ACCORD 12/0405 PRODIGE 2 randomized trial in rectal cancer. *J Clin Oncol* 2012 Dec 20; 30(36): 4558–65.

93 Aschele C, Cionini L, Lonardi S, Pinto C, Cordio S, Rosati G, et al. Primary tumor response to preoperative chemoradiation with or without oxaliplatin in locally advance rectal cancer: pathologic results of the STAR-01 randomized phase II trial. *J Clin Oncol* 2011 Jul 10; 29(20): 2773–80.

94 Weiss C, Arnold D, Dellas K, Liersch T, Hipp M, Fietkau R, et al. Preoperative radiotherapy of advanced rectal cancer with capecitabine and oxaliplatin with or without

cetuximab: a pooled analysis of three prospective phase I–II trials. *Int J Radiat Oncol Biol Phys* 2010 Oct 1; 78(2): 472–8.
95 Kosinski L, Habr-Gama A, Ludwig K, Perez R. Shifting concepts in rectal cancer management. *CA: A Cancer Journal for Clinicians* 2012 Apr 9; 62(3): 173–202.
96 Barker AD, Sigman CC, Kelloff GJ, Hylton NM, Berry DA, Esserman LJ. I-SPY 2: An adaptive breast cancer trial design in the setting of neoadjuvant chemotherapy. *Clin Pharmacol Ther* 2009 May 13; 86(1): 97–100.
97 Kim ES, Herbst RS, Wistuba II, Lee JJ, Blumenschein GR Jr, Tsao A, et al. The BATTLE trial: personalizing therapy for lung cancer. *Cancer Discov* 2011 Jun; 1(1): 44–53.

ANSWERS TO MULTIPLE-CHOICE QUESTIONS

1 D
2 B

CHAPTER 11

Long- versus short-course radiotherapy for rectal cancer

Manisha Palta, Christopher G. Willett & Brian G. Czito
Duke University Medical Center, Durham, NC, USA

KEY POINTS

- Short-course radiotherapy is generally defined as 25 Gy in 5 fractions *without* the concurrent administration of chemotherapy and is a standard treatment approach throughout much of northern Europe
- Long-course radiotherapy is generally defined as 45–50.4 Gy in 25–28 fractions *with* the administration of concurrent 5-FU based chemotherapy and is a standard treatment approach in other parts of Europe and the United States.
- Two randomized control trials, the Polish and Australian Intergroup studies, have compared outcomes between patients receiving short-course RT versus long-course CRT. Additional studies are ongoing.
- There continues to be much debate regarding the optimal neoadjuvant regimen for resectable rectal cancer.

CASE STUDY

A 54-year-old healthy female presents with rectal bleeding. Colonoscopy reveals a polypoid, ulcerative, bleeding mass at 8 cm from the anal verge, and biopsy demonstrates invasive adenocarcinoma. Endoscopic ultrasound demonstrates uT3N1 disease at 8 cm from the anal verge and CT of the chest, abdomen, and pelvis shows no evidence of metastatic disease. The patient is evaluated by a surgical oncologist, medical oncologist, and radiation oncologist.

Colorectal Cancer: Diagnosis and Clinical Management, First Edition. Edited by John H. Scholefield and Cathy Eng.

TIPS / TRICKS / KEY PITFALLS

A preoperative approach using either short-course radiation therapy alone or long-course chemoradiotherapy in potentially resectable rectal cancer patients is supported by randomized trials. Each approach has its relative advantages and disadvantages. Ongoing studies should help further define the roles of both approaches.

Introduction

There is significant debate regarding the optimal neoadjuvant regimen for resectable rectal cancer patients. In many Northern European countries, the use of short-course preoperative radiotherapy (RT) alone (25 Gy in 5 fractions) followed by total mesorectal excision (TME) approximately 1 week later has become standard practice, supported by multiple randomized control trials comparing TME alone to preoperative short-course RT preceding surgery. In the United States and other parts of Europe, the use of long-course conventionally fractionated radiotherapy (45–50.4 Gy in 25–28 fractions) with concurrent administration of fluoropyrimidine-based chemotherapy is favored. At present, two randomized control trials have compared outcomes of short- to long-course RT. This chapter presents current data and respective advantages of each approach.

Short-course radiotherapy

Numerous randomized control trials have compared short-course RT followed by surgery to surgery alone for resectable rectal cancer (Table 11.1). These trials were conducted in Europe where short-course RT has become a standard treatment approach for patients with resectable rectal cancer. Early trials conducted in Sweden demonstrated superiority of preoperative short-course RT prior to surgery over surgery alone in terms of local control [1–4].

The Swedish Rectal Cancer trial included 1168 patients with resectable, Dukes A–C rectal cancer. Patients were randomized to receive 25 Gy in 5 fractions delivered over 1 week followed by surgery 1 week later versus surgery alone. The surgery was considered curative if margins were uninvolved. The study was powered to detect both differences in local control and overall survival (OS). The 5-year local recurrence (LR) (11% vs. 27%) and OS (58% vs. 48%) rates were superior with preoperative short-course RT compared to surgery alone [5]. A statistically significant tumor downstaging effect was seen

Table 11.1 Select randomized trials of preoperative short-course radiotherapy.

Trial	LR	DFS	OS
Swedish (n = 1186) [6]	(13 yr)	(13 yr)	(13 yr)
TME alone	26%	62%	30%
RT + TME	9%	72%	38%
Dutch (n = 1861) [15]	(10 yr)	(10 yr)	(10 yr)
TME alone	11%	73%	49%
RT + TME	5%	80%	48%
MRC (n = 1350) [19]	(3 yr)	(3 yr)	(3 yr)
TME + select postop CRT	10.6%	71.5%	78.6%
RT + TME	4.4%	77.5%	80.3%

TME: total mesorectal excision, RT: radiotherapy, CRT: chemo-radiotherapy, LR: local recurrence, DFS: disease-free survival, OS: overall survival

in those patients receiving preoperative RT. The LR and OS benefit persisted with long-term follow-up. At a median 13-year follow-up, LR (9% vs. 26%) and OS (38% vs. 30%) rates were both in favor of preoperative radiotherapy, with all stages benefiting [6].

Historically, the high LR of disease following standard abdominoperineal resection (APR) or low anterior resection (LAR) (15–30%) has been judged to be due to blunt dissection that violates the planes of the mesorectal circumference [7]. Lateral spread of disease has been shown to occur not only at the level of the tumor but distally within the mesorectum [8]. Heald et al. recommended *en bloc* removal of the tumor within the envelope of the endopelvic fascia to obtain adequate lateral clearance of disease and reduce the likelihood of LR [9;10]. This requires sharp dissection along the plane that separates the visceral from the parietal pelvic fascia with complete *en bloc* removal of the rectum so that all of the rectal mesentery remains within the envelope of the specimen, termed a total mesorectal excision (TME) [11].

A Dutch (CKVO 95–04) multicenter, phase III study of 1861 patients with operable rectal cancer was undertaken to evaluate the role of short-course preoperative RT with TME. Patients were randomized to TME alone versus 25 Gy in 5 fractions followed by TME. No fixed tumors were included in the study and approximately half of enrolled patients had T1/T2 disease. Postoperative RT was administered in those patients who underwent surgery and had a positive circumferential radial margin (CRM). The 2-year OS was 82% in both arms of the study; however, the 2-year LR was 8.2% in the TME-only arm compared to 2.4% in the preoperative RT arm. This highlighted the value of radiation treatment, despite the use of TME. The sphincter preservation rate was the same in both arms, and there was no clear evidence of downstaging effect [12]. The perineal complication rate was slightly higher in the preoperative RT arm of 26% versus 18% in the TME alone arm [13;14]. Ten-year follow-up indicates persistent benefit in LR of 5% with RT versus 11% with TME alone [15]. Updated toxicity analysis shows a higher incidence of sexual dysfunction and slower recovery of bowel function, more fecal incontinence, and poorer quality of life with short-course preoperative RT compared to TME alone [16;17].

In the era of improved surgical technique (with TME), preoperative staging, and histological assessment, the MRC CR07 trial re-evaluated the role of RT. Patients with resectable rectal cancer were randomized to preoperative radiotherapy (25 Gy in 5 fractions) or upfront resection with selective postoperative chemoradiotherapy (CRT) (45 Gy in 25 fractions with concurrent 5-fluorouracil (5-FU)) in patients with a ≤1 mm circumferential resection margin. All 1350 patients had central pathological review [18]. At median follow-up of 4 years, LR was significantly lower in the preoperative radiotherapy group (4.4% vs. 10.6%). Although 3-year disease-free survival (DFS) was improved in the preoperative RT group (77.5% vs. 71.5%), there was no difference in OS [19]. In sum, attempts to identify patients at high risk of recurrence after postoperative resection and administering selective CRT were inferior to nonselective upfront preoperative short-course radiotherapy.

Long-course radiotherapy

By the 1990s, postoperative chemoradiation had become the standard treatment for resectable rectal cancer, with studies demonstrating a 10–15% survival advantage with the addition of chemotherapy to adjuvant RT [20;21]. A number of subsequent phase III trials compared preoperative with postoperative CRT (Table 11.2). The National Surgical Adjuvant Breast and Bowel Project (NSABP) R-03 study was originally designed to accrue 900 patients, but closed prematurely after only accruing 267. In this study, individuals with operable T3/T4 and/or node positive adenocarcinoma of the rectum were randomized (and stratified based on age and sex) to surgery followed by 1 cycle of 5-FU/leucovorin (LV) and then concurrent bolus (weeks 1 and 5) 5-FU/leucovorin (LV) with radiation treatment versus 5-FU/LV for 1 cycle then concurrent CRT treatment followed by surgery. All patients received adjuvant 5-FU and LV for 4 cycles. Although the study was underpowered, 5-year DFS was superior in the preoperative therapy group: 64.7% versus 53.4%.

Table 11.2 Randomized trials of postoperative versus preoperative chemoradiotherapy.

Trial	LR	DFS	OS	pCR	Sphincter Preservation
NSABP R-03 (n = 267) [22]	(5 yr)	(5 yr)	(5 yr)		(5 yr)
Postop CRT	10.7%	53.4%	65.6%		24.2%
Preop CRT	10.7%	64.7%	74.5%	15%	33.9%
Korea (n = 240) [23]	(5 yr)	(5 yr)	(5 yr)		(<5cm from verge)
Postop CRT	6%	74%	85%		42%
Preop CRT	5%	73%	83%	17%	68%
German(n = 823) [24]	(5 yr)	(5 yr)	(5 yr)		(felt to require APR pre-tx)
Postop CRT	13%	65%	74%		19%
Preop CRT	6%	68%	76%	8%	39%

NSABP: National Surgical Adjuvant Breast and Bowel Project, CRT: chemoradiotherapy, LR: local recurrence, DFS: disease free survival, OS: overall survival, pCR: pathological complete response

There was a trend, though not statistically significant, of improved 5-year OS with preoperative therapy: 74.5% versus 65.6%. A pCR was seen in 15% of patients undergoing preoperative therapy [22].

A Korean trial randomized 240 patients with locally advanced (cT3/T4 and/or N+) rectal cancer to preoperative or postoperative CRT. CRT consisted of 50 Gy in 25 fractions with concurrent capecitabine (1650 mg/m^2/day). The standard surgical procedure was TME. Patients received 4 cycles of adjuvant chemotherapy with capecitabine (2500 mg/m^2/day for 14 days followed by 1 week break) or bolus 5-FU (375 mg/m^2/day)/ LV (20 mg/m2/day) for 5 days every 4 weeks. The 5-year DFS, OS, and LR rates were no different between the two arms. Patients with low-lying rectal tumors (<5cm from anal verge) had higher rates of sphincter preservation in the preoperative arm (68% vs. 42%) [23].

The definitive phase III study in favor of preoperative CRT was the CAO/ARO/AIO-94 study performed by the German Rectal Cancer Group. The results of this trial resulted in a subsequent paradigm shift to preoperative CRT. Eight hundred-twenty three Clinically staged T3/T4 and/or node-positive rectal cancers were randomized to receive preoperative CRT followed by TME 6 weeks later or TME followed by postoperative CRT. The radiation dose was 50.4 Gy in 28 fractions in all patients with a 5.4 Gy small volume boost in the postoperative arm. 5-FU (1 g/m^2 per day) was administered during the 1st and 5th weeks of radiotherapy as a 120-hour continuous infusion. Both arms received 4 additional cycles of 5-FU (500 mg/m^2 per day for 5 days every 4 weeks). All surgeons were trained in the use of TME and were asked prior to treatment to evaluate the possibility of sphincter preservation. The

5-year results revealed a pelvic recurrence rate of 6% versus 13% ($p = 0.02$) in favor of the preoperative arm. The distant recurrence rate was 36% versus 38% (p = NSS), DFS was 68% versus 65% (p = NSS), and OS was 76% versus 74% (p = NSS) for preoperative versus postoperative radiation therapy, respectively. There was significant tumor downstaging after preoperative CRT with an 8% pCR. Nodal positivity was 25% in the preoperative versus 40% in the postoperative arm. The sphincter preservation rate in 188 patients with low-lying tumors (declared by the surgeon prior to randomization to require an APR) revealed that 39% versus 19% had a sphincter-preserving low anterior resection ($p = 0.004$) in the preoperative versus the postoperative arm. There were fewer acute (27% vs. 40%) and late toxicities (14% vs. 24%) in the preoperative-treatment group. Thus, preoperative CRT resulted in half the LF and doubled the sphincter preservation rate compared to postoperative therapy. In addition, compliance rates were significantly improved in the preoperative arm. Importantly, there was no difference in OS or DFS between the two arms [24]. This local relapse benefit is sustained with long term follow up; 7% compared to 10% local relapse rate at 10 years with preoperative therapy. PMID: 22529255.

Randomized control trials of long- versus short-course radiotherapy

A number of trials have attempted or are currently assessing the question of whether long-course CRT or short-course RT is superior (Table 11.3). The Polish rectal trial randomized 312 patients to preoperative short-course RT (25 Gy in 5 fractions) followed by surgery within 7 days or preoperative CRT (50.4 Gy in 28 fractions with concurrent bolus 5-FU/LV weeks 1 and 5), with surgery 4–6 weeks after completion. The trial included patients with T3/T4 resectable disease with no evidence of sphincter involvement but with a lower margin of tumor accessible by DRE. The standard surgical procedure was TME and postoperative chemotherapy was optional. Prior to study initiation, workshops were organized for participating surgeons, pathologists, and radiation oncologists in an effort for standardization. The study was designed with 80% power to detect a 15% difference in sphincter preservation rates. After median follow-up of 48 months, there was no benefit from protracted course of CRT for sphincter preservation (the primary endpoint – 61% short-course vs. 58% CRT), DFS (58.4% short-course vs. 55.6% CRT), or OS (67.2% short-course vs. 66.2% CRT). There was a non-significant lower rate of actuarial LR in the short-course RT arm (10.6% vs. 15.6%), despite a higher rate of pCR in the

Table 11.3 Randomized trials of short-course radiotherapy versus long-course chemoradiotherapy.

Trial	Grade III/IV Acute Toxicity	pCR	Sphincter Preservation	LR	DFS	OS	Grade III/IV Late Toxicity
Polish Trial (n = 312) [25]				(4 yr)	(4yr)	(4yr)	
Short-course	3.2%	0.7%	61.2%	10.6%	58.4%	67.2%	10.1%
Long-course	18.2%	16.1%	58.0%	15.6%	55.6%	66.2%	7.1%
Australian Trial (n = 326)				(3 yr)		(5 yr)	(5 yr)
[26;27 (ref PMID 23008301Z)]	1.9%	1%	63%	7.5%	NR	74%	5.8%
Short-course	28%	15%	69%	4.4%	NR	70%	8.2%
Long-course							

pCR: pathological complete response; NR: not reported; LR: local recurrence; DFS: disease-free survival; OS: overall survival.

CRT arm (1% short-course vs. 16% CRT). Acute Grade III/IV toxicity rates were significantly higher in the CRT arm (3.2% vs. 18.2% p <0.001), with 2 toxicity related deaths in the CRT arm. There was no difference in severe late toxicities (10.1% short-course vs. 7.1% CRT) [25].

The results of this trial have raised a number of concerns and criticisms. With power to detect a 15% difference in sphincter preservation, smaller differences between short- and long-course RT would not be apparent. In addition, a prime concern of larger dose per fraction radiotherapy is the potential manifestation of normal tissue late toxicities. With a median of 4 years of follow-up, this duration is too short for assessment of long-term late toxicity. Although only patients with T3/T4 disease were included, nearly 40% of patients in the short-course arm had pathological T1/T2 disease. Despite the use of TME, the LR rates in the Polish trial were higher than those reported in other studies utilizing this surgical technique [13;19]. The authors comment that this difference may be a function of TME being a relatively new technique for some surgeons resulting in suboptimal quality [25]. Similarly, no centralized review of radiotherapy or pathological assessment was performed. Although the decision regarding sphincter preservation was to be made at the time of surgery, surgeons may not have been as familiar with the potential downstaging effect of CRT and hence more reluctant to proceed with sphincter sparing procedures. Another confounding factor is that 15% of patients randomized to the CRT did not receive the assigned intervention [25].

The Australian Intergroup Trial randomized 326 patients with cT3N 0-2 M0 rectal cancer within 12 cm of the anal verge were randomized to short-course RT (25 Gy in 5 fractions) with surgery within 1 week or long-course CRT (50.4 Gy in 28 fractions with continuous infusion 5-FU 225 mg/m^2), with surgery 4–6 weeks following completion of CRT. Both regimens were followed by adjuvant 5-FU-based chemotherapy. The primary endpoint of this study was to compare LR rates at 3 years. Over 90% of patients were clinically staged with pelvic MRI or EUS. With median follow-up of 5.9 years, there was no difference in 3-year LR (7.5% short-course vs. 4.4% CRT), 5-year OS (74% short-course vs. 70% CRT), or Grade III/IV late toxicity (5.8% short-course vs. 8.2% CRT) Despite tumor downstaging, there was no difference in rates of sphincter sparing surgery. PMID reference 23008301. Acute toxicity results presented at a prior meeting demonstrated higher rates of Grade III/IV acute toxicity (1.9% short-course vs. 28% CRT, p<0.001)(27).

Two additional studies are accruing patients and awaiting mature results. The Stockholm III study seeks to answer the question of optimal fractionation regimen and timing of surgery. A trial of 840 patients with resectable rectal cancer 15 cm from the anal verge is planned with randomization to 1 of 3 arms: preoperative short-course RT (25 Gy in 5 fractions) with surgery within 1 week; preoperative short-course RT (25 Gy in 5 fractions) with surgery after 4–8 weeks of completion; or preoperative long-course RT (50 Gy in 25 fractions), with surgery in 4–8 weeks following after completion. The primary study endpoint is time to LR. Interim analysis after randomization of the initial 303 patients demonstrated no difference in rates of Grade III/IV acute toxicity or postoperative complications. However, patients in the long-course arm had the lowest rates of postoperative complications and re-operations. The proportion of patients undergoing APR was lower, though not statistically significant, in the long-course arm compared to either short-course RT groups ($p = 0.070$). One criticism of the trial is that hospitals could choose to participate in randomizing to all 3 arms or 2 arms (early vs. delayed surgery with short-course RT). This hospital directed randomization was an effort to boost accrual but could lead to potential randomization bias. Given that LR rates have improved, particularly with wider implementation and experience with TME, this study is likely underpowered to meet its primary endpoint, though continued accrual and final analysis is pending [28].

The Berlin Rectal Cancer Trial commenced in 2004. In this study, patients with cT2N+/T3Nany rectal cancer staged by EUS or CT/MRI are randomized to short-course RT (25 Gy in 5 fractions) or CRT (50.4 Gy in 28 fractions with CI 5-FU 225 mg/m2). Both groups are scheduled to undergo TME and 12 weeks of additional adjuvant 5-FU-based chemotherapy. The working hypothesis is that CRT is superior to short-course radiotherapy in terms of 5-year LR. Secondary outcomes are OS, DFS, quality of life, R0 resection rate, sphincter preservation, and acute and late toxicity rates [29]. At present the Polish Rectal Trial and Australian Intergroup trial are the only fully published studies addressing the question of short- versus long-course RT. The Stockholm III and Berlin Rectal Cancer trials will add to the literature, and hopefully clarify the optimal preoperative fractionation regimen for rectal cancer.

Advantages of short-course radiotherapy

Lower rates of acute toxicity

Both the Polish and Australian trials demonstrated higher rates of Grade III/IV acute toxicity within the CRT arms [25;30]. Despite improved rates of local control and significant tumor downstaging, a number of neoadjuvant trials demonstrate that the addition of chemotherapy increases rates of severe acute toxicity compared to radiotherapy alone [31;32]. These higher rates of toxicity are not observed with short-course radiotherapy, particularly when surgery is performed within 1 week of RT completion, given that the rectum is surgically removed prior to the manifestation of acute RT effects. In randomized trials of short-course RT, typically only Grade I/II gastrointestinal (GI) acute toxicity is observed [14;33]. Aside from gastrointestinal effects, transient neurologic symptoms, such as sacral/leg pain, have been reported in 10% of patients, possibly related to the higher dose per fraction to neurologic structures. In only 2.5% of patients was that pain severe enough to interrupt treatment [14].

Better compliance

Lower rates of acute toxicity with short-course radiotherapy seem to be associated with higher rates of compliance. In the Polish trial, 98% of patients receiving short-course radiotherapy completed the assigned treatment compared to 69% in the CRT arm. In the Australian trial, 100% of patients completed short-course radiotherapy, while only 77% completed CRT per protocol [27].

Improved costs/convenience

Short-course radiotherapy has been the standard of care in many northern European countries, with the majority of randomized controlled trials evaluating the 25 Gy in 5 fraction regimen conducted in the Netherlands, Scandinavia, and the United Kingdom [34]. Given a centralized healthcare system, these more hypofractionated, shorter courses of radiotherapy allow patients to be treated more quickly and proceed to surgery. This regimen is particular advantageous in countries with more limited resources, centers with long waiting lists, and for patients who have to travel further distances to undergo RT treatment. Similarly, short-course RT may be economically more cost-effective.

Advantages of long-course radiotherapy

Sphincter preservation

A prime rationale for long-course RT is the potential for sphincter preservation as a result of tumor downstaging. In European trials of short-course radiotherapy, APR rates of 35–58% were reported [5;13]. Minimal tumor downstaging is seen with short-course RT and patients determined to need APR prior to treatment commencement will likely be committed to this surgical procedure [12]. Recent data suggest a decline in APR rates in the United States to approximately 20% [35;36]. APR has been associated with a slightly higher morbidity and mortality versus LAR with a worse quality of life related to changes in body image and depression due to the presence of a colostomy [35;37;38].

In the Polish trial, no difference was seen in sphincter preservation rates (61.2% short-course vs. 58% long-course) [25]. The lack of difference may be a function of surgeons not being as familiar with the potential downstaging effect of CRT (as short-course RT was more common) and hence less willing to alter planned surgical procedure. Similarly no difference was seen in sphincter preservation in the Australian Intergroup trial despite tumor downstaging. (ref PMID 23008301Z). In trials of pre- versus postoperative CRT, higher rates of sphincter preservation have been seen with preoperative long-course CRT. In the German rectal cancer trial, patients were assessed prior to treatment to determine the type of surgery (APR vs. LAR) required and patients were stratified by surgeon. Of the patients deemed to require APR prior to treatment, 19% of patients receiving postoperative CRT were able to undergo a sphincter sparing procedure compared to 39% in the preoperative CRT arm [24]. The randomized Korean trial showed similar results in patients with low lying tumors, with a significantly higher rate of sphincter preservation was seen in patients undergoing preoperative CRT compared to postoperative CRT (68% vs. 42% $p = 0.008$) (23). In the NSABP-R03, there was no difference in preoperative or postoperative CRT patients who maintained their sphincter and were free of disease at 5 years (33.9% vs. 24.2% respectively), though this may be a function of failure to meet accrual goals and subsequent lack of statistical power to detect differences [22].

Tumor downstaging/improved resectability

Tumor downstaging is commonly seen with CRT, resulting in improved resectability (R0 resection rates) and sphincter preservation. Data from short-course RT regimens indicates that minimal tumor downstaging occurs [12]. Long-course CRT results in pCR rates of 8–30% [22–24;31;39–41]. Patients with pCR have improved long-term outcomes compared to non-responders and may be able to avoid surgery in highly selected situations [42–46]. Even if pCR is not achieved, tumor downstaging can facilitate R0 resection.

The principal reason for LR in resected rectal cancer appears to be related to the anatomic constraints in obtaining wide radial margins, despite adequate proximal and distal margins [47]. Quirke et al., using whole mount specimens, found that in 27% (14/52) of patients disease had spread to the lateral radial margin, even though the margins appeared negative with standard pathological assessment. Eighty-six percent of those with positive margins developed local regional recurrence of disease as compared to only 3% without lateral resection margin involvement [48]. In addition, pathological assessment in the MRC-07 trial found that the plane of surgery (mesorectal, intramesorectal, or muscularis propria planes) predicted for LR. Three-year LR was 4% in patients undergoing complete mesorectal excision, compared with 7% and 13% in the intramesorectal and muscularis propria groups respectively [18]. A positive radial margin is not only a predictor of LR, but inferior survival rates as well [49].

The R0 resection rate in the Swedish and Dutch trials was roughly 77%, despite inclusion criteria of only patients with mobile/resectable rectal cancers, compared to the more than 85% R0 resection rates in trials implementing CRT [5;13;23;24;31;32]. In the Korean randomized trial, all 105 patients randomized to preoperative CRT underwent complete resection [23]. Similar pathological outcomes have been seen in the Polish rectal trial, with fewer positive CRMs in patients receiving long-course CRT (4% vs. 13%), with considerable reduction in tumor size seen of an average 1.9 cm [25].

Although minimal tumor downstaging or pCR is seen with short-course RT, this may be a function of the timing of surgery (within 1 week of radiation completion). Data from the Lyon R90-01 trial suggests that tumor cells may be present but nonviable following short-course RT, as tumor regression and necrosis takes time to occur [50]. With long-course CRT, there is sufficient time to see evidence of this phenomenon. The Stockholm III trial will shed further light on this, as one aim of the trial is short-course RT with delayed surgery at 4–8 weeks [28].

Fewer postoperative complications

With short-course RT there is a concern of increased postoperative complications. An analysis of the Dutch TME trial demonstrated that irradiated patients experienced higher rates of blood loss and perineal wound complications (in cases of APR TME alone 18% vs. RT + TME 29%) [14]. In the German rectal cancer trial, roughly 10% of patients experienced delayed sacral wound healing, which was similar to the 8% rate in the postoperative arm [24]. Similarly, in the Polish trial, the number of postoperative complications was higher in the short-course arm, at 31% compared with 21% in the long-course CRT group [51].

Lower late toxicity

A primary concern of short-course RT utilization (with the delivery of higher radiation doses per fraction) is potential late effects. Basic radiobiological principles dictate that larger fraction size carries a higher risk of late toxicities. Although there was no difference in late effects in the Polish and Australian Intergroup trials at a median follow-up of roughly 6 years, this is entirely sufficient to detect late toxicities [25;(ref PMID 23008301Z)]. Longer follow-up is needed to adequately assess for differences in short- and long-course RT.

Long-term data from European randomized trials of short-course radiotherapy highlight some concerns for late effect development. Review of hospital records of patients treated in Sweden demonstrated higher small bowel obstruction and abdominal pain admissions, chronic neuropathy, and femoral neck/pelvic fractures in patients treated with short-course RT compared to surgery alone [52–55]. Many of these complications may result from older radiotherapy techniques, including larger fields with inclusion of lumbar vertebral bodies, AP/PA (rather than multi-field) techniques, and no normal tissue blocking. Evaluation of late effects in the Dutch TME trial irradiated patients reported higher rates of fecal incontinence (62% vs. 38%), pad wearing as a result of incontinence (56% vs. 33%), anal blood loss (11% vs. 3%), and mucus loss (27% vs. 15%). Irradiated patients also reported more sexual dysfunction and lower satisfaction of bowel function [16;17].

Addition of chemotherapy

A variety of disease sites have demonstrated the synergistic effects of systemic therapies with radiotherapy, particularly radiosensitization with concurrent 5-FU based chemotherapy. Early adjuvant RT trials in rectal cancer demonstrated the superiority of concurrent CRT, resulting in a significant survival benefit [20;56]. Although neoadjuvant trials evaluating RT alone versus CRT have not shown a survival benefit, the addition of chemotherapy results in higher rates of local control and pCR/tumor downstaging [31;32]. With short-course RT, the high dose per fraction generally prohibits the concurrent administration of radiosensitizing chemotherapy.

Conclusion

The optimal neoadjuvant approach for resectable rectal cancer is far from clear. Both short-course RT (25 Gy in 5 fractions) and long-course CRT (50.4 Gy in 28 fractions with concurrent 5-FU based chemotherapy) represent reasonable therapeutic options. As data from randomized control trials comparing short- with long-course RT emerge, the optimal neoadjuvant therapy regimen will be more clearly defined.

MULTIPLE-CHOICE QUESTIONS

1 Which of the following is not an advantage of short-course radiotherapy?
- **A.** Lower rate of acute toxicity
- **B.** Tumor downstaging
- **C.** Reduced healthcare expense
- **D.** Convenience for patient
- **E.** Higher rate of compliance

2 Which of the following is not a potential advantage of long-course radiotherapy?
- **A.** Higher rates of sphincter preservation
- **B.** Lower rates of involved margins
- **C.** Lower late toxicity rates
- **D.** Lower acute toxicity rates
- **E.** Tumor downstaging

3 Which of the following statements regarding randomized controlled trials of short- versus long-course radiotherapy is false?
- **A.** No improvement in sphincter preservation was seen in the Polish rectal trial
- **B.** No difference in pCR was seen in the Polish rectal trial
- **C.** No statistically significant difference in late toxicities was seen in the Polish or Australian Intergroup trials
- **D.** Higher rates of acute toxicity are seen with long-course RT in both the Polish and Australian Intergroup trials

References

1 Stockholm Colorectal Cancer Study Group. Preoperative short-term radiation therapy in operable rectal carcinoma. A prospective randomized trial. *Cancer* 1990; 66(1): 49–55.

2 Cedermark B, Johansson H, Rutqvist LE, Wilking N. The Stockholm I trial of preoperative short-term radiotherapy in operable rectal carcinoma. A prospective randomized trial. Stockholm Colorectal Cancer Study Group. *Cancer* 1995; 75(9): 2269–75.

3 Stockholm Rectal Cancer Study Group. Randomized study on preoperative radiotherapy in rectal carcinoma. *Ann Surg Oncol* 1996; 3(5): 423–30.

4 Martling A, Holm T, Johansson H, Rutqvist LE, Cedermark B. The Stockholm II trial on preoperative radiotherapy in rectal carcinoma: long-term follow-up of a population-based study. *Cancer* 2001; 92(4): 896–902.

5 Swedish Rectal Cancer Trial. Improved survival with preoperative radiotherapy in resectable rectal cancer. *New Eng J Med* 1997; 336(14): 980–7.

6 Folkesson J, Birgisson H, Pahlman L, Cedermark B, Glimelius B, Gunnarsson U. Swedish Rectal Cancer Trial: long lasting benefits from radiotherapy on survival and local recurrence rate. *J Clin Oncol* 2005; 23(24): 5644–50.

7 Enker WE, Thaler HT, Cranor ML, Polyak T. Total mesorectal excision in the operative treatment of carcinoma of the rectum. *J Am Coll Surg* 1995; 181(4): 335–46.

8 Cawthorn SJ, Parums DV, Gibbs NM, A'Hern RP, Caffarey SM, Broughton CI, et al. Extent of mesorectal spread and involvement of lateral resection margin as prognostic factors after surgery for rectal cancer. *Lancet* 1990; 335(8697): 1055–9.

9 Heald RJ, Husband EM, Ryall RD. The mesorectum in rectal cancer surgery–the clue to pelvic recurrence? *Br J Surg* 1982; 69(10): 613–6.

10 Heald RJ, Moran BJ, Ryall RD, Sexton R, MacFarlane JK. Rectal cancer: the Basingstoke experience of total mesorectal excision, 1978–1997. *Arch Surg* 1998; 133(8): 894–9.

11 MacFarlane JK, Ryall RD, Heald RJ. Mesorectal excision for rectal cancer. *Lancet* 1993; 341(8843): 457–60.

12 Marijnen CA, Nagtegaal ID, Klein Kranenbarg E, Hermans J, van de Velde CJ, Leer JW, et al. No downstaging after short-term preoperative radiotherapy in rectal cancer patients. *J Clin Oncol* 2001; 19(7): 1976–84.

13 Kapiteijn E, Marijnen CA, Nagtegaal ID, Putter H, Steup WH, Wiggers T, et al. Preoperative radiotherapy combined with total mesorectal excision for resectable rectal cancer. *New Eng J Med* 2001; 345(9): 638–46.

14 Marijnen CA, Kapiteijn E, van de Velde CJ, Martijn H, Steup WH, Wiggers T, et al. Acute side effects and complications after short-term preoperative radiotherapy combined with total mesorectal excision in primary rectal cancer: report of a multicenter randomized trial. *J Clin Oncol* 2002; 20(3): 817–25.

15 van Gijn W, Marijnen CA, Nagtegaal ID, Kranenbarg EM, Putter H, Wiggers T, et al. Preoperative radiotherapy combined with total mesorectal excision for resectable rectal cancer: 12-year follow-up of the multicentre, randomised controlled TME trial. *Lancet Oncol* 2011; 12(6): 575–82.

16 Peeters KC, van de Velde CJ, Leer JW, Martijn H, Junggeburt JM, Kranenbarg EK, et al. Late side effects of short-course preoperative radiotherapy combined with total mesorectal excision for rectal cancer: increased bowel dysfunction in irradiated patients – a Dutch colorectal cancer group study. *J Clin Oncol* 2005; 23(25): 6199–206.

17 Marijnen CA, van de Velde CJ, Putter H, van den Brink M, Maas CP, Martijn H, et al. Impact of short-term preoperative radiotherapy on health-related quality of life and sexual functioning in primary rectal cancer: report of a multicenter randomized trial. *J Clin Oncol* 2005; 23(9): 1847–58.

18 Quirke P, Steele R, Monson J, Grieve R, Khanna S, Couture J, et al. Effect of the plane of surgery achieved on local recurrence in patients with operable rectal cancer: a prospective study using data from the MRC CR07 and NCIC-CTG CO16 randomised clinical trial. *Lancet* 2009; 373(9666): 821–8.

19 Sebag-Montefiore D, Stephens RJ, Steele R, Monson J, Grieve R, Khanna S, et al. Preoperative radiotherapy versus selective postoperative chemoradiotherapy in patients with rectal cancer (MRC CR07 and NCIC-CTG C016): a multicentre, randomised trial. *Lancet* 2009; 373(9666): 811–20.

20 Thomas PR, Lindblad AS. Adjuvant postoperative radiotherapy and chemotherapy in rectal carcinoma: a review of the Gastrointestinal Tumor Study Group experience. *Radiother Oncol* 1988; 13(4): 245–52.

21 Krook JE, Moertel CG, Gunderson LL, Wieand HS, Collins RT, Beart RW, et al. Effective surgical adjuvant therapy for high-risk rectal carcinoma. *New Eng J Med* 1991; 324(11): 70–15.

22 Roh MS, Colangelo LH, O'Connell MJ, Yothers G, Deutsch M, Allegra CJ, et al. Preoperative multimodality therapy improves disease-free survival in patients with carcinoma of the rectum: NSABP R-03. *J Clin Oncol* 2009; 27(31): 5124–30.

23 Park JH, Yoon SM, Yu CS, Kim JH, Kim TW, Kim JC. Randomized phase 3 trial comparing preoperative and postoperative chemoradiotherapy with capecitabine for locally advanced rectal cancer. *Cancer* 2011; 117(16): 3703–12.

24 Sauer R, Becker H, Hohenberger W, Rodel C, Wittekind C, Fietkau R, et al. Preoperative versus postoperative chemoradiotherapy for rectal cancer. *New Eng J Med* 2004; 351(17): 1731–40.

25 Bujko K, Nowacki MP, Nasierowska-Guttmejer A, Michalski W, Bebenek M, Kryj M. Long term results of a randomized trial comparing preoperative short-course radiotherapy with preoperative conventionally fractionated chemoradiation for rectal cancer. *Br J Surg* 2006; 93(10): 1215–23.

26 Ngan SW, Burmeister B, Fisher RL, et al. Randomized trial of short-course radiotherapy versus long-course chemoradiation comparing rates of local recurrence in patients with T3 rectal cancer: trans-tasman radiation oncology group trial 01.04. *J Clin Oncol* 2012; 30: 3827–33.

27 Ngan S, Fisher R, Mackay J. Acute adverse events in a randomised trial of short-course versus long-course preoperative radiotherapy for T3 adenocarcinoma of the rectum: A Trans-Tasman Radiation Oncology Group trial (TROG 01.04) *Eur J Cancer* 2007; 4 suppl 5: 237.

28 Pettersson D, Cedermark B, Holm T, Radu C, Pahlman L, Glimelius B, et al. Interim analysis of the Stockholm III trial of preoperative radiotherapy regimens for rectal cancer. *Br J Surg* 2010; 97(4): 580–7.

29 Siegel R, Burock S, Wernecke KD, Kretzschmar A, Dietel M, Loy V, et al. Preoperative short-course radiotherapy versus combined radiochemotherapy in locally advanced rectal cancer: a multi-centre prospectively randomised study of the Berlin Cancer Society. *BMC Cancer* 2009; 9: 50.

30 Ngan SR, Fisher D, Goldstein M, Solomon B, Burmeister SP, Ackland DJ, et al. A randomized trial comparing local recurrence (LR) rates between short-course (SC) and long-course (LC) preoperative radiotherapy (RT) for clinical T3 rectal cancer: An intergroup trial. *J Clin Oncol* 2010; 28: 15s (suppl: abstr 3509).

31 Gerard JP, Conroy T, Bonnetain F, Bouche O, Chapet O, Closon-Dejardin MT, et al. Preoperative radiotherapy with or without concurrent fluorouracil and leucovorin in T3-4 rectal cancers: results of FFCD 9203. *J Clin Oncol* 2006; 24(28): 4620–5.

32 Bosset JF, Collette L, Calais G, Mineur L, Maingon P, Radosevic-Jelic L, et al. Chemotherapy with preoperative radiotherapy in rectal cancer. *New Eng J Med* 2006; 355(11): 1114–23.

33 Bujko K, Nowacki MP, Nasierowska-Guttmejer A, Michalski W, Bebenek M, Pudelko M, et al. Sphincter preservation following preoperative radiotherapy for rectal cancer: report of a randomised trial comparing short-term radiotherapy vs. conventionally fractionated radiochemotherapy. *Radiother Oncol* 2004; 72(1): 15–24.

34 Minsky BD. Counterpoint: long-course chemoradiation is preferable in the neoadjuvant treatment of rectal cancer. *Seminars Rad Oncol* 2011; 21(3): 228–33.

35 Jessup JM, Stewart AK, Menck HR. The National Cancer Data Base report on patterns of care for adenocarcinoma of the rectum, 1985–95. *Cancer* 1998; 83(11): 2408–18.

36 You YN, Baxter NN, Stewart A, Nelson H. Is the increasing rate of local excision for stage I rectal cancer in the United States justified? A nationwide cohort study from the National Cancer Database. *Ann Surg* 2007; 245(5): 726–33.
37 Grumann MM, Noack EM, Hoffmann IA, Schlag PM. Comparison of quality of life in patients undergoing abdominoperineal extirpation or anterior resection for rectal cancer. *Ann Surg* 2001; 233(2): 149–56.
38 Williams NS, Durdey P, Johnston D. The outcome following sphincter-saving resection and abdominoperineal resection for low rectal cancer. *Br J Surg* 1985; 72(8): 595–8.
39 Aschele C, Cionini L, Lonardi S, Pinto C, Cordio S, Rosati G, et al. Primary tumor response to preoperative chemoradiation with or without oxaliplatin in locally advanced rectal cancer: pathologic results of the STAR-01 randomized phase III trial. *J Clin Oncol* 2011; 29(20): 2773-80.
40 Gerard JP, Azria D, Gourgou-Bourgade S, Martel-Laffay I, Hennequin C, Etienne PL, et al. Comparison of two neoadjuvant chemoradiotherapy regimens for locally advanced rectal cancer: results of the phase III trial ACCORD 12/0405-Prodige 2. *J Clin Oncol* 2010; 28(10): 1638–44.
41 Mohiuddin M, Winter K, Mitchell E, Hanna N, Yuen A, Nichols C, et al. Randomized phase II study of neoadjuvant combined-modality chemoradiation for distal rectal cancer: Radiation Therapy Oncology Group Trial 0012. *J Clin Oncol* 2006; 24(4): 650–5.
42 Stipa F, Chessin DB, Shia J, Paty PB, Weiser M, Temple LK, et al. A pathologic complete response of rectal cancer to preoperative combined-modality therapy results in improved oncological outcome compared with those who achieve no downstaging on the basis of preoperative endorectal ultrasonography. *Ann Surg Oncol* 2006; 13(8): 1047–53.
43 Hughes R, Glynne-Jones R, Grainger J, Richman P, Makris A, Harrison M, et al. Can pathological complete response in the primary tumour following pre-operative pelvic chemoradiotherapy for T3-T4 rectal cancer predict for sterilisation of pelvic lymph nodes, a low risk of local recurrence and the appropriateness of local excision? *Intl J Colorect Dis* 2006; 21(1): 11–7.
44 Capirci C, Valentini V, Cionini L, De Paoli A, Rodel C, Glynne-Jones R, et al. Prognostic value of pathologic complete response after neoadjuvant therapy in locally advanced rectal cancer: long-term analysis of 566 ypCR patients. *Intl J Rad Oncol Biol Phys* 2008; 72(1): 99–107.
45 Habr-Gama A, Perez RO, Nadalin W, Sabbaga J, Ribeiro U, Jr., Silva e Sousa AH, Jr., et al. Operative versus non-operative treatment for stage 0 distal rectal cancer following chemoradiation therapy: long-term results. *Ann Surg* 2004; 240(4): 711–7; discussion 7–8.
46 Maas M, Beets-Tan RG, Lambregts DM, Lammering G, Nelemans PJ, Engelen SM, et al. Wait-and-see policy for clinical complete responders after chemoradiation for rectal cancer. *J Clin Oncol* 2011; 29(35): 4633–40.
47 Nelson H, Petrelli N, Carlin A, Couture J, Fleshman J, Guillem J, et al. Guidelines 2000 for colon and rectal cancer surgery. *J Nat Cancer Inst* 2001; 93(8): 583–96.
48 Quirke P, Durdey P, Dixon MF, Williams NS. Local recurrence of rectal adenocarcinoma due to inadequate surgical resection. Histopathological study of lateral tumour spread and surgical excision. *Lancet* 1986; 2(8514): 996–9.
49 Nagtegaal ID, Quirke P. What is the role for the circumferential margin in the modern treatment of rectal cancer? *J Clin Oncol* 2008; 26(2): 303–12.

50 Francois Y, Nemoz CJ, Baulieux J, Vignal J, Grandjean JP, Partensky C, et al. Influence of the interval between preoperative radiation therapy and surgery on downstaging and on the rate of sphincter-sparing surgery for rectal cancer: the Lyon R90-01 randomized trial. *J Clin Oncol* 1999; 17(8): 2396.

51 Bujko K, Nowacki MP, Kępka L, Olędzki J, Bębenek M, Kryj M, et al. Postoperative complications in patients irradiated pre-operatively for rectal cancer: report of a randomised trial comparing short-term radiotherapy vs chemoradiation. *Colorect Dis* 2005; 7(4): 410–6.

52 Birgisson H, Pahlman L, Gunnarsson U, Glimelius B. Adverse effects of preoperative radiation therapy for rectal cancer: long-term follow-up of the Swedish Rectal Cancer Trial. *J Clin Oncol* 2005; 23(34): 8697–705.

53 Birgisson H, Pahlman L, Gunnarsson U, Glimelius B. Late gastrointestinal disorders after rectal cancer surgery with and without preoperative radiation therapy. *Br J Surg* 2008; 95(2): 206–13.

54 Frykholm GJ, Sintorn K, Montelius A, Jung B, Påhlman L, Glimelius B. Acute lumbosacral plexopathy during and after preoperative radiotherapy of rectal adenocarcinoma. *Radiother Oncol* 1996; 38(2): 12–30.

55 Holm T, Singnomklao T, Rutqvist LE, Cedermark B. Adjuvant preoperative radiotherapy in patients with rectal carcinoma. Adverse effects during long-term follow-up of two randomized trials. *Cancer* 1996; 78(5): 968–76.

56 Prolongation of the disease-free interval in surgically treated rectal carcinoma. Gastrointestinal Tumor Study Group. *New Eng J Med* 1985; 312(23): 1465–72.

ANSWERS TO MULTIPLE-CHOICE QUESTIONS

1 B
2 D
3 B

CHAPTER 12

More treatment is not necessarily better – limited options for chemotherapeutic radiosensitization

Daedong Kim
The University of Texas MD Anderson Cancer Centre, Houston, TX, USA

KEY POINTS

- The combination of RT with CT has proved to be a successful concept in rectal cancer treatment and provided the rationale for chemoradiotherapy (CRT) in the clinical setting.
- The combination of capecitabine with RT in the neoadjuvant setting is tolerable and demonstrates similar pathological complete remission (pCR) rates to that of infusional 5-FU studies.
- Irinotecan is usually administered in combination with 5-FU or capecitabine. Although higher pCR rates were achieved, the major dose-limiting toxicity (DLT) was grade 3/4 diarrhea.
- The combination of oxaliplatin with 5-FU or capecitabine significantly increased grade 3/4 toxicities without significantly improving the pCR rate.
- Bevacizumab has demonstrated favorable pCR rates but perioperative safety concerns have been raised.
- Cetuximab in conjunction with 5-FU and RT demonstrated disappointing pCR rate, without synergistic or unexpected toxicities.
- The combination of erlotinib and bevacizumab with 5-FU or capecitabine is well tolerated with promising pCR rates and warrants further investigation.

Colorectal Cancer: Diagnosis and Clinical Management, First Edition. Edited by John H. Scholefield and Cathy Eng.

Introduction

The combination of radiotherapy (RT) with chemotherapy (CT) has proved to be a successful concept in rectal cancer treatment and provides the rationale for chemoradiotherapy (CRT) in the clinical setting. After the Gastrointestinal Tumor Study Group demonstrated the benefits of chemoradiation, postoperative adjuvant CRT has been recommended to improve outcomes and reduce recurrence rates in locally advanced rectal cancer (LARC), when compared with surgery alone or surgery plus RT or CT alone [1–4].

The German CAO/ARO/AIO-94 study investigated preoperative 5-FU-based CRT versus postoperative CRT for stage II/III rectal cancer and demonstrated that rates of compliance, local regional control, and sphincter preservation, as well as acute/late toxicity were improved, but noted no difference in 5-year survival rates [5]. These findings have validated the advantages of preoperative CRT and led to a new standard of care in the use of neoadjuvant chemoradiation treatment of LARC.

Despite considerable reduction of local recurrence rates, lack of improvement in overall survival (OS) and the risk of distant metastases remain significant problems in LARC. In an attempt to improve the efficacy of downstaging, as well as the control of the distant spread of LARC, the integration of novel cytotoxic drugs and biological targeted agents, such as capecitabine, irinotecan, oxaliplatin, bevacizumab, and cetuximab, in combined therapy has been explored. The main goal of such intensive CRT is to achieve higher rates of local control with lower rates of distant metastasis to improve patients' outcomes. However, novel schedules for CRT addressing which chemotherapeutic drugs should be used in what combination and sequence are questions that remain unanswered.

Integration of cytotoxic drugs

Continuous infusion 5-FU concomitant to preoperative RT is generally used, and based on 5-FU pharmacokinetics, sensitization and pCR is more likely to be achieved with prolonged infusions (12–18%) rather than bolus infusions (5–10%) [6–12]. The pCR rate of 5-FU alone as a radiation sensitizer is 5–20% and thus sets the bar for all other radiation sensitizers to surpass.

Capecitabine is a oral pro-drug of 5-FU and was believed to provide more selective delivery to tumor tissue because of its enzymatic conversion and increased levels of thymidine phosphorylase (TP) in tumors relative to normal tissues. However, this preclinical finding does not seem to have a bearing in human subjects. Thus far, in the adjuvant and metastatic settings, capecitabine has been determined as non-inferior for systemic treatment. In a similar fashion, the combination of capecitabine with RT versus continuous infusion 5-FU in the neoadjuvant setting is tolerable with similar pCR rates (13–24%) [13–15].

Irinotecan is a topoisomerase-1 inhibitor and was investigated in combination with continuous infusion 5-FU in neoadjuvant CRT for LARC. Higher pCR rates (26–37%) were achieved in combination with 5-FU [16–19]. As expected, the major DLT was grade 3/4 diarrhea (30%) and these results did not translate into any additive or synergistic clinical effect compared with 5-FU-based CRT in a larger randomized Phase II trial [17].

The combination of oxaliplatin with 5-FU or capecitabine yielded promising pCR rates (14–28%) in small-Phase I/II trials [20–22]. Unexpectedly, in two randomized Phase III trials, STAR-01 and ACCORD 12, adding oxaliplatin to fluorouracil-based preoperative CRT versus single agent treatment, significantly increased grade 3/4 toxicities without significantly improving the pCR rate (16% and 19%, respectively) [23;24].

In addition, the Radiation Oncology Group (RTOG) 0247 completed a small randomized Phase II trial of preoperative capecitabine with irinotecan (CAPEIRI) or oxaliplatin (CAPOX) with RT, to evaluate both the pCR rate and the toxicity, and to determine if one regimen was superior. Although not significant, the CAPOX regimen had a higher pCR rate (20.8% vs. 10.4%) with a similar incidence of toxicity. Preliminary results from the NSABP R-04 trial reported similarly increased toxicities but noted no benefit to early outcomes. Definitive analysis of tumor control will be presented in 2013 [25]. Other studies, including the Pan-European Trials in Adjuvant Colon Cancer (PETACC)-6 study, are randomizing patients to compare neoadjuvant CRT using fluoropyrimidine-based CT, with or without oxaliplatin. Such studies will help reveal the efficacy of intensive CRT using various neoadjuvant regimens.

Integration of biologic targeted agents

Bevacizumab, the anti-angiogenic agent, in combination with 5-FU- or capecitabine-based CRT regimens demonstrated a promising 16% and 32% pCR rate, respectively. Toxicities were generally mild, although wound dehiscence was seen in 12% of patients [26;27]. Phase I/II trials, using preoperative CRT with CAPOX plus bevacizumab, have revealed pCR rates of

18%, but important safety concerns about perioperative toxicity have been raised [7;28].

Cetuximab in conjunction with 5-FU and RT demonstrated mixed results, without synergistic or unexpected toxicities, but was disappointing with respect to the clinical end-point of pCR. According to a meta-anaysis, the addition of cetuximab to fluoropyrimidine-based CRT suggests an overall pCR of 9.1% [29]. EXPERT-C is a randomized Phase II trial in high risk rectal cancer patients (identified as T3-4, N2, or close circumferential margins by MRI of the rectum) investigating induction CAPOX-C, capecitabine/cetuximab, during radiation therapy, and followed by adjuvant chemotherapy; results demonstrated impressive radiographic response rates and noted an improvement in OS when compared to the CAPOX arm [30]. pCR rates after neoadjuvant CT and CRT were 18% versus 15% (11% vs. 7% in KRAS/BRAF wild-type), respectively [31]. Although the primary end-point of improved pCR was not met, the concept of induction CT may optimize the delivery of drugs in the preoperative setting, similar to other studies [32;33].

The tyrosine kinase inhibitors of the epidermal growth factor (EGFR) receptor, gefitinib and erlotinib, have also been investigated as potential radiosensitizers. Gefitinib was combined with CRT and demonstrated enhanced cytotoxicity in human CRC cell lines [34;35]. A Phase I trial combining gefitinib, capecitabine, and RT resulted in significant toxicities, including medication-refractory diarrhea and arterial thrombosis [36]. However, in two separate studies, the combinations of RT with either concurrent capecitabine plus erlotinib and bevacizumab, or 5-FU plus erlotinib and bevacizumab, were well tolerated with promising pCR rates (44% and 47%, respectively) [37;38]. As such, the use of erlotinib as a radiosensitizer warrants further investigation.

Conclusion

Although some studies suggest a higher pCR rate with the addition of new agents compared with 5-FU or capecitabine alone, this increased pCR rate is associated with an increase in acute toxicity. Furthermore, early end-points in terms of efficacy may not be coupled to longer-term end-points such as disease-free survival (DFS) and OS. More rationally designed preclinical and translational studies with recognized predictive factors such as KRAS mutations might help select appropriate patients, and determine the optimal sequence of chemotherapy and biological combinations.

CASE STUDY

The patient is a 57-year-old female with a history of rectal fullness for several months. Diagnostic colonoscopy revealed a non-obstructing circumferential rectal mass, measuring approximately 6 cm in length, extending to 2 cm from the dentate line. Biopsy and imaging confirmed corresponding wall thickening of the involved rectum as well as enlarged regional lymph nodes without evidence of metastatic disease. Baseline staging confirmed T3, N1 rectal cancer via MRI. She was recommended neoadjuvant chemoradiation therapy and completed therapy under protocol for a total dose of 50.4 Gy in 28 fractions.

TIPS AND TRICKS / KEY PITFALLS

- Although pCR rates can be used to compare the efficacy of different studies, observed pCR is influenced by the time interval between CRT and surgery, tumor stage, and the intensity of CRT [39;40]. Furthermore, pCR rates after preoperative CRT have not yet been validated as a surrogate for disease recurrence or as an end-point for long-term outcomes such as DFS or OS. Prolonged delays in radiation therapy may result in suboptimal outcomes and the use of adjuvant CRT postoperatively will result in reduced adherence to adjuvant chemotherapy and greater acute toxicities.
- Biomarkers to predict response to CRT are required to better discern which patients at high risk of relapse would benefit from additional intensified treatment in addition to standard 5-FU-based CRT. Presently, no predictive biomarkers have been established or validated in rectal cancer. In the near future, based on the results of these analyses, the individual patient will ideally be stratified into different alternative treatment concepts.

MULTIPLE CHOICE QUESTIONS

(You may include questions with one or multiple correct answers. If applicable, you may wish to include a feedback paragraph to explain the correct answer.)

1 Which chemotherapeutic agent is considered as a basic drug for CRT in rectal cancer treatment?

A. Bevacizumab
B. Irinotecan
C. Oxaliplatin
D. Fluoropyrimidine
E. Cetuximab

2 If she decided to receive CRT using the basic agent described in Question 1, which toxicity will be the most common for this patient during chemoradiation?

A. Neuropathy
B. Diarrhea

C. Wound dehiscence
D. Thromboembolism
E. Neutropenia

3 If she wanted to add an anti-angiogenic agent into her regimen, which expected adverse effect would be a major concern after chemoradiation?
A. Neuropathy
B. Diarrhea
C. Wound dehiscence
D. Nausea
E. Neutropenia

References

1 Krook JE, Moertel CG, Gunderson LL, et al. Effective surgical adjuvant therapy for high-risk rectal carcinoma. *N Engl J Med* 1991; 324: 709–15.

2 Gastrointestinal Tumor Study Group. Prolongation of the disease-free interval in surgically treated rectal carcinoma. *N Engl J Med* 1985 Jun 6; 312(23): 1465–72.

3 Wolmark N, Wieand HS, Hyams DM, Colangelo L, Dimitrov NV, Romond EH, et al. Randomized trial of postoperative adjuvant chemotherapy with or without radiotherapy for carcinoma of the rectum: National Surgical Adjuvant Breast and Bowel Project Protocol R-02. *J Natl Cancer Inst* 2000 Mar 1; 92(5): 388–96.

4 NIH Consensus Conference. Adjuvant therapy for patients with colon and rectal cancer. *JAMA* 1990; 264: 1444–50.

5 Sauer R, Becker H, Hohenberger W, Rödel C, Wittekind C, Fietkau R, et al. Preoperative versus postoperative chemoradiotherapy for rectal cancer. *N Engl J Med* 2004 Oct 21; 351(17): 1731–40.

6 Byfield JE, Calabro-Jones P, Klisak I, Kulhanian F. Pharmacologic requirements for obtaining sensitization of human tumor cells in vitro to combined 5-fluorouracil or ftorafur and X rays. *Int J Radiat Oncol Biol Phys* 1982; 8: 1923–33.

7 Hartley A, Ho KF, McConkey C, et al. Pathological complete response following preoperative chemoradiotherapy in rectal cancer: analysis of phase II/III trials. *Br J Radiol* 2005; 78: 934–8.

8 Chari RS, Tyler DS, Anscher MS: Preoperative radiation and chemotherapy in the treatment of adenocarcinoma of the rectum. *Ann Surg* 1995; 221: 778–86.

9 Pucciarelli S, Friso ML, Toppan P et al. Preoperative combined radiotherapy and chemotherapy for middle and lower rectal cancer: preliminary results. *Ann Surg Oncol* 2000; 7: 38–44.

10 Rich TA, Skibber JM, Ajani JA: Preoperative infusional chemoradiation therapy for stage T3 rectal cancer. *Int J Radiat Oncol Biol Phys* 1995; 32: 1025–9.

11 Mohiuddin M, Regine WF, John WJ, Hagihara PF, McGrath PC, Kenady DE, et al. Preoperative chemoradiation in fixed distal rectal cancer: dose time factors for pathological complete response. *Int Radiat Oncol Biol Phys* 2000; 46(4): 883–8.

12 Bosset JF, Pavy JJ, Hamers HP, Horiot JC, Fabri MC, Rougier P, et al. Determination of the optimal dose of 5-fluorouracil when combined with low dose D,L-leucovorin and

irradiation in rectal cancer: results of three consecutive phase II studies. EORTC Radiotherapy Group. *Eur J Cancer* 1993; 29(10): 140610.

13 Krishnan S, Janjan N, Skibber J, Rodriguez-Bigas MA, Wolff RA, Das P. Phase II study of capecitabine (Xeloda) and concomitant boost radiotherapy in patients with locally advanced cancer. *Int J Radiat Oncol Biol Phys* 2006; 66: 762–71.

14 Kim JC, Kim TW, Kim JH, Yu CS, Kim HC, Chang HM, et al. Preoperative concurrent radiotherapy with capecitabine before total mesorectal excision in locally advanced rectal cancer. *Int J Radiat Oncol Biol Phys* 2005; 63: 346–53.

15 De Paoli A, Chiara S, Luppi G, Friso ML, Beretta GD, Del Prete S, et al. Capecitabine in combination with preoperative radiation therapy in locally advanced resectable, rectal cancer: a multicentric phase II study. *Ann Oncol* 2006; 17: 246–51.

16 Mehta V, Cho C, Ford J, et al. Phase II trial of preoperative 3D conformal radiotherapy, protracted venous infusion 5-fluorouracil, in weekly CPT-11, followed by surgery for ultrasound stage T3 rectal cancer. *Int J Radiat Oncol Biol Phys* 2003; 55: 132–7.

17 Mohiuddin M, Winter K, Mitchell E, et al. Randomized phase II study of neoadjuvant combined-modality chemoradiation for distal rectal cancer. Radiation Therapy Oncology Group Trial 0012. *J Clin Oncol* 2006; 24: 650–5.

18 Willeke F, Horisberge K, Kraus-Tiefenbacher U, et al. A phase II study of capecitabine and irinotecan in combination with concurrent pelvic radiotherapy (Capiri-RT) as neoadjuvant treatment of locally advanced rectal cancer. *Br J Cancer* 2007; 96: 912–17.

19 Klautke G, Feyerherd P, Ludwig K, Prall F, Foitzik T, Fietkau R. Intensified concurrent chemoradiotherapy with 5-fluorouracil and irinotecan as neoadjuvant treatment in patients with locally advanced rectal cancer. *Br J Cancer* 2005; 92: 1190–7.

20 Gérard JP, Chapet O, Nemoz C, Romestaing P, Mornex F, Coquard R, et al. Preoperative concurrent chemoradiotherapy in locally advanced rectal cancer with high-dose radiation and oxaliplatin-containing regimen: the Lyon R0-04 phase II trial. *J Clin Oncol* 2003 Mar 15; 21(6): 1119–24.

21 Aschele C, Friso ML, Pucciarelli S, Lonardi S, Sartor L, Fabris G, et al. A phase I–II study of weekly oxaliplatin, 5-fluorouracil continuous infusion and preoperative radiotherapy in locally advanced rectal cancer. *Ann Oncol* 2005 Jul; 16(7): 1140–6.

22 Machiels JP, Duck L, Honhon B, Coster B, Coche JC, Scalliet P, et al. Phase II study of preoperative oxaliplatin, capecitabine and external beam radiotherapy in patients with rectal cancer: the RadiOxCape study. *Ann Oncol* 2005 Dec; 16(12): 1898–905.

23 Aschele C, Cionini L, Lonardi S, Pinto C, Cordio S, Rosati G, et al. Primary tumor response to preoperative chemoradiation with or without oxaliplatin in locally advanced rectal cancer: pathologic results of the STAR-01 randomized phase III trial. *J Clin Oncol* 2011 Jul 10; 29(20): 2773–80.

24 Gérard JP, Azria D, Gourgou-Bourgade S, Martel-Lafay I, Hennequin C, Etienne PL, et al. Clinical outcome of the ACCORD 12/0405 PRODIGE 2 randomized trial in rectal cancer. *J Clin Oncol.* 2012 Dec 20; 30(36): 4558–65.

25 Roh MS, Yothers GA, O'Connell MJ, Beart RW, Pitot HC, Shields AF, et al. The impact of capecitabine and oxaliplatin in the preoperative multimodality treatment in patients with carcinoma of the rectum: NSABP R-04. 2011 ASCO Annual Meeting. *J Clin Oncol* 29: 2011 (suppl: abstr 3503).

26 Willett CG, Duda DG, di Tomaso E, et al. Efficacy, safety, and biomarkers of neoadjuvant bevacizumab, radiation therapy, and fluorouracil in rectal cancer: a multidisciplinary phase II study. *J Clin Oncol* 2009; 27: 3020–6.

27 Crane CH, Eng C, Feig BW et al. Phase II trial of neoadjuvant bevacizumab, capecitabine, and radiotherapy for locally advanced rectal cancer. *Int J Radiat Oncol Biol Phys* 2010; 76: 824–30.

28 Czito BG, Bendell JC, Willett CG,et al. Bevacizumab, oxaliplatin, and capecitabine with radiation therapy in rectal cancer: Phase I trial results. *Int J Radiat Oncol Biol Phys* 2007; 68: 472–8.

29 Glynne-Jones R, Mawdsley S, Harrison M. Cetuximab and chemoradiation for rectal cancer – is the water getting muddy? *Acta Oncol* 2010 Apr; 49(3): 278–86.

30 Wong SJ, Winter K, Meropol NJ, Anne PR, Kachnic L, Rashid A, et al. Radiation Therapy Oncology Group 0247: a randomized Phase II study of neoadjuvant capecitabine and irinotecan or capecitabine and oxaliplatin with concurrent radiotherapy for patients with locally advanced rectal cancer. *Int J Radiat Oncol Biol Phys* 2012 Mar 15; 82(4): 1367–75.

31 Dewdney A, Cunningham D, Tabernero J, Capdevila J, Glimelius B, Cervantes A, et al. Multicenter randomized Phase II clinical trial comparing neoadjuvant oxaliplatin, capecitabine, and preoperative radiotherapy with or without cetuximab followed by total mesorectal excision in patients with high-risk rectal cancer (EXPERT-C). *J Clin Oncol* 2012 May 10; 30(14): 1620–7.

32 Chau I, Brown G, Cunningham D, et al. Neoadjuvant capecitabine and oxaliplatin followed by synchronous chemoradiation and total mesorecta lexcision in magnetic resonance imaging: Defined poor-risk rectal cancer. *J Clin Oncol* 2006; 24: 668–74.

33 Fernandez-Martos C, Pericay C, Aparicio J, Salud A, Safont M, Massuti B, et al. Phase II randomized study of concomitant chemoradiotherapy followed by surgery and adjuvant capecitabine plus oxaliplatin (CAPOX) compared with induction CAPOX followed by concomitant chemoradiotherapy and surgery in Magnetic Resonance Imaging-defined, locally advanced rectal cancer: Grupo Cancer de Recto 3 study. *J Clin Oncol* 2010; 28: 859–65.

34 Ciardiello F, Caputo R, Bianco R, Damiano V, Pomatico G, De Placido S, et al. Antitumor effect and potentiation of cytotoxic drugs activity in human cancer cells by ZD-1839 (Iressa), an epidermal growth factor receptor-selective tyrosine kinase inhibitor. *Clin Cancer Res* 2000; 6: 2053–63.

35 Williams K, Telfer B, Stratford I, Wedge SR. ZD1839 ('Iressa'), a specific oral epidermal growth factor receptor-tyrosine kinase inhibitor, potentiates radiotherapy in a human colorectal cancer xenograft model. *Br J Cancer* 2002; 86: 1157–61.

36 Czito B, Willett C, Bendell JC, Morse MA, Tyler DS, Fernando NH, et al. Increased toxicity with gefitinib, capecitabine and radiation therapy in pancreatic and rectal cancer: Phase I trial results. *J Clin Oncol* 2006; 24: 656–62.

37 Blaszkowsky LS, Hong TS, Zhu AX, Kwak EL, Mamon HJ, Shellito PC, et al. A phase I/II study of bevacizumab, erlotinib, and 5-fluorouracil with concurrent external beam radiation therapy in locally advanced rectal cancer. 2009 ASCO Annual Meeting. *J Clin Oncol* 27: 15s, 2009 (suppl: abstr 4106).

38 Das P, Eng C, Rodriguez-Bigas MA, Chang GJ, Skibber JM, et al. Preoperative radiation therapy with concurrent capecitabine, bevacizumab, and erlotinib for rectal adenocarcinoma: a Phase I trial. 2012 Gastrointestinal Cancers Symposium. *J Clin Oncol* 30, 2012 (suppl 4: abstr 544).

39 Hartley A, Ho KF, McConkey C, Geh JL. Pathological complete response following preoperative chemoradiotherapy in rectal cancer: analysis of phase II/III trials. *Br J Radiol* 2005; 78: 934–8.

40 Wiltshire KL, Ward IG, Swallow C, Oza AM, Cummings B, Pond GR, et al. Preoperative radiation with concurrent chemotherapy for resectable rectal cancer: effect of dose escalation on pathologic complete response, local recurrence-free survival, disease-free survival, and overall survival. *Int J Radiat Oncol Biol Phys* 2006; 64: 709–16.

ANSWERS TO MULTIPLE-CHOICE QUESTIONS

1 D
2 B
3 C

CHAPTER 13

Controversies in advanced disease – surgical approaches for metastatic resection

Amanda B. Cooper, Thomas A. Aloia, Jean-Nicolas Vauthey & Steven A. Curley
The University of Texas MD Anderson Cancer Center, Houston, TX, USA

KEY POINTS

- Although CT is the best overall colorectal cancer staging modality, MRI is the preferred modality for preoperative identification and characterization of liver metastases when available. Intraoperative ultrasound provides an important final evaluation for metastases not detected by preoperative imaging.
- Portal vein embolization may induce hypertrophy that improves the safety of extended liver resections in patients who would otherwise have a marginal functional liver remnant.
- The extent of hypertrophy seen after portal vein embolization is highly predictive of the degree of post-resection regeneration that can be expected.
- Peri-operative chemotherapy improves recurrence-free and progression-free survival and may improve overall survival for patients with metastatic colorectal cancer involving the liver.
- The number of liver metastases and the presence of resectable extrahepatic metastatic disease are no longer considered absolute contraindications to surgical treatment of colorectal liver metastases.
- Radiofrequency ablation can be a useful adjunctive therapy in cases where small liver metastases are unresectable due to location or the volume of surrounding parenchyma that would be resected.

Colorectal Cancer: Diagnosis and Clinical Management, First Edition. Edited by John H. Scholefield and Cathy Eng.

CASE STUDY

A 54-year-old male presents to your office with an asymptomatic rectal adenocarcinoma (involving <50% of the rectal lumen) and a 6 cm liver metastasis abutting the right and middle hepatic veins near the junction with the inferior vena cava.

He is diabetic and obese, but has no history of alcohol use or viral hepatitis. He has hypertension, but no other significant medical comorbidities. His performance status is good.

Review of his MRI with a radiologist does not show any additional metastases, but does show a small left liver.

TIPS AND TRICKS / KEY PITFALLS

- For patients with synchronous presentation of liver metastases and an asymptomatic colorectal cancer, a reverse approach to treatment sequencing may be employed whereby the liver metastases are resected with or without neoadjuvant chemotherapy prior to treatment of the primary tumor.
- Simultaneous resection of the primary tumor and the liver metastases should only be undertaken in patients requiring either a low-risk colon resection and/or a minor liver resection.
- Patients previously treated with either oxaliplatin (sinusoidal obstruction syndrome) or irinotecan (steatohepatitis) may have chemotherapy-induced liver injury. These patients may be at increased risk of post-hepatectomy liver failure and so may require a greater than 20% functional liver remnant.
- The risk of disappearing liver metastases can be minimized with early involvement of a liver surgeon and careful limitation of the number of cycles of neoadjuvant chemotherapy.
- A significant number of disappearing liver metastases that are not resected will ultimately recur, so any such lesions should be resected and/or closely monitored.

Epidemiology and background

Colorectal cancer is the third most common cancer and has the third highest cancer-related mortality rate in both American men and women [1]. As many as 50% of patients with colorectal cancer will either present with or subsequently develop liver metastases. Liver metastases represent the most common cause of death for patients affected by colorectal cancer [2–4]. Margin-negative surgical resection is a necessary component of therapy if cure and long-term survival is to be achieved in these patients. Contemporary multimodality therapy allows 20–30% of patients with liver metastases to ultimately undergo surgical resection, with resulting 5 year survival rates of 47–58% [3;5;6].

Imaging and staging work-up

When available, the 2012 Americas Hepato-Pancreato-Biliary Association/Society of Surgical Oncology/Society for Surgery of the Alimentary Tract Consensus Statement on the Multidisciplinary Management of Colorectal Cancer Liver Metastases recommends magnetic resonance imaging (MRI) with gadoxetate disodium (Eovist; Bayer Healthcare Pharmaceuticals) delayed images and diffusion-weighted images as the preferred imaging modality for the detection and characterization of liver metastases [5]. This recommendation is based primarily on the superior sensitivity of MRI for categorizing intrahepatic lesions smaller than 1 cm and for the detection of metastases within a steatotic liver; it should be kept in mind, however, that while MRI has greater sensitivity for intrahepatic disease, CT provides superior detection of extrahepatic disease [7].

PET/CT has been recommended by some authors for its ability to detect extrahepatic metastatic disease, which may help reduce non-therapeutic laparotomy rates in patients with liver metastases [8]. A retrospective British study found that PET/CT was superior to contrast-enhanced CT scan for the detection of extrahepatic metastatic disease, but had a similar sensitivity and specificity to liver MRI for the detection of liver metastases, with MRI having a greater accuracy for the detection of subcentimeter lesions [9]. However, a survival benefit has never been demonstrated with the use of PET/CT. Tumors of less than 1 cm and mucinous tumors are also often not detected by PET/CT. PET positive lesions are nonspecific, particularly in the setting of inflammation, and the sensitivity of PET is low in patients who have been previously treated with chemotherapy [7]. Given these limitations of PET/CT, it is not currently recommended for routine staging or surveillance of colorectal cancer [10].

Intra-operative ultrasound represents a key aspect of the surgical management of patients with colorectal liver metastases. It may identify lesions not seen on CT scan in up to 27% of patients undergoing resection of primary or metastatic liver tumors, with even higher rates of detection of occult lesions as the number of tumors increases [11]. Detection of additional lesions by intra-operative ultrasound may necessitate a change in the surgical plan.

Resectability and operability

Both resectability and operability should be evaluated prior to planning a liver resection for metastatic colorectal cancer. *Operability* is the ability of the patient to tolerate hepatic resection [12] and is based on factors such as performance status and comorbidities. A tumor's *resectability* encompasses both technical and oncologic factors [12]. Technically resectable metastatic disease is that which can be entirely removed with negative margins while sparing a minimum of two adjacent liver segments and preserving adequate inflow, outflow, and biliary drainage of the remnant with adequate parenchyma to support vital liver functions (i.e. at least 20% of the estimated total liver volume in patients with normal liver parenchyma) [7;13].

Although in the past, oncologic factors such as the presence of more than three metastases or extrahepatic metastatic disease have been considered at least relative contraindications to hepatectomy for colorectal metastases, recent data has suggested that this thinking should be revised [14;15]. Two retrospective studies have reported reasonable long-term survival in patients with four or more metastases after complete resection [16;17]. In one of these studies, the presence of multiple tumor nodules was an independent predictor of lower overall survival rates, but not of lower disease-free survival rates [15]. In the second study, patients with more than three metastases had a 21.5% 5-year actuarial disease-free survival rate with a 50.9% overall survival rate after multimodality therapy [17]. Other studies have also recently reported favorable survival in patients with resectable liver metastases and limited sites of resectable extrahepatic disease, including lung [18], limited peritoneal disease, and portal lymph nodes [19;20]. One oncologic factor which is still considered a contraindication to hepatectomy is progression while on chemotherapy in the form of development of new liver metastases or new sites of extrahepatic disease [12]. Such patients should show a response to an alternative line of systemic therapy before surgical resection is undertaken.

Response to therapy

Recent studies suggest that approximately 5–10% of patients may have a pathological complete response after treatment with oxaliplatin- or irinotecan-based chemotherapy [21;22]. In these studies, pathological complete response was shown to be an independent predictor of improved overall survival on multivariate analysis, with major pathologic response (<50% viable tumor cells) having a higher hazard ratio than previously established predictors of survival, such as disease-free interval, tumor size, and tumor multiplicity [22]. A study from the MD Anderson Cancer Center has suggested that the morphologic response to chemotherapy may also predict overall survival, with the 'optimal' morphologic response consisting of an homogeneous low attenuation lesion with a thin, sharply defined tumor-liver interface [23]. In this study, 47% of patients treated with bevacizumab had an optimal morphological response versus 12% of those not treated with bevacizumab [23]. Patients with an optimal morphologic response had 3- and 5-year overall survival rates of 82% and 74%, respectively, versus 60% and 45% ($p < 0.001$) for patients with a less than optimal response [23].

Synchronous metastases and treatment sequencing

For the approximately 25% of colorectal cancer patients who are diagnosed with synchronous liver metastases, three different management strategies may be considered [24]. The classic approach to management of these patients has involved primary tumor resection followed by resection of the liver metastases. The downsides to this approach include potential progression of the liver metastases before the patient receives any systemic therapy and possible delay in or even omission of systemic therapy and/or liver resection due to postoperative complications following resection of the primary tumor. In an effort to avoid these potential problems, two alternative management strategies have been developed. The first alternative strategy proposed was combined resection of the primary tumor and the liver metastases as a single operation. Several retrospective studies have described the use of this approach with morbidity and mortality rates that are no worse than those with sequential resections [24–27]. The patients included in these studies, however, have been highly selected and in the majority of cases have required a colon resection with a relatively low complication rate (e.g. right hemicolectomy) or if a more complex colorectal resection was indicated, have required a limited liver resection (e.g. wedge resection). For this reason, consideration of this approach is recommended in a limited number of patients [7].

More recently, a second alternative strategy for the management of synchronous metastases has been proposed, whereby liver resection is performed prior to colorectal resection. This strategy is commonly referred to as the reverse approach and may involve neoadjuvant chemotherapy prior to both surgical resections. Utilization of this strategy requires an asymptomatic (i.e. neither obstructing nor bleeding) colorectal primary. With this approach, systemic treatment of the metastatic disease is guaranteed and the likelihood of the liver metastases progressing to an unresectable status is minimized

[28;29]. The primary tumor rarely progresses significantly during the administration of neoadjuvant chemotherapy, but if this does occur, the treatment plan must be altered, so surveillance of the colorectal tumor must be undertaken at regular intervals during the initial phase of treatment [30;31]. Following resection of the liver metastases, the primary tumor can be addressed with appropriate locoregional therapy (e.g. resection of a colon primary or chemoradiation and subsequent resection of a locally advanced rectal tumor). Selection of the appropriate treatment strategy for patients with synchronous colorectal liver metastases requires prioritization based on which site, if either is symptomatic, followed by which site poses the greater oncological risk. These factors can be best evaluated with a multidisciplinary assessment prior to initiation of therapy.

Cautionary notes on neoadjuvant chemotherapy

Chemotherapy-induced liver injury

As use of chemotherapy prior to resection of colorectal liver metastases has become more common, liver surgeons have begun to appreciate that in certain patients the liver may sustain significant damage from the chemotherapy. The earliest reports of such damage described the presence of sinusoidal obstruction and veno-occlusive disease, later termed the sinusoidal obstruction syndrome [32], in as many as 78% of patients treated with oxaliplatin-containing regimens [33–36]. While these histological changes may be observed for months after completion of chemotherapy, they do not seem to correlate with the total dose of oxaliplatin [33;34]. Most studies have not found an association between the presence of the sinusoidal obstruction syndrome and higher rates of postoperative complications; however, one French study [34–36] has described an association with increased length of hospital stay and higher morbidity rates [37], and another study has shown a correlation with higher rates of transfusion [35].

Up to 20% of patients receiving irinotecan-containing chemotherapy regimens may develop steatohepatitis [34;36], which has been associated with increased postoperative mortality rates [34], and potentially increased rates of postoperative hepatic insufficiency [38]. More recent data has shown that steatohepatitis occurs primarily in patients with a high body mass index [39], suggesting that irinotecan may cause progression of steatohepatitis in susceptible patients rather than *de novo* induction of steatohepatitis [38]. Longer durations of preoperative chemotherapy have been associated with higher rates of postoperative complications [35;37;40;41]. The study describing the most conservative breakpoint reported that receipt of fewer than 6 cycles of 5-FU-based preoperative chemotherapy was associated with significantly lower rates of postoperative complications (19% vs. >40%) relative to patients receiving additional cycles of chemotherapy [41].

Disappearing liver metastases

Modern chemotherapy regimens are now so effective that radiographic complete responses, also known as disappearing liver metastases, may occur in up to 25% of patients [42]. Unfortunately, however, these radiographic complete responses do not always correlate with pathological complete responses. One retrospective study reported that nearly 60% of disappearing metastases that were not resected eventually recurred at the same site [42]. However, these local recurrences did not adversely affect overall survival rates. Another retrospective study showed that persistent macroscopic disease could be identified intraoperatively in 30% of disappearing liver metastases and in 80% of resected lesions without macroscopic residual disease, microscopic disease could be identified [43]. In this study, 74% of lesions without macroscopic residual disease, which were not resected, developed local recurrences within a year of surgery. The risk of having liver metastases disappear can be minimized if a liver surgeon evaluates the patient early with an optimal liver imaging study, ideally prior to initiation of chemotherapy and if neoadjuvant chemotherapy is limited to a short duration (e.g. 4 cycles), or until the response has been sufficient for resection to be feasible [5].

Peri-operative chemotherapy

The EORTC Intergroup Trial 40983 was a multicenter randomized trial evaluating the use of peri-operative chemotherapy in patients with resectable colorectal liver metastases [2]. Oxaliplatin-naïve patients were enrolled in this trial and were randomized to either 6 cycles of pre-operative and 6 cycles of postoperative FOLFOX4 or to surgery without adjuvant therapy. Patients in the peri-operative chemotherapy arm of the trial had a 35% relative risk reduction (and a 7% absolute risk reduction) in 3-year progression free survival [2]. These patients also had a significantly higher rate of reversible postoperative complications (25% vs. 16% in the surgery alone arm). Forty percent of patients achieved a partial or complete response as measured by RECIST criteria and on average total tumor diameter decreased by an average of 25% [2].

The use of peri-operative chemotherapy in patients with stage IV colorectal cancer has also been examined in a meta-analysis of randomized trials. This study found no evidence for a survival benefit with hepatic arterial chemotherapy, but did show a survival advantage that approached significance for patients receiving peri-operative systemic chemotherapy (HR 0.74, p = 0.08) [44]. A significant recurrence-free survival benefit, however, was found with both hepatic arterial chemotherapy (HR 0.78, p = 0.01) and systemic peri-operative chemotherapy (HR 0.75, p = 0.003).

Functional liver remnant and portal vein embolization (PVE)

A study of liver volumes in patients without cancer showed that in 75% of patients, segments II and III of the liver contributed less than 20% of the total liver volume and in more than 10% of patients, segments II, III, and IV comprised 25% or less of the total liver volume [45]. In patients such as these, the risk of postoperative liver failure after an extended right hepatectomy, and possibly even after a right hepatectomy, would be dangerously high. In 1990, Makuuchi first introduced the concept of PVE as a means of inducing hypertrophy of the functional liver remnant [46]. This advancement has decreased the risk of postoperative liver insufficiency and allowed surgical resection in many patients who would not otherwise be candidates due to a congenitally small left liver. Since the introduction of PVE, additional studies have expanded upon the indications and techniques for the appropriate use of PVE and have further confirmed the safety of this procedure. Its use is typically recommended when the anticipated functional liver remnant is less than 20–25% of estimated total liver volume [47;48]. The expected average increase in volume of the remnant liver is 12% of the total liver volume [47]. Hypertrophy rates correlate with the increase velocity in portal blood flow in the non-embolized segment on post-procedure day 1 [49]. Elevated portal blood flow in the non-embolized segments can be measured for at least 2 weeks after embolization [49], which is the basis for the recommended 2–4 week waiting period before resection is undertaken [47].

Recently, an alternate approach to the treatment of patients with a marginal or inadequate functional liver remnant has been described. Right portal vein ligation with *in situ* splitting (also known as ALPPS-associating liver partition and portal vein ligation staged hepatectomy) involves two operations (50). During the initial operation, the right portal vein is ligated and the hepatic parenchyma is completely (or nearly-completely) transected. After a period of a few days, the resection is completed at a second operation. Those that advocate this approach believe it achieves more rapid and, perhaps, greater hypertrophy than is seen after PVE [51;52]. Critics of the approach, however, stress the importance of caution given the high morbidity rate (68%), high in-hospital mortality rate (12%), and lack of data on long-term oncologic outcomes following this strategy [50;53].

Repeat hepatectomy

Recurrence eventually develops in approximately 65–85% of patients who undergo hepatectomy for colorectal metastases, with 20–30% of these recurrences isolated to the liver [54]. For such patients, as long as a margin negative resection can be obtained, repeat liver resection results in equivalent long-term survival to patients without recurrence, without significantly higher peri-operative morbidity or mortality rates compared to initial hepatectomy [55–58].

Metachronous metastases – unresectable with downstaging

In retrospective studies, contemporary chemotherapy regimens including oxaliplatin and irinotecan have converted 12.5–38% of patients with initially unresectable liver metastases into surgical candidates [19;59]. Although approximately 80% of such patients will recur, 33–50% will be 5-year survivors and 23% will be 10-year survivors if an aggressive approach resecting recurrent disease is employed [19;59;60].

Second-line chemotherapy

If colorectal patients with marginally resectable or unresectable liver metastases fail to respond to first-line chemotherapy, they may respond to second-line chemotherapy. A retrospective analysis has addressed the question of whether or not liver resection is reasonable in such patients [61]. This study reported, 1-, 3-, and 5-year survival rates of 83%, 41%, and 22%, respectively, with 1- and 3-year disease-free survival rates of 37% and 11%, respectively, with reasonable postoperative morbidity and mortality rates patients responding to second-line chemotherapy.

Biological agents

The addition of biological agents, such as vascular endothelial growth factor (VEGF) inhibitors and epidermal growth factor receptor (EGFR) inhibitors to cytotoxic chemotherapy, often results in treatment responses in patients with metastatic colorectal cancer. Emerging evidence from phase II and III randomized clinical trials suggests that including include biological agents in chemotherapy regimens may increase the chances of converting unresectable liver metastases into resectable ones [62].

Randomized controlled trials of FOLFOX or FOLFIRI with or without bevacizumab, a VEGF inhibitor, have shown significant improvements in overall survival, progression free survival, and rates of response in both previously treated and previously untreated patients with the addition of bevacizumab [63;64]. A retrospective study has shown that the combination of bevacizumab and FOLFOX results in a lower percentage of viable tumor cells in resected specimens, without higher complete pathologic response rates [65]. This study also showed a lower frequency and severity of sinusoidal obstruction syndrome in patients who had received bevacizumab. Another retrospective study described similar results with a decreased severity of the sinusoidal obstruction syndrome, without an improved rate of response by RECIST criteria in patients treated with bevacizumab [66]. Resection rates have never been a pre-specified endpoint in any published randomized controlled trials of bevacizumab for patients with stage IV colorectal cancer.

The EGFR is frequently present on colon cancer cells and is targeted by cetuximab [67]. A retrospective analysis of the data from a randomized phase II trial, of cetuximab plus either FOLFOX or FOLFIRI in patients with unresectable liver metastases from colorectal cancer, showed that partial or complete responses were significantly more common in patients with KRAS-wide type tumors (70%) than in those with KRAS-mutations (41%) [68]. This study also showed that cetuximab increased baseline resectability rates from 32% to 60% ($p < 0.0001$). A randomized phase III trial of FOLFIRI with or without cetuximab in patients with stage IV colorectal cancer (not limited to patients with liver metastases) showed that patients in the cetuximab group had higher rates of surgery for metastases (7% vs. 3.7%) and higher rates of R0 resection (4.8% vs. 1.7%, $p = 0.002$); however, these were not pre-specified endpoints of the study [69].

Radiofrequency ablation

The phase II EORTC 40004 study randomized patients with unresectable liver metastases to systemic therapy, either with or without radiofrequency ablation (RFA) [70]. Although this study reported a non-significant improvement in 30-month overall survival for the RFA group, 3-year progression free survival rates were significantly improved in the patients treated with RFA.

A retrospective study from MD Anderson showed that in patients with colorectal liver metastases, both true local and liver-only recurrence rates were significantly higher in patients treated with RFA than in patients who underwent resection [3]. In this study, patients treated with resection also had significantly higher overall survival rates and those patients treated with RFA had survival rates that were higher than patients treated with chemotherapy only, but not dramatically so. A second retrospective study from the same institution, but limited only to patients with solitary liver metastases, confirmed that patients treated with RFA had significantly lower local recurrence, disease-free, and overall survival rates than patients treated with resection [71]. Subset analysis in this study showed that even for patients with tumors 3 cm or smaller, local recurrence and overall survival rates were lower with RFA than with resection and disease-free survival rates were lower, although this difference did not reach statistical significance. Taken together, these data suggest that for colorectal liver metastases, resection is the preferred treatment if it can be accomplished safely. For patients who are not candidates for resection, treatment with RFA may improve survival over chemotherapy alone, particularly for patients with small (≤3 cm) tumors.

MULTIPLE-CHOICE QUESTIONS

1 The most appropriate treatment approach for this patient would be:
   A. Neoadjuvant chemoradiation followed by low anterior resection and then hepatectomy
   B. Combined hepatic resection and low anterior resection
   C. Immediate hepatic resection followed by treatment of the rectal primary
   D. Neoadjuvant chemotherapy followed by liver resection and then treatment of the rectal primary

2 You counsel the patient that he may require a pre-operative portal vein embolization to minimize his risk of which complication:
   A. Chemotherapy-induced liver injury
   B. Posthepatectomy liver insufficiency
   C. Cirrhosis
   D. Bile leak

3 Given this patient's obesity, use of which chemotherapeutic agent puts him at greatest risk of chemotherapy-induced liver injury and associated postoperative complications:
   A. Bevacizumab
   B. Cetuximab
   C. Irinotecan
   D. Oxaliplatin

References

1 American Cancer Society. *Cancer Facts and Figures 2013.*

2 Nordlinger B, Sorbye H, Glimelius B, Poston GJ, Schlag PM, Rougier P, et al. Perioperative chemotherapy with FOLFOX4 and surgery versus surgery alone for resectable

liver metastases from colorectal cancer (EORTC Intergroup trial 40983): a randomised controlled trial. *Lancet* 2008 Mar 22; 371(9617): 1007–16.

3 Abdalla EK, Vauthey JN, Ellis LM, Ellis V, Pollock R, Broglio KR, et al. Recurrence and outcomes following hepatic resection, radiofrequency ablation, and combined resection/ablation for colorectal liver metastases. *Ann Surg* 2004 Jun; 239(6): 818–25; discussion 25–7.

4 Vibert E, Canedo L, Adam R. Strategies to treat primary unresectable colorectal liver metastases. *Seminars Oncol* 2005 Dec; 32(6 Suppl 8): 33–9.

5 Adams RB, Aloia TA, Loyer E, Pawlik TM, Taouli B, Vauthey JN. Selection for hepatic resection of colorectal liver metastases: expert consensus statement. *HPB* 2013 Feb; 15(2): 91–103.

6 Choti MA, Sitzmann JV, Tiburi MF, Sumetchotimetha W, Rangsin R, Schulick RD, et al. Trends in long-term survival following liver resection for hepatic colorectal metastases. *Ann Surg* 2002 Jun; 235(6): 759–66. PubMed PMID: 12035031.

7 Charnsangavej C, Clary B, Fong Y, Grothey A, Pawlik TM, Choti MA. Selection of patients for resection of hepatic colorectal metastases: expert consensus statement. *Ann Surg Oncol* 2006 Oct; 13(10): 1261–8.

8 Pawlik TM, Assumpcao L, Vossen JA, Buijs M, Gleisner AL, Schulick RD, et al. Trends in nontherapeutic laparotomy rates in patients undergoing surgical therapy for hepatic colorectal metastases. *Ann Surg Oncol* 2009 Feb; 16(2): 371–8.

9 Kong G, Jackson C, Koh DM, Lewington V, Sharma B, Brown G, et al. The use of 18F-FDG PET/CT in colorectal liver metastases – comparison with CT and liver MRI. *Eur J Nuc Med Mol Imag* 2008 Jul; 35(7): 1323–9.

10 NCCN Clinical Practice *Guidelines in Oncology: Colon Cancer Version 3.2013* 2013 [July 22, 2013]. Available from: *http://www.nccn.org/professionals/physician_gls/pdf/colon.pdf*

11 Scaife CL, Ng CS, Ellis LM, Vauthey JN, Charnsangavej C, Curley SA. Accuracy of preoperative imaging of hepatic tumors with helical computed tomography. *Ann Surg Oncol* 2006 Apr; 13(4): 542–6.

12 Tzeng CW, Aloia TA. Colorectal liver metastases. *J Gastro Surg* 2013 Jan; 17(1): 195–201.

13 Ribero D, Abdalla EK, Madoff DC, Donadon M, Loyer EM, Vauthey JN. Portal vein embolization before major hepatectomy and its effects on regeneration, resectability and outcome. *Br J Surg* 2007 Nov; 94(11): 1386–94.

14 Fong Y, Fortner J, Sun RL, Brennan MF, Blumgart LH. Clinical score for predicting recurrence after hepatic resection for metastatic colorectal cancer: analysis of 1001 consecutive cases. *Ann Surg* 1999 Sep; 230(3): 309–18; discussion 18–21.

15 Iwatsuki S, Dvorchik I, Madariaga JR, Marsh JW, Dodson F, Bonham AC, et al. Hepatic resection for metastatic colorectal adenocarcinoma: a proposal of a prognostic scoring system. *J Am Coll Surg* 1999 Sep; 189(3): 291–9.

16 Minagawa M, Makuuchi M, Torzilli G, Takayama T, Kawasaki S, Kosuge T, et al. Extension of the frontiers of surgical indications in the treatment of liver metastases from colorectal cancer: long-term results. *Ann Surg* 2000 Apr; 231(4): 487–99.

17 Pawlik TM, Abdalla EK, Ellis LM, Vauthey JN, Curley SA. Debunking dogma: surgery for four or more colorectal liver metastases is justified. *J Gastro Surg* 2006 Feb; 10(2): 240–8.

18 Brouquet A, Vauthey JN, Contreras CM, Walsh GL, Vaporciyan AA, Swisher SG, et al. Improved survival after resection of liver and lung colorectal metastases compared with liver-only metastases: a study of 112 patients with limited lung metastatic disease. *J Am Coll Surg* 2011 Jul; 213(1): 62–9; discussion 9–71.

19 Adam R, Delvart V, Pascal G, Valeanu A, Castaing D, Azoulay D, et al. Rescue surgery for unresectable colorectal liver metastases downstaged by chemotherapy: a model to predict long-term survival. *Ann Surg* 2004 Oct; 240(4): 644–57; discussion 57–8. PubMed PMID: 15383792.

20 Elias D, Ouellet JF, Bellon N, Pignon JP, Pocard M, Lasser P. Extrahepatic disease does not contraindicate hepatectomy for colorectal liver metastases. *Br J Surg* 2003 May; 90(5): 567–74.

21 Adam R, Wicherts DA, de Haas RJ, Aloia T, Levi F, Paule B, et al. Complete pathologic response after preoperative chemotherapy for colorectal liver metastases: myth or reality? *J Clin Oncol* 2008 Apr 1; 26(10): 1635–41.

22 Blazer DG, 3rd, Kishi Y, Maru DM, Kopetz S, Chun YS, Overman MJ, et al. Pathologic response to preoperative chemotherapy: a new outcome end point after resection of hepatic colorectal metastases. *J Clin Oncol* 2008 Nov 20; 26(33): 5344–51.

23 Shindoh J, Loyer EM, Kopetz S, Boonsirikamchai P, Maru DM, Chun YS, et al. Optimal morphologic response to preoperative chemotherapy: an alternate outcome end point before resection of hepatic colorectal metastases. *J Clin Oncol* 2012 Dec 20; 30(36): 4566–72.

24 Martin R, Paty P, Fong Y, Grace A, Cohen A, DeMatteo R, et al. Simultaneous liver and colorectal resections are safe for synchronous colorectal liver metastasis. *J Am Coll Surg* 2003 Aug; 197(2): 233–41; discussion 41–2.

25 Slupski M, Wlodarczyk Z, Jasinski M, Masztalerz M, Tujakowski J. Outcomes of simultaneous and delayed resections of synchronous colorectal liver metastases. *Can J Surg* 2009 Dec; 52(6): E241–4.

26 Capussotti L, Ferrero A, Vigano L, Ribero D, Lo Tesoriere R, Polastri R. Major liver resections synchronous with colorectal surgery. *Ann Surg Oncol* 2007 Jan; 14(1): 195–201.

27 Lyass S, Zamir G, Matot I, Goitein D, Eid A, Jurim O. Combined colon and hepatic resection for synchronous colorectal liver metastases. *J Surg Oncol* 2001 Sep; 78(1): 17–21.

28 Mentha G, Majno PE, Andres A, Rubbia-Brandt L, Morel P, Roth AD. Neoadjuvant chemotherapy and resection of advanced synchronous liver metastases before treatment of the colorectal primary. *Br J Surg* 2006 Jul; 93(7): 872–8.

29 Mentha G, Roth AD, Terraz S, Giostra E, Gervaz P, Andres A, et al. 'Liver first' approach in the treatment of colorectal cancer with synchronous liver metastases. *Dig Surg* 2008; 25(6): 430–5.

30 Poultsides GA, Servais EL, Saltz LB, Patil S, Kemeny NE, Guillem JG, et al. Outcome of primary tumor in patients with synchronous stage IV colorectal cancer receiving combination chemotherapy without surgery as initial treatment. *J Clin Oncol* 2009 Jul 10; 27(20): 3379–84.

31 Brouquet A, Mortenson MM, Vauthey JN, Rodriguez-Bigas MA, Overman MJ, Chang GJ, et al. Surgical strategies for synchronous colorectal liver metastases in 156 consecutive patients: classic, combined or reverse strategy? *J Am Coll Surg* 2010 Jun; 210(6): 934–41.

32 DeLeve LD, Shulman HM, McDonald GB. Toxic injury to hepatic sinusoids: sinusoidal obstruction syndrome (veno-occlusive disease). *Sem Liver Dis* 2002 Feb; 22(1): 27–42.

33 Rubbia-Brandt L, Audard V, Sartoretti P, Roth AD, Brezault C, Le Charpentier M, et al. Severe hepatic sinusoidal obstruction associated with oxaliplatin-based chemotherapy in patients with metastatic colorectal cancer. *Ann Oncol* 2004 Mar; 15(3): 460–6.

34 Vauthey JN, Pawlik TM, Ribero D, Wu TT, Zorzi D, Hoff PM, et al. Chemotherapy regimen predicts steatohepatitis and an increase in 90-day mortality after surgery for hepatic colorectal metastases. *J Clin Oncol* 2006 May 1; 24(13): 2065–72.
35 Aloia T, Sebagh M, Plasse M, Karam V, Levi F, Giacchetti S, et al. Liver histology and surgical outcomes after preoperative chemotherapy with fluorouracil plus oxaliplatin in colorectal cancer liver metastases. *J Clin Oncol* 2006 Nov 1; 24(31): 4983–90.
36 Pawlik TM, Olino K, Gleisner AL, Torbenson M, Schulick R, Choti MA. Preoperative chemotherapy for colorectal liver metastases: impact on hepatic histology and postoperative outcome. *J Gastrot Surg* 2007 Jul; 11(7): 860–8.
37 Nakano H, Oussoultzoglou E, Rosso E, Casnedi S, Chenard-Neu MP, Dufour P, et al. Sinusoidal injury increases morbidity after major hepatectomy in patients with colorectal liver metastases receiving preoperative chemotherapy. *Ann Surg* 2008 Jan; 247(1): 118–24.
38 Bilchik AJ, Poston G, Curley SA, Strasberg S, Saltz L, Adam R, et al. Neoadjuvant chemotherapy for metastatic colon cancer: a cautionary note. *J Clin Oncol* 2005 Dec 20; 23(36): 9073–8.
39 Fernandez FG, Ritter J, Goodwin JW, Linehan DC, Hawkins WG, Strasberg SM. Effect of steatohepatitis associated with irinotecan or oxaliplatin pretreatment on resectability of hepatic colorectal metastases. *J Am Coll Surg* 2005 Jun; 200(6): 845–53.
40 Kishi Y, Zorzi D, Contreras CM, Maru DM, Kopetz S, Ribero D, et al. Extended preoperative chemotherapy does not improve pathologic response and increases postoperative liver insufficiency after hepatic resection for colorectal liver metastases. *Ann Surg Oncol* 2010 Nov; 17(11): 2870–6.
41 Karoui M, Penna C, Amin-Hashem M, Mitry E, Benoist S, Franc B, et al. Influence of preoperative chemotherapy on the risk of major hepatectomy for colorectal liver metastases. *Ann Surg* 2006 Jan; 243(1): 1–7. PubMed PMID: 16371728.
42 van Vledder MG, de Jong MC, Pawlik TM, Schulick RD, Diaz LA, Choti MA. Disappearing colorectal liver metastases after chemotherapy: should we be concerned? *J Gastro Surg* 2010 Nov; 14(11): 1691–700.
43 Benoist S, Brouquet A, Penna C, Julie C, El Hajjam M, Chagnon S, et al. Complete response of colorectal liver metastases after chemotherapy: does it mean cure? *J Clin Oncol* 2006 Aug 20; 24(24): 3939–45. PubMed PMID: 16921046.
44 Wieser M, Sauerland S, Arnold D, Schmiegel W, Reinacher-Schick A. Peri-operative chemotherapy for the treatment of resectable liver metastases from colorectal cancer: A systematic review and meta-analysis of randomized trials. *BMC Cancer* 2010; 10: 309.
45 Abdalla EK, Denys A, Chevalier P, Nemr RA, Vauthey JN. Total and segmental liver volume variations: implications for liver surgery. *Surgery* 2004 Apr; 135(4): 404–10.
46 Makuuchi M, Thai BL, Takayasu K, Takayama T, Kosuge T, Gunven P, et al. Preoperative portal embolization to increase safety of major hepatectomy for hilar bile duct carcinoma: a preliminary report. *Surgery* 1990 May; 107(5): 521–7.
47 Abdalla EK, Hicks ME, Vauthey JN. Portal vein embolization: rationale, technique and future prospects. *Br J Surg* 2001 Feb; 88(2): 165–75.
48 Abdalla EK, Barnett CC, Doherty D, Curley SA, Vauthey JN. Extended hepatectomy in patients with hepatobiliary malignancies with and without preoperative portal vein embolization. *Arch Surg* 2002 Jun; 137(6): 675–80; discussion 80–1.
49 Goto Y, Nagino M, Nimura Y. Doppler estimation of portal blood flow after percutaneous transhepatic portal vein embolization. *Ann Surg* 1998 Aug; 228(2): 209–13.

50 Schnitzbauer AA, Lang SA, Goessmann H, Nadalin S, Baumgart J, Farkas SA, et al. Right portal vein ligation combined with *in situ* splitting induces rapid left lateral liver lobe hypertrophy enabling 2-staged extended right hepatic resection in small-for-size settings. *Ann Surg* 2012 Mar; 255(3): 405–14.
51 Alvarez FA, Ardiles V, Sanchez Claria R, Pekolj J, de Santibanes E. Associating liver partition and portal vein ligation for staged hepatectomy (ALPPS): Tips and tricks. *J Gastro Surg* 2012 Nov 27.
52 de Santibanes E, Clavien PA. Playing Play-Doh to prevent postoperative liver failure: the 'ALPPS' approach. *Ann Surg* 2012 Mar; 255(3): 415–7.
53 Aloia TA, Vauthey JN. Associating liver partition and portal vein ligation for staged hepatectomy (ALPPS): what is gained and what is lost? *Ann Surg* 2012 Sep; 256(3): e9; author reply e16–9.
54 Wanebo HJ, Chu QD, Avradopoulos KA, Vezeridis MP. Current perspectives on repeat hepatic resection for colorectal carcinoma: a review. *Surgery* 1996 Apr; 119(4): 361–71.
55 Neeleman N, Andersson R. Repeated liver resection for recurrent liver cancer. *Br J Surg* 1996 Jul; 83(7): 893–901.
56 Antoniou A, Lovegrove RE, Tilney HS, Heriot AG, John TG, Rees M, et al. Meta-analysis of clinical outcome after first and second liver resection for colorectal metastases. *Surgery* 2007 Jan; 141(1): 9–18.
57 Adair RA, Young AL, Cockbain AJ, Malde D, Prasad KR, Lodge JP, et al. Repeat hepatic resection for colorectal liver metastases. *Br J Surg* 2012 Sep; 99(9): 1278–83.
58 Andreou A, Brouquet A, Abdalla EK, Aloia TA, Curley SA, Vauthey JN. Repeat hepatectomy for recurrent colorectal liver metastases is associated with a high survival rate. *HPB* 2011 Nov; 13(11): 774–82.
59 Giacchetti S, Itzhaki M, Gruia G, Adam R, Zidani R, Kunstlinger F, et al. Long-term survival of patients with unresectable colorectal cancer liver metastases following infusional chemotherapy with 5-fluorouracil, leucovorin, oxaliplatin and surgery. *Ann Oncol* 1999 Jun; 10(6): 663–9.
60 Bismuth H, Adam R, Levi F, Farabos C, Waechter F, Castaing D, et al. Resection of nonresectable liver metastases from colorectal cancer after neoadjuvant chemotherapy. *Ann Surg* 1996 Oct; 224(4): 509–20; discussion 20–2.
61 Brouquet A, Overman MJ, Kopetz S, Maru DM, Loyer EM, Andreou A, et al. Is resection of colorectal liver metastases after a second-line chemotherapy regimen justified? *Cancer* 2011 Oct 1; 117(19): 4484–92.
62 Nordlinger B, Van Cutsem E, Gruenberger T, Glimelius B, Poston G, Rougier P, et al. Combination of surgery and chemotherapy and the role of targeted agents in the treatment of patients with colorectal liver metastases: recommendations from an expert panel. *Ann Oncol* 2009 Jun; 20(6): 985–92.
63 Hurwitz H, Fehrenbacher L, Novotny W, Cartwright T, Hainsworth J, Heim W, et al. Bevacizumab plus Irinotecan, Fluorouracil, and Leucovorin for metastatic colorectal cancer. *New Eng J Med* 2004 Jun 3; 350(23): 2335–42.
64 Giantonio BJ, Catalano PJ, Meropol NJ, O'Dwyer PJ, Mitchell EP, Alberts SR, et al. Bevacizumab in combination with Oxaliplatin, Fluorouracil, and Leucovorin (FOLFOX4) for previously treated metastatic colorectal cancer: results from the Eastern Cooperative Oncology Group Study E3200. *J Clin Oncol* 2007 Apr 20; 25(12): 1539–44.
65 Ribero D, Wang H, Donadon M, Zorzi D, Thomas MB, Eng C, et al. Bevacizumab improves pathologic response and protects against hepatic injury in patients treated

with Oxaliplatin-based chemotherapy for colorectal liver metastases. *Cancer* 2007 Dec 15; 110(12): 2761–7.

66 Klinger M, Eipeldauer S, Hacker S, Herberger B, Tamandl D, Dorfmeister M, et al. Bevacizumab protects against sinusoidal obstruction syndrome and does not increase response rate in neoadjuvant XELOX/FOLFOX therapy of colorectal cancer liver metastases. *Eur J Surg Oncol* 2009 May; 35(5): 515–20.

67 Cunningham D, Humblet Y, Siena S, Khayat D, Bleiberg H, Santoro A, et al. Cetuximab monotherapy and cetuximab plus irinotecan in irinotecan-refractory metastatic colorectal cancer. *New Eng J Med* 2004 Jul 22; 351(4): 337–45.

68 Folprecht G, Gruenberger T, Bechstein WO, Raab HR, Lordick F, Hartmann JT, et al. Tumor response and secondary resectability of colorectal liver metastases following neoadjuvant chemotherapy with cetuximab: the CELIM randomised phase 2 trial. *Lancet Oncol* 2010 Jan; 11(1): 38–47.

69 Van Cutsem E, Kohne CH, Hitre E, Zaluski J, Chang Chien CR, Makhson A, et al. Cetuximab and chemotherapy as initial treatment for metastatic colorectal cancer. *New Eng J Med* 2009 Apr 2; 360(14): 1408–17.

70 Ruers T, Punt C, Van Coevorden F, Pierie JP, Borel-Rinkes I, Ledermann JA, et al. Radiofrequency ablation combined with systemic treatment versus systemic treatment alone in patients with non-resectable colorectal liver metastases: a randomized EORTC Intergroup phase II study (EORTC 40004). *Ann Oncol* 2012 Oct; 23(10): 2619–26.

71 Aloia TA, Vauthey JN, Loyer EM, Ribero D, Pawlik TM, Wei SH, et al. Solitary colorectal liver metastasis: resection determines outcome. *Arch Surg* 2006 May; 141(5): 460–6; discussion 6–7.

ANSWERS TO MULTIPLE-CHOICE QUESTIONS

1 D
2 B
3 C

CHAPTER 14

Controversies in chemotherapy in advanced colorectal cancer

Ludmila Katherine Martin & Tanios Bekaii-Saab
The Ohio State University Comprehensive Cancer Center, Columbus, OH, USA

KEY POINTS

- Combination chemotherapy remains the standard for untreated mCRC; however, sequential therapy may be considered for select patients.
- There is no data on optimal sequencing of biological agents in the treatment of KRAS wild-type patients.
- Metastatectomy for patients with limited hepatic metastatic disease can prolong survival and potentially cure a small subset of patients.
- Conversion therapy should be limited to 3–4 months to limit potential hepatotoxicity.
- Chemotherapy-free intervals may be reasonable in select patients with mCRC.

Introduction

In the United States, colorectal cancer is the third leading cause of cancer death [1]. Approximately 50% of patients with colorectal cancer will develop metastatic disease (mCRC.) Availability of multiple therapies has improved survival to more than 24 months [2–18], which has generated debate over the most effective use of these agents. This chapter addresses some of the controversies in the treatment of mCRC, including sequential versus combination chemotherapy, management of KRAS wild-type patients, conversion therapy, and chemotherapy-free intervals. Unless otherwise specified, all data pertains to first-line therapy.

Colorectal Cancer: Diagnosis and Clinical Management, First Edition. Edited by John H. Scholefield and Cathy Eng.

Sequential versus combination chemotherapy

The addition of either irinotecan or oxaliplatin to fluoropyrimidines improves response and survival in mCRC [2;4] at the expense of added toxicity. Irinotecan [19–21] and 5-FU [22–28] have activity as single agents in colorectal cancer, while oxaliplatin is relatively inactive alone [29]. Evidence suggests improved outcomes when patients receive all three active agents during their disease course [29;30]. In the palliative setting, it is reasonable to question whether an aggressive approach using up-front combination chemotherapy is truly necessary.

The MRC FOCUS trial

The FOCUS trial evaluated the optimal sequencing of 5-FU, oxaliplatin and irinotecan [31]. Patients received one of three treatment strategies. Strategy A was 5-FU continued until disease progression, and second-line irinotecan every 3 weeks. Strategy B involved first-line 5-FU until progression, with second-line 5-FU with either oxaliplatin or irinotecan. Strategy C was first-line 5-FU plus either irinotecan or oxaliplatin. The primary endpoint was survival, with secondary analysis for non-inferiority between strategies B and C subsequently added.

The number of patients treated was 2135. Forty-nine percent of patients received additional therapy following removal from study, but only 23% of patients received all 3 agents. Grade 3–4 toxicities were more common in Strategy C. Median survival was lower than expected for all groups. The survival difference between Strategies C and A was statistically significant, but did not satisfy the pre-specified requirement of $p < 0.01$ to confirm superiority. However, comparison of patients on Strategy C receiving irinotecan to Strategy A revealed a significant survival advantage for FOLFIRI over sequential 5-FU and irinotecan, and ORR and PFS were significantly improved for Strategy C. Non-inferiority was confirmed between strategies B and C, with no difference in survival between oxaliplatin-containing regimens and irinotecan-containing regimens. The authors concluded that a strategy of up-front single-agent 5-FU followed by combination therapy at progression did not compromise overall survival.

The DCCG CAIRO trial

On the CAIRO trial [32], patients received either sequential treatment with first-line capecitabine, second-line irinotecan, and third-line capecitabine plus oxaliplatin, or combination therapy with first-line capecitabine plus irinotecan, and second-line capecitabine plus oxaliplatin. The primary endpoint was survival. The number of patients treated was 803. The median time on treatment was significantly longer for sequential versus combination treatment. Grade 3–4 toxicities were increased with combination therapy. There was no survival difference between the two arms. For first-line but not second-line therapy, response and disease control were significantly higher for combination therapy, as was progression-free survival. The authors concluded that combination therapy was more toxic and no more effective than sequential therapy.

Discussion

The FOCUS and CAIRO trials failed to show survival benefit for up-front combination therapy. Both trials show that combination chemotherapy is more toxic, but also improves response and progression-free survival. These benefits are important in patients with symptomatic disease or those with limited metastatic disease that may be convertible to a resectable state. A recent retrospective analysis from the US Intergroup 9741 trial suggests achieving a complete response with first-line therapy is an independent predictor of survival [33], further supporting an aggressive combination approach to initial treatment. Finally, as demonstrated in FOCUS, many patients receiving sequential therapy will not be exposed to all three agents, which may improve survival [34].

In conclusion, the evidence suggests that the majority of patients with untreated mCRC should receive combination chemotherapy, although sequential therapy may be appropriate for select patients. Sequential therapy should be avoided in symptomatic patients or patients who have potentially curable limited metastatic disease. Patients who have pre-existing toxicities or comorbid conditions precluding the safety of combination therapy may be appropriate for sequential therapy.

Management of patients with KRAS wild-type tumors

Phase III data confirm that the addition of biological therapy to combination chemotherapy improves clinical outcomes in mCRC. For patients with KRAS wild-type tumors, multiple biological therapies are available, including the anti-VEGF monoclonal antibody bevacizumab, and the anti-EGFR monoclonal antibodies cetuximab and panitumumab; however, the best way to sequence these agents is unknown.

EGFR-Targeted Agents in KRAS wild-type mCRC

Several phase III studies have examined the role of adding cetuximab or panitumumab to combination chemotherapy. Updated analyses from the CRYSTAL trial demonstrate that adding cetuximab to irinotecan-based therapy (FOLFIRI) significantly improves overall and progression-free survival in previously untreated patients [15;17]. In contrast, two studies have failed to demonstrate benefit from adding cetuximab to oxaliplatin-based first-line therapy. Arm B of the 3-arm COIN study evaluated the effect on survival of cetuximab combined with either 5-FU (34% of patients) or capecitabine (66% of patients) plus oxaliplatin. Cetuximab did not improve outcome when compared to FOLFOX or XELOX (Arm A) [35]. Similarly, the recently published NORDIC VII study showed no improvement in the primary outcome measure of PFS or survival for the addition of cetuximab to bolus 5FU plus oxaliplatin (FLOX) [36].

On the other hand, PRIME study reached its primary endpoint (PFS), suggesting a clinical benefit from adding panitumumab to FOLFOX, although no significant improvement in overall survival was observed [9]. In the second-line setting, panitumumab significantly improved progression-free survival and response when combined with FOLFIRI [18].

VEGF-targeted agents

In untreated, unselected patients, bevacizumab improves survival and delays progression in combination with 5FU and irinotecan [6;13;37], and modestly prolongs progression-free survival when added to FOLFOX or XELOX [5]. In the second-line setting, the E3200 study demonstrated significant overall and progression-free survival benefit from the addition of bevacizumab to FOLFOX in irinotecan-refractory patients [12]. Finally, recently presented data from the phase III VELOUR study show significant overall and progression-free survival benefit for the addition of the VEGF-trap aflibercept to FOLFIRI in oxaliplatin-refractory patients [38]. Additional analyses of patients treated with bevacizumab, irinotecan, and 5FU [13] reveal that bevacizumab provides clinical benefit regardless of KRAS mutational status [39].

Discussion

There is no clear consensus to help define the optimal sequencing of biological agents in the treatment of KRAS wild-type patients. Both bevacizumab and anti-EGFR agents (cetuximab and panitumumab) provide benefit in this patient population. In the coming year, results of studies such as CALGB 80405 and AIO KRK-0306 will provide more information on how to best sequence these therapies. At this time, based on reasonable amount of data, NCCN guidelines support the use of irinotecan-based therapy combinations with EGFR inhibitors or bevacizumab, or oxaliplatin-based combinations with either bevacizumab or panitumumab as up-front therapy. Available data suggest a lack of synergy between oxaliplatin and cetuximab and these agents should not be used in combination.

Conversion chemotherapy for patients with limited metastatic disease

Roughly two-thirds of patients will develop liver metastases during their disease course but only 10–15% will be candidates for metastatectomy [40;41]. Although most of these patients will experience disease recurrence, a small percentage can be cured [42]. Five-year survival after R0 resection of liver metastases is between 30% and 35% [43], versus les than 9% for unresectable stage IV disease.

Involvement of critical structures may limit initial resectability of liver metastases. Chemotherapy and biological therapy are being increasingly utilized in am effort to convert unresectable liver metastases to a completely resectable state. This approach, termed 'conversion therapy', can allow between 12% and 33% of patients to undergo R0 (complete) resection [43–50].

Combination chemotherapy

The most effective approach to conversion chemotherapy is unclear; however, strategy should attempt to achieve a high response rate. Additional factors including time from adjuvant chemotherapy, pre-existing liver injury, or residual toxicities should also be taken into consideration.

Table 14.1 provides a summary of ORR and resection rates, when available, reported in phase III trials. Combining a fluoropyrimidine with oxaliplatin or irinotecan results in ORR of 36–59% [3;5;9;16;51–55] and 39–56% [6;10;15;54], respectively. In studies reporting secondary surgery outcomes, 2–24% of patients with unresectable liver disease were able to undergo surgery following chemotherapy and up to 14% of patients achieved R0 resection with median survival up to 39 months [2;15;54;56].

A recent phase III trial compared chemotherapy with 5-FU, oxaliplatin, and irinotecan (FOLFOXIRI) to FOLFIRI [10], with increased toxicity but significant improvement in ORR and R0 hepatic metastatectomy rate. An analysis of pooled data from 3 trials of preoperative FOLFOXIRI observed a 19%

Table 14.1 Summary of phase III trials of first-line chemotherapy that included patients with unresectable liver metastases.

Study	Year	Treatment	N	ORR (%)	Resection rate (%)	R0 resection rate (%)	mOS (m)
[2]	2000	FOLFOX	420	50.7	6.7	—	16.2
		5-FU		22.3	3.3	—	14.7
[4]	2000	IFL	683	50/39**	—	—	14.8
		5-FU		28/21**	—	—	12.6
		Irinotecan		21/18**	—	—	12
[8]	2000	IFL	387	49	—	—	17.4
		5-FU		31	—	—	14.1
[13]	2004	IFL	411	34.8	—	—	15.6
[3]	2004	FOLFOX	795	45	—	—	19.5
		IFL		31	—	—	15
		IROX		35	—	—	17.4
[37]	2004	FOLFOX	220	54	24	14	20.6
		FOLFIRI		56	9	7	21.5
[23]	2006	FOLFOX		58.5	17.7	11.3	19.3/38.9*
[10]	2007	FOLFOXIRI	244	66	36	15	22.6
		FOLFIRI		41	12	6	16.7
[35]	2007	FOLFOX	686	57	—	—	16.7
		FOLFIRI		49	—	—	15.4
[36]	2007	XELIRI	398	46	2	—	17.4
[6]	2007	FOLFIRI	430	47.2	—	—	23.1
		IFL		43.3	—	—	17.6
		XELIRI		38.6**	—	—	18.9
[58]	2008	FOLFOX	634	48	—	—	19.6
		XELOX		47	—	—	19.8
[16]	2009	FOLFOX	168	36	—	2.4	—
[15]	2009	FOLFIRI	602	38.7	3.7	1.7	18.6
[9]	2010	FOLFOX	550	48	9.4	7	19.7
[25]	2011	FOLFOX/XELOX	815	46	—	—	19.6

*Survival in all patients/patients undergoing hepatic metastatectomy
**Unconfirmed/confirmed
– Not reported

R0 resection rate and 5-year survival of 42%. No severe liver injury or post-operative mortality was observed [44].

Significantly higher incidence of liver injury has been reported in patients who have received chemotherapy prior to surgery [57;58]. Hepatic sinusoidal injury is reported in up to 78% of liver specimens following preoperative oxaliplatin [58;59] within 4 months of therapy [60]. In addition, nodular regenerative hyperplasia preventing liver resection has been observed with oxaliplatin [61]. Irinotecan is associated with increased incidence of steatohepatitis after a median of 16 weeks of therapy, which can affect the ability to safely perform large liver resections [60;62;63]. Data regarding the effect of chemotherapy-induced liver toxicity on perioperative morbidity and mortality are mixed [60;62–68], but suggest that more than 12–16 weeks of preoperative treatment and less than 4 weeks between chemotherapy and surgery are associated with increased postsurgical complications [69;70].

Chemotherapy plus biologic therapy

The addition of targeted agents to chemotherapy has been studied in phase III trials, with variable improvement in response. Data regarding response rates and resection rates on phase III trials of chemotherapy plus biologics are summarized in Table 14.2.

Table 14.2 Summary of phase III trials of first-line chemotherapy plus biologics.

Study	Year	Treatment	N	ORR (%)	Resection rate (%)	R0 resection rate (%)	mOS (m)
[13]	2004	IFL + bevacizumab	402	44.8	—	—	20.3
[14]	2005	5-FU + bevacizumab	313	40	—	—	18.3
[16]	2007	FOLFOX + cetuximab	169/61**	61**	—	9.8**	—
[6, 7]	2007	FOLFIRI + bevacizumab	117	57.9	—	—	NR*
		IFL+ bevacizumab		53.3	—	—	19.2
[5]	2008	FOLFOX + bevacizumab	349	38***	8.4***	—	21.2
		XELOX + bevacizumab	350				21.4
[15]	2009	FOLFIRI + cetuximab	599/172**	59.3**	7	4.8	24.9**
[9]	2010	FOLFOX + panitumumab	593/325**	55**	10.5**	8.3**	23.9**
[55]	2012	XELOX + bevacizumab	239	47%	12	9.2	23.2

–Not reported
*Not reached
**KRAS WT population only
***Patients receiving bevacizumab regardless of FOLFOX or XELOX

Anti-EGFR monoclonal antibodies

Data suggest that patients with KRAS mutation do not benefit from these agents [9;15;16] and their use is restricted to patients with confirmed KRAS wild-type tumors. On the CRYSTAL trial, FOLFIRI plus cetuximab improved ORR in KRAS wild-type patients, and increased the percentage of patients able undergo surgery and R0 resection [15]. Based on the PRIME study, panitumumab results in a trend toward improved objective response when added to FOLFOX in KRAS wild-type patients [9]. There is no benefit to the addition of cetuximab to FOLFOX [35;36].

Bevacizumab

Phase III studies have evaluated the addition of the anti-VEGF monoclonal antibody bevacizumab to combination chemotherapy. Bevacizumab improved ORR to 45% or 58% when added to IFL [13] or FOLFIRI [6] in phase III studies (rates of resection were not reported); however, adding bevacizumab to FOLFOX or XELOX did not improve response rate [5]. These data suggest that in the setting of conversion therapy, the combination of FOLFIRI and bevacizumab is an appropriate option, whereas the role of bevacizumab added to FOLFOX is unclear. Evaluation of the addition of bevacizumab to FOLFOXIRI versus FOLFIRI in the phase III setting is ongoing (NCT00719797).

Several bevacizumab-related toxicities may adversely impact postsurgical outcome. The evidence is inconsistent to clearly define a relationship between bevacizumab and postoperative morbidity (71–74); however, data from the observational BRiTE study demonstrate an incidence of serious wound complications in only 2% in patients who discontinued bevacizumab ≥8 weeks prior to surgery, compared to 10% in those who received bevacizumab within 2 weeks of surgery [71;75]. Based on the 21-day half-life of bevacizumab, it is recommended to discontinue its use 6–8 weeks prior to hepatic resection, to allow adequate clearance and reduce the risk of potential complications [73–75].

Discussion

Recommended chemotherapy regimens for conversion therapy include FOLFOX/XELOX with or (preferably) without bevacizumab, FOLFOX with panitumumab (KRAS wild-type only), FOLFIRI with anti-EGFR therapy (KRAS wild-type only), FOLFIRI with bevacizumab, or FOLFOXIRI. The role of new biological agents, such as aflibercept and regorafenib in conversion therapy, remains to be determined. Bevacizumab should be discontinued 6–8 weeks prior to surgery to decrease the risk of postoperative complications.

When administering preoperative chemotherapy, clinicians must be cognizant of the potential for development of chemotherapy-induced liver injury and underlying predisposing factors such as body mass index. The minimum duration of chemotherapy (ideally ≤4 cycles) should be provided in the neoadjuvant setting to achieve required tumor regression prior to surgery.

The role of chemotherapy-free intervals

Advances in therapy have transformed mCRC into a chronic disease for many patients. In the setting of palliation of incurable disease, maintaining the balance between quality of life and disease control is an extremely relevant and often challenging task. Chemotherapy-free intervals are therefore an important component of the management of advanced colorectal cancer.

The MRC CR06 trial

The MRC CR06 trial evaluated the effect of chemotherapy-free interval (CFI) on survival when compared to continuous 5-FU administered until disease progression [76]. Patients received continuous treatment with 5-FU or treatment for 3 months followed by CFI with chemotherapy reintroduction at disease progression. The trial closed early and was underpowered to assess the primary endpoint of survival.

Patients on the CFI arm had a median CFI of 2.8 months but only roughly one-third of patients restarted chemotherapy, mostly due to disease progression (80%). Patients not restarting original chemotherapy either received no further therapy (42%) or an alternate chemotherapy regimen (21%). There was no survival difference between the two arms and no delay in progression with continuous chemotherapy. Patients on continuous therapy reported more chemotherapy-specific side effects. The authors concluded that no clear benefit could be demonstrated for continuous chemotherapy, and that CFI following 12 weeks of chemotherapy was safe and did not compromise survival.

The Gercor OPTIMOX trials

In the OPTIMOX-1 trial, the investigators demonstrated that oxaliplatin could be safely discontinued after 6 cycles of FOLFOX, with less sensory neuropathy and without adverse effects on clinical outcome [53]. To compare complete discontinuation of chemotherapy to the OPTIMOX method, the OPTIMOX-2 study was conducted [77]. Patients were treated with 6 cycles (3 months) of modified (m) FOLFOX7 and either maintenance therapy (Arm 1-reference) with simplified LV5FU2, or a chemotherapy-free interval (CFI,

Arm 2-OPTIMOX-2). In both arms, mFOLFOX7 was reintroduced at tumor regrowth to original size. The primary endpoint was duration of disease control (DDC), defined as the sum of progression-free survivals while receiving mFOLFOX7 and maintenance therapy/CFI. The planned sample size was decreased when bevacizumab was approved for first-line therapy, resulting in an underpowered study.

The number of patients treated was 216 and roughly 80% of eligible patients on each arm underwent reintroduction of mFOLFOX7. Toxicities were similar on each arm after reintroduction of mFOLFOX7. Median DDC was and PFS were both significantly longer on arm 1 versus arm 2. Overall survival and ORR were similar. ORR after first FOLFOX reintroduction was 20.4% in Arm 1 and 30.3% in Arm 2 and 90% of patients who experienced partial response at FOLFOX reintroduction had experienced partial response with initial therapy. Median PFS at FOLFOX reintroduction was not significantly different between the arms. The authors concluded that CFI adversely affects DDC; however, chemotherapy discontinuation may still be an appropriate option for select patients, such as those who experience complete or near complete response to therapy.

The MRC COIN trial

In the MRC COIN study [78], 1630 patients were randomized to receive continuous chemotherapy with investigator choice of capecitabine or 5-FUand oxaliplatin until progression or toxicity (Arm A), or 12 weeks of chemotherapy followed by cessation until progressive disease, at which time chemotherapy was reintroduced (Arm C). The primary endpoint of the study was non-inferiority of OS between the arms.

The cumulative dose-intensity of chemotherapy was greater on Arm A; however, the dose intensity of chemotherapy was greater in Arm C during on-therapy periods. Grade 3–4 hand/foot syndrome and peripheral neuropathy were more frequent on Arm A. 63% of patients on Arm B began a CFI, and the median length of CFI prior to progression was 3.7 months, with 64% of those patients restarting a second chemotherapy course. As in OPTIMOX, best response was typically seen in the first 3 months of treatment. Seventy percent of patients on Arm C restarting chemotherapy after progression on CFI achieved disease control. Significantly fewer patients received second-line therapy on Arm C compared to Arm A (52% vs. 62%). In both populations, the upper bound of the confidence interval for OS was higher than the predefined non-inferiority boundary, so the primary endpoint was not met. Post-hoc analyses identified patients with elevated platelet count (≥400,000/μL) as a subpopulation for which CFI may be harmful. Quality of life analyses revealed significant benefit favoring CFI for multiple parameters. The investigators concluded that although this was a negative study and intermittent chemotherapy cannot be routinely recommended, patients with normal baseline platelet count may benefit from this approach.

Discussion

Taken together, the results of published studies suggest CFI should not be routinely offered to all patients; however, there may be a population of patients that is appropriate for intermittent chemotherapy. For example, patients who had a partial response or prolonged disease control with initial chemotherapy may have a similar degree of response on chemotherapy re-initiation. Criteria for consideration of CFI can include intolerable toxicity, complete response, or prolonged stable disease (≥12 months), achievement of best objective response, or completion of a predefined number of chemotherapy cycles.

TIPS AND TRICKS / KEY PITFALLS

- Combination chemotherapy with 5-FU, oxaliplatin, and irinotecan (FOLFOXIRI) causes significant gastrointestinal and hematologic toxicity.
- Bevacizumab should be discontinued at least 6–8 weeks prior to hepatic surgery and should not be re-initiated for at least 6 weeks post-operatively.
- Oxaliplatin-based therapy should not be combined with cetuximab in KRAS wild-type patients.

CASE STUDY AND MULTIPLE-CHOICE QUESTIONS

Case 1

A 45-year-old man was treated for stage IIIB colon cancer with colectomy and 6 months of adjuvant FOLFOX. After 2 years from initial diagnosis, a CT scan of the abdomen shows a 4-cm liver lesion. Biopsy reveals metastatic adenocarcinoma with a mutation in KRAS. His surgical oncologist felt the lesion is borderline resectable. He has no residual chemotherapy-related toxicities.

1 Which of the following are appropriate chemotherapy regimens for this patient (more than 1 answer may be correct)?

   A. FOLFOX plus cetuximab

   B. FOLFOXIRI

   C. FOLFIRI plus bevacizumab

   D. FOLFOX

   E. Single-agent 5-FU

Case 2

A 69-year-old woman with mCRC received mFOLFOX6 plus bevacizumab for 12 months with a partial response for the last 10 months. She required dose-reduction of oxaliplatin for persistent grade 2 neuropathy. She now has difficulty with self-care activities of daily living.

2 Which of the following represent reasonable modifications to this patient's therapy (more than 1 answer may be correct)?

A. Continue 5-FU and oxaliplatin and bevacizumab at the current doses.

B. Discontinue oxaliplatin and continue maintenance 5-FU and bevacizumab until disease progression or resolution of neurotoxicity, at which time oxaliplatin can be reintroduced.

C. Completely discontinue chemotherapy and begin close surveillance with the plan to restart chemotherapy at evidence of progression.

D. Further dose-reduce oxaliplatin to 45 mg/m^2 and continue therapy.

References

1 Jemal A, Siegel R, Xu J, Ward E. Cancer statistics, 2010. CA *Cancer J Clin* 2010 Sep–Oct; 60(5): 277–300.

2 de Gramont A, Figer A, Seymour M, Homerin M, Hmissi A, Cassidy J, et al. Leucovorin and fluorouracil with or without oxaliplatin as first-line treatment in advanced colorectal cancer. *J Clin Oncol* 2000 Aug; 18(16): 2938–47.

3 Goldberg RM, Sargent DJ, Morton RF, Fuchs CS, Ramanathan RK, Williamson SK, et al. A randomized controlled trial of fluorouracil plus leucovorin, irinotecan, and oxaliplatin combinations in patients with previously untreated metastatic colorectal cancer. *J Clin Onco*l 2004 Jan 1; 22(1): 23–30.

4 Saltz LB, Cox JV, Blanke C, Rosen LS, Fehrenbacher L, Moore MJ, et al. Irinotecan plus fluorouracil and leucovorin for metastatic colorectal cancer. Irinotecan Study Group. *N Engl J Med* 2000 Sep 28; 343(13): 905–14.

5 Saltz LB, Clarke S, Diaz-Rubio E, Scheithauer W, Figer A, Wong R, et al. Bevacizumab in combination with oxaliplatin-based chemotherapy as first-line therapy in metastatic colorectal cancer: a randomized phase III study. *J Clin Oncol* 2008 Apr 20; 26(12): 2013–19.

6 Fuchs CS, Marshall J, Mitchell E, Wierzbicki R, Ganju V, Jeffery M, et al. Randomized, controlled trial of irinotecan plus infusional, bolus, or oral fluoropyrimidines in first-line treatment of metastatic colorectal cancer: results from the BICC-C Study. *J Clin Oncol* 2007 Oct 20; 25(30): 4779–86.

7 Fuchs CS, Marshall J, Barrueco J. Randomized, controlled trial of irinotecan plus infusional, bolus, or oral fluoropyrimidines in first-line treatment of metastatic colorectal cancer: updated results from the BICC-C study. *J Clin Oncol* 2008 Feb 1; 26(4): 689–90.

8 Douillard JY, Cunningham D, Roth AD, Navarro M, James RD, Karasek P, et al. Irinotecan combined with fluorouracil compared with fluorouracil alone as first-line treatment

for metastatic colorectal cancer: a multicentre randomised trial. *Lancet* 2000 Mar 25; 355(9209): 1041–7.

9 Douillard JY, Siena S, Cassidy J, Tabernero J, Burkes R, Barugel M, et al. Randomized, phase III trial of panitumumab with infusional fluorouracil, leucovorin, and oxaliplatin (FOLFOX4) versus FOLFOX4 alone as first-line treatment in patients with previously untreated metastatic colorectal cancer: the PRIME study. *J Clin Oncol* 2010 Nov 1; 28(31): 4697–705.

10 Falcone A, Ricci S, Brunetti I, Pfanner E, Allegrini G, Barbara C, et al. Phase III trial of infusional fluorouracil, leucovorin, oxaliplatin, and irinotecan (FOLFOXIRI) compared with infusional fluorouracil, leucovorin, and irinotecan (FOLFIRI) as first line treatment for metastatic colorectal cancer: the Gruppo Oncologico Nord Ovest. *J Clin Oncol* 2007 May 1; 25(13): 1670–6.

11 Fyfe GA, Hurwitz H, Fehrenbacher L, Cartwright T, Hainsworth J, Heim W, et al. Bevacizumab plus irinotecan/5-FU/leucovorin for treatment of metastatic colorectal cancer results in survival benefit in all pre-specified subgroups. *J Clin Oncol* 2004; 22(14S).

12 Giantonio BJ, Catalano PJ, Meropol NJ, O'Dwyer PJ, Mitchell EP, Alberts SR, et al. Bevacizumab in combination with oxaliplatin, fluorouracil, and leucovorin (FOLFOX4) for previously treated metastatic colorectal cancer: results from the Eastern Cooperative Oncology Group Study E3200. *J Clin Oncol* 2007 Apr 20; 25(12): 1539–44.

13 Hurwitz H, Fehrenbacher L, Novotny W, Cartwright T, Hainsworth J, Heim W, et al. Bevacizumab plus irinotecan, fluorouracil, and leucovorin for metastatic colorectal cancer. *N Engl J Med* 2004 Jun 3; 350(23): 2335–42.

14 Hurwitz HI, Fehrenbacher L, Hainsworth JD, Heim W, Berlin J, Holmgren E, et al. Bevacizumab in combination with fluorouracil and leucovorin: an active regimen for first-line metastatic colorectal cancer. *J Clin Oncol* 2005 May 20; 23(15): 3502–8.

15 Van Cutsem E, Kohne CH, Hitre E, Zaluski J, Chang Chien CR, Makhson A, et al. Cetuximab and chemotherapy as initial treatment for metastatic colorectal cancer. *N Engl J Med* 2009 Apr 2; 360(14): 1408–17.

16 Bokemeyer C, Bondarenko I, Makhson A, Hartmann JT, Aparicio J, de Braud F, et al. Fluorouracil, leucovorin, and oxaliplatin with and without cetuximab in the first-line treatment of metastatic colorectal cancer. *J Clin Oncol* 2009 Feb 10; 27(5): 663–71.

17 Van Cutsem E, Kohne CH, Lang I, Folprecht G, Nowacki MP, Cascinu S, et al. Cetuximab plus irinotecan, fluorouracil, and leucovorin as first-line treatment for metastatic colorectal cancer: updated analysis of overall survival according to tumor KRAS and BRAF mutation status. *J Clin Oncol* 2011 Apr 18.

18 Peeters M, Price TJ, Cervantes A, Sobrero AF, Ducreux M, Hotko Y, et al. Randomized phase III study of panitumumab with fluorouracil, leucovorin, and irinotecan (FOLFIRI) compared with FOLFIRI alone as second-line treatment in patients with metastatic colorectal cancer. *J Clin Oncol* 2010 Nov 1; 28(31): 4706–13.

19 Rougier P, Van Cutsem E, Bajetta E, Niederle N, Possinger K, Labianca R, et al. Randomised trial of irinotecan versus fluorouracil by continuous infusion after fluorouracil failure in patients with metastatic colorectal cancer. *Lancet* 1998 Oct 31; 352(9138): 1407–12.

20 Cunningham D, Pyrhonen S, James RD, Punt CJ, Hickish TF, Heikkila R, et al. Randomised trial of irinotecan plus supportive care versus supportive care alone after fluorouracil failure for patients with metastatic colorectal cancer. *Lancet* 1998 Oct 31; 352(9138): 1413–18.

21 Kim GP, Sargent DJ, Mahoney MR, Rowland KM, Jr, Philip PA, Mitchell E, et al. Phase III non-inferiority trial comparing irinotecan with oxaliplatin, fluorouracil, and leucovorin in patients with advanced colorectal carcinoma previously treated with fluorouracil: N9841. *J Clin Oncol* 2009 Jun 10; 27(17): 2848–54.

22 Aranda E, Diaz-Rubio E, Cervantes A, Anton-Torres A, Carrato A, Massuti T, et al. Randomized trial comparing monthly low-dose leucovorin and fluorouracil bolus with weekly high-dose 48-hour continuous-infusion fluorouracil for advanced colorectal cancer: a Spanish Cooperative Group for Gastrointestinal Tumor Therapy (TTD) study. *Ann Oncol* 1998 Jul; 9(7): 727–31.

23 Jager E, Heike M, Bernhard H, Klein O, Bernhard G, Lautz D, et al. Weekly high-dose leucovorin versus low-dose leucovorin combined with fluorouracil in advanced colorectal cancer: results of a randomized multicenter trial. Study Group for Palliative Treatment of Metastatic Colorectal Cancer Study Protocol 1. *J Clin Oncol* 1996 Aug; 14(8): 2274–9.

24 Buroker TR, O'Connell MJ, Wieand HS, Krook JE, Gerstner JB, Mailliard JA, et al. Randomized comparison of two schedules of fluorouracil and leucovorin in the treatment of advanced colorectal cancer. *J Clin Oncol* 1994 Jan; 12(1): 14–20.

25 de Gramont A, Bosset JF, Milan C, Rougier P, Bouche O, Etienne PL, et al. Randomized trial comparing monthly low-dose Leucovorin and fluorouracil bolus with bimonthly high-dose leucovorin and fluorouracil bolus plus continuous infusion for advanced colorectal cancer: a French intergroup study. *J Clin Oncol* 1997 Feb; 15(2): 808–15.

26 Poon MA, O'Connell MJ, Moertel CG, Wieand HS, Cullinan SA, Everson LK, et al. Biochemical modulation of Fluorouracil: evidence of significant improvement of survival and quality of life in patients with advanced colorectal carcinoma. *J Clin Oncol* 1989 Oct; 7(10): 1407–18.

27 Hoff PM, Ansari R, Batist G, Cox J, Kocha W, Kuperminc M, et al. Comparison of oral capecitabine versus intravenous fluorouracil plus leucovorin as first-line treatment in 605 patients with metastatic colorectal cancer: results of a randomized phase III study. *J Clin Oncol* 2001 Apr 15; 19(8): 2282–92.

28 Van Cutsem E, Twelves C, Cassidy J, Allman D, Bajetta E, Boyer M, et al. Oral capecitabine compared with intravenous fluorouracil plus leucovorin in patients with metastatic colorectal cancer: results of a large phase III study. *J Clin Oncol* 2001 Nov 1; 19(21): 4097–106.

29 Rothenberg ML, Oza AM, Bigelow RH, Berlin JD, Marshall JL, Ramanathan RK, et al. Superiority of oxaliplatin and fluorouracil-leucovorin compared with either therapy alone in patients with progressive colorectal cancer after irinotecan and fluorouracil-leucovorin: interim results of a phase III trial. *J Clin Oncol* 2003 Jun 1; 21(11): 2059–69.

30 Grothey A, Sargent D, Goldberg RM, Schmoll HJ. Survival of patients with advanced colorectal cancer improves with the availability of fluorouracil-leucovorin, irinotecan, and oxaliplatin in the course of treatment. *J Clin Oncol* 2004 Apr 1; 22(7): 1209–14.

31 Seymour MT, Maughan TS, Ledermann JA, Topham C, James R, Gwyther SJ, et al. Different strategies of sequential and combination chemotherapy for patients with poor prognosis advanced colorectal cancer (MRC FOCUS): a randomised controlled trial. *Lancet* 2007 Jul 14; 370(9582): 143–52.

32 Koopman M, Antonini NF, Douma J, Wals J, Honkoop AH, Erdkamp FL, et al. Sequential versus combination chemotherapy with capecitabine, irinotecan, and oxaliplatin in advanced colorectal cancer (CAIRO): a phase III randomised controlled trial. *Lancet* 2007 Jul 14; 370(9582): 135–42.

33 Dy GK, Krook JE, Green EM, Sargent DJ, Delaunoit T, Morton RF, et al. Impact of complete response to chemotherapy on overall survival in advanced colorectal cancer: results from Intergroup N9741. *J Clin Oncol* 2007 Aug 10; 25(23): 3469–74.

34 Grothey A, Sargent D, Goldberg RM, Schmoll HJ. Survival of patients with advanced colorectal cancer improves with the availability of fluorouracil-leucovorin, irinotecan, and oxaliplatin in the course of treatment. *J Clin Oncol* 2004 Apr 1; 22(7): 1209–14.

35 Maughan TS, Adams RA, Smith CG, Meade AM, Seymour MT, Wilson RH, et al. Addition of cetuximab to oxaliplatin-based first-line combination chemotherapy for treatment of advanced colorectal cancer: results of the randomised phase 3 MRC COIN trial. *Lancet* 2011 Jun 18; 377(9783): 2103–14.

36 Tveit KM, Guren T, Glimelius B, Pfeiffer P, Sorbye H, Pyrhonen S, et al. Phase III trial of cetuximab with continuous or intermittent fluorouracil, leucovorin, and oxaliplatin (Nordic FLOX) versus FLOX alone in first-line treatment of metastatic colorectal cancer: The NORDIC-VII Study. *J Clin Oncol* 20 May 2012; 30(15): 1755–62.

37 Fuchs CS, Marshall J, Barrueco J. Randomized, controlled trial of irinotecan plus infusional, bolus, or oral fluoropyrimidines in first-line treatment of metastatic colorectal cancer: updated results from the BICC-C study. *J Clin Oncol* 2008 Feb 1; 26(4): 689–90.

38 Van Cutsem E, Tabernero J, Lakomy R, Prausova J, Ruff P, Van Hazel G, et al. Intravenous (IV) aflibercept versus placebo in combination with irinotecan/5-FU (FOLFIRI) for second-line treatment of metastatic colorectal cancer (mCRC): results of a multinational phase III trial (EFC10262-VELOUR). *Ann Oncol* 2011; 22(5s).

39 Hurwitz HI, Yi J, Ince W, Novotny WF, Rosen O. The clinical benefit of bevacizumab in metastatic colorectal cancer is independent of K-ras mutation status: analysis of a phase III study of bevacizumab with chemotherapy in previously untreated metastatic colorectal cancer. *Oncologist* 2009 Jan; 14(1): 22–8.

40 Kemeny N. Management of liver metastases from colorectal cancer. *Oncology* 2006 Sep; 20(10): 1161–76, 1179; discussion 1179–80, 1185–6.

41 Alberts SR, Horvath WL, Sternfeld WC, Goldberg RM, Mahoney MR, Dakhil SR, et al. Oxaliplatin, fluorouracil, and leucovorin for patients with unresectable liver-only metastases from colorectal cancer: a North Central Cancer Treatment Group phase II study. *J Clin Oncol* 2005 Dec 20; 23(36): 9243–9.

42 Tomlinson JS, Jarnagin WR, DeMatteo RP, Fong Y, Kornprat P, Gonen M, et al. Actual 10-year survival after resection of colorectal liver metastases defines cure. *J Clin Oncol* 2007 Oct 10; 25(29): 4575–80.

43 Adam R, Wicherts DA, de Haas RJ, Ciacio O, Levi F, Paule B, et al. Patients with initially unresectable colorectal liver metastases: is there a possibility of cure? *J Clin Oncol* 2009 Apr 10; 27(11): 1829–35.

44 Masi G, Loupakis F, Pollina L, Vasile E, Cupini S, Ricci S, et al. Long-term outcome of initially unresectable metastatic colorectal cancer patients treated with 5-fluorouracil/leucovorin, oxaliplatin, and irinotecan (FOLFOXIRI) followed by radical surgery of metastases. *Ann Surg* 2009 Mar; 249(3): 420–5.

45 Nordlinger B, Van Cutsem E, Rougier P, Kohne CH, Ychou M, Sobrero A, et al. Does chemotherapy prior to liver resection increase the potential for cure in patients with metastatic colorectal cancer? A report from the European Colorectal Metastases Treatment Group. *Eur J Cancer* 2007 Sep; 43(14): 2037–45.

46 Alberts SR, Horvath WL, Sternfeld WC, Goldberg RM, Mahoney MR, Dakhil SR, et al. Oxaliplatin, fluorouracil, and leucovorin for patients with unresectable liver-only

metastases from colorectal cancer: a North Central Cancer Treatment Group phase II study. *J Clin Oncol* 2005 Dec 20; 23(36): 9243–9.

47 Barone C, Nuzzo G, Cassano A, Basso M, Schinzari G, Giuliante F, et al. Final analysis of colorectal cancer patients treated with irinotecan and 5-fluorouracil plus folinic acid neoadjuvant chemotherapy for unresectable liver metastases. *Br J Cancer* 2007 Oct 22; 97(8): 1035–9.

48 Ychou M, Viret F, Kramar A, Desseigne F, Mitry E, Guimbaud R, et al. Tritherapy with fluorouracil/leucovorin, irinotecan and oxaliplatin (FOLFIRINOX): a Phase II study in colorectal cancer patients with non-resectable liver metastases. *Cancer Chemother Pharmacol* 2008 Jul; 62(2): 195–201.

49 Bismuth H, Adam R, Levi F, Farabos C, Waechter F, Castaing D, et al. Resection of non-resectable liver metastases from colorectal cancer after neoadjuvant chemotherapy. *Ann Surg* 1996 Oct; 224(4): 509–0; discussion 520–2.

50 Delaunoit T, Alberts SR, Sargent DJ, Green E, Goldberg RM, Krook J, et al. Chemotherapy permits resection of metastatic colorectal cancer: experience from Intergroup N9741. *Ann Oncol* 2005 Mar; 16(3): 425–9.

51 de Gramont A, Figer A, Seymour M, Homerin M, Hmissi A, Cassidy J, et al. Leucovorin and fluorouracil with or without oxaliplatin as first-line treatment in advanced colorectal cancer. *J Clin Oncol* 2000 Aug; 18(16): 2938–47.

52 Cassidy J, Clarke S, Diaz-Rubio E, Scheithauer W, Figer A, Wong R, et al. Randomized Phase III study of capecitabine plus oxaliplatin compared with fluorouracil/folinic acid plus oxaliplatin as first-line therapy for metastatic colorectal cancer. *J Clin Oncol* 2008 Apr 20; 26(12): 2006–12.

53 Tournigand C, Cervantes A, Figer A, Lledo G, Flesch M, Buyse M, et al. OPTIMOX1: a randomized study of FOLFOX4 or FOLFOX7 with oxaliplatin in a stop-and-go fashion in advanced colorectal cancer – a GERCOR study. *J Clin Oncol* 2006 Jan 20; 24(3): 394–400.

54 Tournigand C, Andre T, Achille E, Lledo G, Flesh M, Mery-Mignard D, et al. FOLFIRI followed by FOLFOX6 or the reverse sequence in advanced colorectal cancer: a randomized GERCOR study. *J Clin Oncol* 2004 Jan 15; 22(2): 229–37.

55 Diaz-Rubio E, Gomez-Espana A, Massuti B, Sastre J, Abad A, Valladares M, et al. First-line XELOX plus bevacizumab followed by XELOX plus bevacizumab or single-agent bevacizumab as maintenance therapy in patients with metastatic colorectal cancer: the phase III MACRO TTD study. *Oncologist* 2012 Jan 10; 17(11): 1426–8.

56 Giacchetti S, Perpoint B, Zidani R, Le Bail N, Faggiuolo R, Focan C, et al. Phase III multicenter randomized trial of oxaliplatin added to chronomodulated fluorouracil-leucovorin as first-line treatment of metastatic colorectal cancer. *J Clin Oncol* 2000 Jan; 18(1): 136–47.

57 Karoui M, Penna C, Amin-Hashem M, Mitry E, Benoist S, Franc B, et al. Influence of preoperative chemotherapy on the risk of major hepatectomy for colorectal liver metastases. *Ann Surg* 2006 Jan; 243(1): 1–7.

58 Aloia T, Sebagh M, Plasse M, Karam V, Levi F, Giacchetti S, et al. Liver histology and surgical outcomes after preoperative chemotherapy with fluorouracil plus oxaliplatin in colorectal cancer liver metastases. *J Clin Oncol* 2006 Nov 1; 24(31): 4983–90.

59 Rubbia-Brandt L, Audard V, Sartoretti P, Roth AD, Brezault C, Le Charpentier M, et al. Severe hepatic sinusoidal obstruction associated with oxaliplatin-based chemotherapy in patients with metastatic colorectal cancer. *Ann Oncol* 2004 Mar; 15(3): 460–6.

60 Vauthey JN, Pawlik TM, Ribero D, Wu TT, Zorzi D, Hoff PM, et al. Chemotherapy regimen predicts steatohepatitis and an increase in 90-day mortality after surgery for hepatic colorectal metastases. *J Clin Oncol* 2006 May 1; 24(13): 2065–72.

61 Hubert C, Sempoux C, Horsmans Y, Rahier J, Humblet Y, Machiels JP, et al. Nodular regenerative hyperplasia: a deleterious consequence of chemotherapy for colorectal liver metastases? *Liver Int* 2007 Sep; 27(7): 938–43.

62 Kooby DA, Fong Y, Suriawinata A, Gonen M, Allen PJ, Klimstra DS, et al. Impact of steatosis on perioperative outcome following hepatic resection. *J Gastrointest Surg* 2003 Dec; 7(8): 1034–44.

63 Pawlik TM, Olino K, Gleisner AL, Torbenson M, Schulick R, Choti MA. Preoperative chemotherapy for colorectal liver metastases: impact on hepatic histology and postoperative outcome. *J Gastrointest Surg* 2007 Jul; 11(7): 860–8.

64 Hubert C, Fervaille C, Sempoux C, Horsmans Y, Humblet Y, Machiels JP, et al. Prevalence and clinical relevance of pathological hepatic changes occurring after neoadjuvant chemotherapy for colorectal liver metastases. *Surgery* 2010 Feb; 147(2): 185–94.

65 Nakano H, Oussoultzoglou E, Rosso E, Casnedi S, Chenard-Neu MP, Dufour P, et al. Sinusoidal injury increases morbidity after major hepatectomy in patients with colorectal liver metastases receiving preoperative chemotherapy. *Ann Surg* 2008 Jan; 247(1): 118–24.

66 Scoggins CR, Campbell ML, Landry CS, Slomiany BA, Woodall CE, McMasters KM, et al. Preoperative chemotherapy does not increase morbidity or mortality of hepatic resection for colorectal cancer metastases. *Ann Surg Oncol* 2009 Jan; 16(1): 35–41.

67 Cucchetti A, Ercolani G, Cescon M, Di Gioia P, Peri E, Brandi G, et al. Safety of hepatic resection for colorectal metastases in the era of neo-adjuvant chemotherapy. *Br J Surg* 2011 Aug; 98(8): 1147–54.

68 Choti MA. Chemotherapy-associated hepatotoxicity: do we need to be concerned? *Ann Surg Oncol* 2009 Sep; 16(9): 2391–4.

69 Welsh FK, Tilney HS, Tekkis PP, John TG, Rees M. Safe liver resection following chemotherapy for colorectal metastases is a matter of timing. *Br J Cancer* 2007 Apr 10; 96(7): 1037–42.

70 Kishi Y, Zorzi D, Contreras CM, Maru DM, Kopetz S, Ribero D, et al. Extended preoperative chemotherapy does not improve pathologic response and increases postoperative liver insufficiency after hepatic resection for colorectal liver metastases. *Ann Surg Oncol* 2010 Nov; 17(11): 2870–6.

71 Grothey A, Sugrue E, Hedrick E, Purdie D, Yi J, Dong W, et al. Association between exposure to bevacizumab (BV) beyond first progression (BBP) and overall survival (OS) in patients (pts) with metastatic colorectal cancer (mCRC): Results from a large obesrvational study (BRiTE). *J Clin Oncol* 2007; 25(18S).

72 Kesmodel SB, Ellis LM, Lin E, Chang GJ, Abdalla EK, Kopetz S, et al. Preoperative bevacizumab does not significantly increase postoperative complication rates in patients undergoing hepatic surgery for colorectal cancer liver metastases. *J Clin Oncol* 2008 Nov 10; 26(32): 5254–60.

73 D'Angelica M, Kornprat P, Gonen M, Chung KY, Jarnagin WR, DeMatteo RP, et al. Lack of evidence for increased operative morbidity after hepatectomy with perioperative use of bevacizumab: a matched case-control study. *Ann Surg Oncol* 2007 Feb; 14(2): 759–65.

74 Reddy SK, Morse MA, Hurwitz HI, Bendell JC, Gan TJ, Hill SE, et al. Addition of bevacizumab to irinotecan- and oxaliplatin-based preoperative chemotherapy regimens does

not increase morbidity after resection of colorectal liver metastases. *J Am Coll Surg* 2008 Jan; 206(1): 96–106.

75 Kozloff M, Yood MU, Berlin J, Flynn PJ, Kabbinavar FF, Purdie DM, et al. Clinical outcomes associated with bevacizumab-containing treatment of metastatic colorectal cancer: the BRiTE observational cohort study. *Oncologist* 2009 Sep; 14(9): 862–70.

76 Maughan TS, James RD, Kerr DJ, Ledermann JA, Seymour MT, Topham C, et al. Comparison of intermittent and continuous palliative chemotherapy for advanced colorectal cancer: a multicentre randomised trial. *Lancet* 2003 Feb 8; 361(9356): 457–64.

77 Chibaudel B, Maindrault-Goebel F, Lledo G, Mineur L, Andre T, Bennamoun M, et al. Can chemotherapy be discontinued in unresectable metastatic colorectal cancer? The GERCOR OPTIMOX2 Study. *J Clin Oncol* 2009 Dec 1; 27(34): 5727–33.

78 Adams RA, Meade AM, Seymour MT, Wilson RH, Madi A, Fisher D, et al. Intermittent versus continuous oxaliplatin and fluoropyrimidine combination chemotherapy for first-line treatment of advanced colorectal cancer: results of the randomised phase 3 MRC COIN trial. *Lancet Oncol* 2011 July; 12(7): 642–53.

ANSWERS TO MULTIPLE-CHOICE QUESTIONS

1 B, C, D
2 B, C

PART 5
Outcomes

CHAPTER 15

What is the role of surveillance for colorectal cancer?

Daedong Kim
The University of Texas MD Anderson Cancer Center, Houston, TX, USA

KEY POINTS

- The primary aim of surveillance is to detect locoregional recurrence, metastases, or metachronous primary disease at an early, asymptomatic stage
- Several randomized controlled trials (RCTs) evaluating different follow-up strategies showed no significant differences in survival between more intensive versus less intensive surveillance programs
- The ongoing GILDA, FACS, and COLOFOL trials are more likely to reflect any advances in modern surgical techniques and the use of adjuvant therapies.

Introduction

Approximately two-thirds of patients with colorectal cancer (CRC) will present with potentially curable disease by radical surgery and/or adjuvant chemotherapy. Of these, 30–50% will subsequently develop recurrent disease [1;2]. Relapse most often presents within 5 years after the resection of primary disease, with 80% of recurrences occurring within the first 3 years [3]. The most common sites of recurrence are the liver, the lungs, and the original site of resection [4–6].

After definitive treatment is completed, it is common clinical practice to monitor patients for several years with follow-up strategies designed to detect tumor recurrence at a stage when further curative procedures can be used. Despite this widespread practice, there is considerable controversy about the

Colorectal Cancer: Diagnosis and Clinical Management, First Edition. Edited by John H. Scholefield and Cathy Eng.

optimal frequency, the kinds of essential tests, and the duration of surveillance to detect recurrence.

The primary aim of surveillance in patients with CRC treated by curative surgery is to detect locoregional recurrence, metastases, or metachronous primary disease at an early, asymptomatic stage. Compared with those who are symptomatic, patients identified with recurrence as a result of surveillance programs have a higher rate of curative salvage resection and better rates of survival than those whose recurrences present with symptoms [7;8].

Randomized controlled trials and meta-analyses

Several randomized controlled trials (RCTs) evaluating different follow-up strategies showed no significant differences in survival between more intensive versus less intensive surveillance programs, with the exception of two trials [7;9–15]. However, even in these two trials, the improved survival is attributed not only to curative surgery, as in the case of resectable liver metastases, but also to additional (4–11%) attributions of other factors, including increased psychosocial support, promotion of beneficial dietary and lifestyle factors, and improved treatment of co-morbidity [16;17].

Four meta-analyses reported a 20–33% reduction in the hazard ratio and an absolute risk reduction of 7% for 5-year mortality with intensive follow-up, although no improvement was seen in the cancer-specific survival rate [9;12;14;18].

It is important to note that in a meta-analysis, small sample sizes, the inclusion of both colon and rectal cancers, and significant heterogeneity in the surveillance programs, including combinations in types of procedures and frequency, make it impossible to infer the best combination and frequency of visits, blood tests, endoscopic procedures, and radiologic investigations. Furthermore, the studies in meta-analyses are often performed over a broad span of time, during which the introduction of more efficacious chemotherapy, more sensitive CT scans, and more aggressive liver resection strategies need to be accounted for.

Follow-up tests and procedures

Although a significant number of recurrences are detected by symptoms, it is hard to discern early hepatic, lung, or anastomotic recurrences using solely history-taking and physical examination. In one meta-analysis, more follow-up was found to be statistically insignificant, but was favored to reduce mortality and incurable recurrence over no follow-up at all [19].

Carcinoembryonic antigen (CEA) forms the backbone of surveillance and CEA titers are elevated in 60% of patients with recurrence [8;20–22]. However, CEA is most sensitive for hepatic and retroperitoneal metastases and least sensitive for local recurrences and peritoneal or pulmonary disease [22]. Therefore, the primary intent of serial CEA measurement is to detect asymptomatic hepatic metastases and it can be an optimal tool in those patients whose CEA is elevated preoperatively [23]. Although the utility of serial CEA testing has been questioned, it helps to detect asymptomatic and curable recurrence and seems to have a positive effect on survival [24;25].

Chest-imaging is recommended as part of the evaluation. Furthermore, as these metastases are located at peripheral sites they are more amenable to resection; in fact, more than 70% of pulmonary recurrences found on chest CT are treatable by curative resection. Annual chest CT was therefore included in the American Society of Clinical Oncology (ASCO) recommendations for high-risk patients [8;18].

Ultrasonography and CT scans of the abdomen can assist in detecting recurrences in conjunction with elevated CEA titers, because CEA monitoring can detect hepatic recurrences prior to or at the same time as detection by liver imaging [26]. Such follow-up was associated with earlier detection of hepatic recurrences susceptible to curative surgical resection and a reduction in cancer related mortality [24;27].

18F-fluorodeoxyglucose-positron emission tomography (FDG-PET) is limited to use as an adjunctive tool combined with CT, where it can be useful for patients who have an elevated CEA level accompanying a normal CT scan to determine the location and extent of an otherwise occult disease recurrence (28). However, the use of systematic FDG-PET as a regular part of a surveillance strategy is dubious because of several limitations, including the normal physiologic uptake of FDG in certain organs, the poor uptake in mucinous cancers, the inability to detect small lesions (<1 cm), and high cost [29].

Colonoscopy can be used to detect anastomotic recurrences or metachronous cancers during surveillance, and the resectability of recurrences detected by colonoscopy was higher than in other modalities [8;9;30]. However, the incidences of such recurrences were reported to be low (1.1–6.3%) and there was no evidence of a survival benefit with the detection of intraluminal recurrent disease [24;25]. The optimal interval between colonoscopies is unknown but the first postoperative examination is recommended after 1 year and subsequent studies are recommended at 3- to

5-yearly intervals, unless intervening events occur, such as the identification of high risk polyps (villous adenoma, tubular adenoma >1cm, or high grade dysplasia) [31].

The current guidelines of major health organizations

Existing data suggest a regimen of intensive surveillance, though guidelines produced by major health organizations vary, as illustrated in Table 15.1.

Promising future trials

The Gruppo Italiano di Lavoro per la Diagnosi Anticipata (GILDA) group of investigators is currently conducting a randomized trial of 'intensive' versus 'minimal' follow-up in patients with stage II or III colorectal cancer. Major outcomes being investigated include OS, a better timing profile of recurrence diagnosis, quality of life, and financial costs. An interim analysis did not demonstrate any improvement in OS between two groups; however, the follow-up time was short [32].

The FACS trial from the UK has explored the effect of CEA monitoring in primary care and intensive hospital follow-up with CT and ultrasound scanning. The primary outcome is the number of recurrences treated with curative intensive surgery, but enrollment remains slow.

In the multi-centre COLOFOL study, participants are randomized to either a 'low frequency' or a 'high frequency' follow-up. The only difference between regimens is the interval between follow-up test, performed at 1 and 3 years for the low frequency and at 6 month intervals in the high frequency group. The primary outcomes are OS and disease-specific survival.

Note that these trials are more likely to reflect any advances in modern surgical techniques and in the use of adjuvant therapies to treat CRC. Future randomized trials need to focus on larger sample sizes, and to identify the contribution of the specific elements of surveillance to outcomes in detail. One of the most intriguing concepts in surveillance is adapting the intensity of surveillance to the patient's risk of recurrence. Clearly, patients who are considered at a higher risk of recurrence experience greater benefits from surveillance than lower risk patients. Individualized risk stratification empowers patients, enhancing their ability to make meaningful choices and ultimately improving outcomes.

Table 15.1 Summary of guidelines regarding surveillance produced by major health organizations.

Guideline	ASCRS(2004)(35)	ASCO(2005)(18)	ACPGBI(2007)(36)	NCCN(2009)(37)	ESMO(2009)(38)
History and Physical Examination	3 mo for minimum 2 yr	3–6 mo for 3 yr then 6 mo for 2 yr	NR for frequency	3–6 mo for 2 yr then 6 mo for 3 yr	3–6 mo for 3 yr then 6 mo for 2 yr
CEA	3 mo for minimum 2 yr	3 mo for 3 yr in stage II or III	NR	3–6 mo for 2 yr then 6 mo for 3 yr	3–6 mo for 3 yr then 6 mo for 2 yr (if initially elevated)
Imaging	NR	CT of chest/abd/pelvis annually for 3 yr (high risk)	CT of chest/abd, within first 2 yr	CT of abd/pelvis annually for 3 yr (high risk)	CT of chest/abd/pelvis 6 mo for 3 yr (high risk) then annually for 2 yr
Colonoscopy	Every 3 yr	At 3 yr postop, then every 5 yr or clinically indicated	Every 5 yr	At 1 yr postop. Then clinically indicated	At 1 yr postop, then every 3 yr (colon) or 5 yr (rectum)

ASCRS, American Society of Colon and Rectal Surgeons; ASCO, American Society of Clinical Oncology; ACPGBI, Association of Coloproctology of Great Britain & Ireland; NCCN, National Comprehensive Cancer Network; ESMO, European Society of Medical Oncology; CT, computed tomography; NR, not recommended

CASE STUDY

The patient was diagnosed with sigmoid colon cancer and underwent a laparoscopic anterior resection in May 2010 for a T3 N2, poorly differentiated colon cancer with 7/15 lymph nodes positive for disease. The patient underwent 6 months of adjuvant chemotherapy with FOLFOX until November 2010 and was placed on surveillance. There were no abnormalities in physical examination and all other reviews of systems were negative, but her CEA rose from 1.8 ng/ml to 10.7 ng/ml in a follow-up examination in May 2011. She then had an abdominal CT scan which revealed a mass lesion measuring 3.2 cm in the left lobe of the liver, and a 2.4 cm lesion in the right ovary suspicious for malignancy. She underwent surgery in July 2011 for left lobectomy with bilateral salpingo-oophorectomy.

TIPS AND TRICKS / KEY PITFALLS

- There is no evidence of the usefulness of complete blood cell (CBC) counts, liver function tests, or other tumor markers such as CA19-9 in surveillance, and none of these tests are currently recommended in the published guidelines.
- Benign conditions which can elevate CEA include smoking, infections, inflammatory bowel disease, pancreatitis, liver cirrhosis, and some benign epithelial tumors [33;34]. A temporary rise in CEA after chemotherapy and radiotherapy can be attributed to the death of tumor cells and release of CEA into the blood stream. However, in benign diseases, this is usually not elevated above 10 ng/ml.
- One of the RCTs reported that recurrences, which occurred in patients who received intensive follow-up, were more likely to undergo a curative resection and have a significant survival benefit, but this finding was limited to a subgroup analysis (stage II colon cancer and those with rectal tumors) [9].

MULTIPLE-CHOICE QUESTIONS

(You may include questions with one or multiple correct answers. If applicable, you may wish to include a feedback paragraph to explain the correct answer.)

1 What is not the primary aim of surveillance in patients with CRC treated by curative intent surgery?

A. Detect locoregional recurrence
B. Detect metastases
C. Detect synchronous primary disease
D. Detect metachronous primary disease
E. None of above

2 What is the best additional test to discern the possibility of ovarian metastasis in this patient?
 A. Repeated CEA level monitoring
 B. Gynecologic physical examination
 C. Pelvic ultrasonography
 D. Positron Emission Tomography (PET)
 E. Pelvic MRI

3 What makes it impossible to infer the best combination and frequency of surveillance tests from the meta-analyses of the RCTs evaluating follow-up strategies of CRC?
 A. Significant heterogeneity in the surveillance programs
 B. They were performed over a broad span of time
 C. Inclusion of both colon and rectal cancers
 D. Small sample sizes
 E. All of above

References

1 Rao AR, Kagan AR, Chan PM, Gilbert HA, Nussbaum H, Hintz BL. Patterns of recurrence following curative resection alone for adenocarcinoma of the rectum and sigmoid colon. *Cancer* 1981; 48: 1492–5.

2 Böhm B, Schwenk W, Hucke HP, Stock W. Does methodic long-term follow-up affect survival after curative resection of colorectal carcinoma? *Dis Colon Rectum* 1993; 36(3): 280–6.

3 Sargent DJ, Wieand HS, Haller DG, Gray R, Benedetti JK, Buyse M, et al. Disease-free survival versus overall survival as a primary end point for adjuvant colon cancer studies: individual patient data from 20,898 patients on 18 randomized trials. *J Clin Oncol* 2005 Dec 1; 23(34): 8664–70.

4 Taylor WE, Donohue JH, Gunderson LL, Nelson H, Nagorney DM, Devine RM, et al. The Mayo Clinic experience with multimodality treatment of locally advanced or recurrent colon cancer. *Ann Surg Oncol* 2002; 9: 177–85.

5 Manfredi S, Bouvier AM, Lepage C, Hatem C, Dancourt V, Faivre J. Incidence and patterns of recurrence after resection for cure of colonic cancer in a well defined population. *Br J Surg* 2006; 93: 1115–22.

6 Kievit J. Follow-up of patients with colorectal cancer: numbers needed to test and treat. *Eur J Cancer* 2002; 38: 986–99.

7 Wang T, Cui Y, Huang WS, Deng YH, Gong W, Li CJ, et al. The role of postoperative colonoscopic surveillance after radical surgery for colorectal cancer: a prospective, randomized clinical study. *Gastrointest Endosc* 2009; 69(3): 609–15.

8 Chau I, Allen MJ, Cunningham D, Norman AR, Brown G, Ford HE, et al. The value of routine serum carcino-embryonic antigen measurement and computed tomography in the surveillance of patients after adjuvant chemotherapy for colorectal cancer. *J Clin Oncol* 2004; 22: 1420–9.

9 Rodríguez-Moranta F, Saló J, Arcusa A, Boadas J, Piñol V, Bessa X, et al. Postoperative surveillance in patients with colorectal cancer who have undergone curative resection: a prospective, multicenter, randomized, controlled trial. *J Clin Oncol* 2006; 24: 386–93.

10 Mākelā JT, Laitinen SO, Kairaluoma MI. Five-year follow-up after radical surgery for colorectal cancer: results of a prospective randomized trial. *Arch Surg* 1995; 130: 1062–7.

11 Ohlsson B, Breland U, Ekberg H, Graffner H, Tranberg KG. Follow-up after curative surgery for colorectal carcinoma: randomized comparison with no follow-up. *Dis Colon Rectum* 1995; 38: 619–26.

12 Kjeldsen BJ, Kronborg O, Fenger C, Jörgensen OD. A prospective randomized study of follow-up after radical surgery for colorectal cancer. *Br J Surg* 1997; 84: 666–9.

13 Schoemaker D, Black R, Giles L, Toouli J. Yearly colonoscopy, liver CT, and chest radiography do not influence 5-year survival of colorectal cancer patients. *Gastroenterology* 1998; 114: 7–14.

14 Secco GB, Fardelli R, Gianquinto D, Bonfante P, Baldi E, Ravera G, et al. Efficacy and cost of risk adapted follow-up in patients after colorectal cancer surgery: a prospective, randomized and controlled trial. *Eur J Surg Oncol* 2002; 28: 418–23.

15 Pietra N, Sarli L, Costi R, Ouchemi C, Grattarola M, Peracchia A. Role of follow-up in management of local recurrences of colorectal cancer: a prospective, randomized study. *Dis Colon Rectum* 1998; 41: 1127–33.

16 Kievit J. Follow-up of patients with colorectal cancer: numbers needed to test and treat. *Eur J Cancer* 2002; 38: 986–99.

17 Renehan AG, Egger M, Saunders MP, O'Dwyer ST. Mechanisms of improved survival from intensive follow up in colorectal cancer: a hypothesis. *Br J Cancer* 2005; 92: 430–3.

18 Desch CE, Benson AB III, Somerfield MR, Flynn PJ, Krause C, Loprinzi CL, et al. American Society of Clinical Oncology. Colorectal cancer surveillance: 2005 update of an American Society of Clinical Oncology practice guideline. *J Clin Oncol* 2005; 23(33): 8512–19.

19 Jeffery M, Hickey B, Hider P: Follow-up strategies for patients treated for non-metastatic colorectal cancer. *Cochrane Database Syst Rev* 2007, 1: CD002200.

20 Graham RA, Wang S, Catalano PJ, Haller DG. Postsurgical surveillance of colon cancer: preliminary cost analysis of physician examination, carcinoembryonic antigen testing, chest X-ray, and colonoscopy. *Ann Surg* 1998; 228: 59–63.

21 Zeng Z, Cohen AM, Urmacher C. Usefulness of carcinoembryonic antigen monitoring despite normal preoperative values in node-positive colon cancer patients. *Dis Colon Rectum* 1993; 36: 1063–8.

22 Moertel CG, Fleming TR, Macdonald JS, Haller DG, Laurie JA, Tangen C. An evaluation of the carcinoembryonic antigen (CEA) test for monitoring patients with resected colon cancer. *JAMA* 1993; 270(8): 943–7.

23 Locker GY, Hamilton S, Harris J, Jessup JM, Kemeny N, Macdonald JS, et al. ASCO 2006 update of recommendations for the use of tumor markers in gastrointestinal cancer. *J Clin Oncol* 2006 Nov 20; 24(33): 5313–27.

24 Tjandra J, Chan M: Follow-up after curative resection of colorectal cancer: a meta-analysis. *Dis Colon Rectum* 2007, 50(11): 1783–99.

25 Renehan AG, Egger M, Saunders MP, O'Dwyer ST. Impact on survival of intensive follow up after curative resection for colorectal cancer: systematic review and meta-analysis of randomised trials. *BMJ* 2002 Apr 6; 324(7341): 813.

26 Sugarbaker PH, Gianola FJ, Dwyer A, et al: A simplified plan for follow-up of patients with colon and rectal cancer supported by prospective studies of laboratory and radiologic test results. *Surgery* 1987; 102: 79–87.

27 Jeffery M, Hickey B, Hider P: Follow-up strategies for patients treated for non-metastatic colorectal cancer. *Cochrane Database Syst Rev* 2007, 1: CD002200.

28 Libutti SK, Alexander HR Jr, Choyke P, Bartlett DL, Bacharach SL, Whatley M, et al. A prospective study of 2-[18F] fluoro-2-deoxy-D-glucose/positron emission tomography scan, 99mTc-labeled arcitumomab (CEA-scan), and blind second-look laparotomy for detecting colon cancer recurrence in patients with increasing carcinoembryonic antigen levels. *Ann Surg Oncol* 2001 Dec; 8(10): 779–86.

29 Kamel IR, Cohade C, Neyman E, Fishman EK, Wahl RL. Incremental value of CT in PET/CT of patients with colorectal carcinoma. *Abdom Imaging* 2004 Nov–Dec; 29(6): 663–8.

30 Min BW, Urn JW, Moon HY. Role of regular follow-up after curative surgery for colorectal cancer. *Hepatogastroenterology* 2007; 54: 63–6.

31 Winawer S, Fletcher R, Rex D, Bond J, Burt R, Ferrucci J, et al. Colorectal cancer screening and surveillance: clinical guidelines and rationale-Update based on new evidence. *Gastroenterology* 2003 Feb; 124(2): 544–60.

32 Grossmann EM, Johnson FE, Virgo KS, Longo WE, Fossati R. Follow-up of colorectal cancer patients after resection with curative intent – the GILDA trial. *Surg Oncol* 2004; 13: 119–24.

33 van der Schouw YT, Verbeek AL, Wobbes T, Segers MF, Thomas CM. Comparison of four serum tumour markers in the diagnosis of colorectal carcinoma. *Br J Cancer* 1992; 66(1): 148–54.

34 George PK, Loewenstein MS, O'Brien MJ, Bronstein B, Koff RS, Zamcheck N. Circulating CEA levels in patients with fulminant hepatitis. *Dig Dis Sci* 1982; 27(2): 139–42.

35 Anthony T, Simmang C, Hyman N, et al. Practice parameters for the surveillance and follow-up of patients with colon and rectal cancer. *Dis Colon Rectum* 2004; 47: 807–17.

36 The Association of Coloproctology of Great Britain and Ireland (ACPGBI). Guidelines for the management of colorectal cancer, 2007. Available from: URL: *http://www.acpgbi.org.uk/assets/documents/COLO_guides.pdf*

37 Engstrom PF, Arnoletti JP, Benson AB III, et al. NCCN Clinical Practice Guidelines in Oncology: colon cancer. *J Natl Compr Canc Net* 2009; 7: 778–831.

38 Van Cutsem E, Oliveira J; ESMO Guidelines Working Group. Primary colon cancer: ESMO clinical recommendations for diagnosis, adjuvant treatment and follow-up. *Ann Oncol* 2009; 20(suppl 4): 49–50.

ANSWERS TO MULTIPLE-CHOICE QUESTIONS

1 C
2 D
3 E

PART 6
Vignettes

CHAPTER 16

The young patient with colorectal cancer – genetic counseling discussion

Sarah Bannon, Maureen E. Mork & Miguel A. Rodriguez-Bigas
The University of Texas MD Anderson Cancer Center, Department of Surgical Oncology, Houston, TX, USA

Clinical Vignette #1

A 40-year-old male presents for genetic consultation. He was recently diagnosed with a hepatic flexure adenocarcinoma with mucinous features on colonoscopy following episodes of hematochezia. His family history is significant for his paternal grandmother who was diagnosed with uterine cancer in her 50s and a paternal uncle who died of colorectal cancer in his 40s. The patient's father died in his 50s in an accident, and the patient's mother is living in her 60s. The patient has one sister, age 30, and has two children, ages 5 and 10. The patient's referring physician ordered microsatellite instability (MSI) and immunohistochemistry (IHC) testing on the patient's biopsy. MSI testing reveals a MSI-high tumor with loss of staining of *MSH2* and *MSH6* and intact staining for *MLH1* and *PMS2*. The patient consents to *MSH2* genetic testing, including sequencing, deletion/duplication testing, and *EPCAM* deletion testing.

Discussion

While the median age of colorectal cancer (CRC) diagnosis is 70 years, approximately 17% of CRC cases are diagnosed in individuals under 50 [1]. Individuals with CRC at a young age, even without a significant family history of CRC, are at increased risk of having an underlying genetic susceptibility, putting them and their family members at significantly increased risk of developing cancer. Approximately 5% of CRC is hereditary, meaning that it is due

Colorectal Cancer: Diagnosis and Clinical Management, First Edition. Edited by John H. Scholefield and Cathy Eng.

to a single mutation in a gene that predisposes an individual to high lifetime risks of CRC and other cancers [2]. Hereditary non-polyposis colorectal cancer (HNPCC), also referred to as Lynch syndrome (LS), accounts for 2–3% of all CRCs. Familial adenomatous polyposis (FAP) and *MUTYH*-associated polyposis (MAP), inherited adenomatous polyposis conditions, account for approximately 2% of CRC cases. Less than 1% of cases of CRC are attributed to the rarer hamartomatous polyposis conditions, specifically Peutz-Jeghers syndrome (PJS), juvenile polyposis syndrome (JPS), and Cowden syndrome (CS) [2]. Detailed management guidelines are proposed by the National Comprehensive Cancer Centers Network® (NCCN®) Guidelines for Colorectal Cancer Screening [3].

Lynch syndrome (LS)

Lynch syndrome, an autosomal dominant condition caused by mutations in the mismatch repair genes (*MLH1*, *MSH2*, *MSH6*, *PMS2*, and rarely, *EPCAM*), is associated with tumors that demonstrate MSI. The majority of cases are inherited from a parent; the *de novo*, or new mutation, rate is not known, although expected to be low (<2%) [4]. LS is primarily characterized by an increased risk for CRC in men and women of 20–80% by age 70, with a preponderance of right-sided tumors. The mean age of CRC diagnosis in individuals with LS is 42–61 years. CRCs associated with LS often show histological evidence of MSI and host immune response, including lymphocytic infiltrates, Crohn's-like lymphocytic reaction, poor differentiation with signet ring cells, medullary (solid/cribriform) growth pattern, and/or mucinous features [5].

Women with LS are also at increased risk of cancers of the endometrium of 20–60% by age 70, with a mean age of diagnosis of 47–55 years [6]. Cancers of the ovary (4–11%), stomach (5–8%), small intestine (~6%), hepatobiliary tract (2–18%), upper urinary tract (8% overall, up to 27% in males), brain/central nervous system (CNS) (4%), and sebaceous neoplasms (1–9%) are also seen at increased frequency compared to the general population [7;8]. Surveillance and management recommendations for CRC and extra-colonic cancers are outlined in the NCCN Guidelines® for Colorectal Cancer Screening, version 2.2012 [3].

The ranges in cancer risk are due to the varying penetrance of the mismatch repair genes. *MLH1* and *MSH2* mutations account for approximately 90% of mutations causing LS; *MSH6* mutations for 7–10%; and *PMS2* mutations in more than 5% [2]. Deletions in the *EPCAM* gene, which result in epigenetic silencing of *MSH2*, account for 1% of families [9]. LS associated with *MLH1*, *MSH2*, and *EPCAM* mutations is considered 'classic' LS, with the highest penetrance of cancer risks. *MSH6* and *PMS2*-associated LS could be considered an attenuated phenotype, with reduced CRC risks (44% in *MSH6*, 20% in *PMS2*) [8].

Evaluation

Age of diagnosis, tumor location, pathology features, presence or absence of polyps, and family history are important criteria to consider when evaluating a patient with CRC diagnosed at less than 50 years. MSI-high histology, regardless of patient age, should prompt evaluation by PCR (polymerase chain reaction) and immunohistochemistry.

CRC less than 50 with no synchronous adenomas

In patients without polyposis, the Revised Bethesda Guidelines help to determine whether a patient is appropriate for MSI analysis [5]. These include:

- CRC diagnosed in a patient <50 years.
- Presence of synchronous or metachronous LS-associated tumors,* regardless of age;
- CRC with MSI-histology** diagnosed in a patient <60 years;
- CRC diagnosed in a patient with one or more first-degree relatives with an LS-associated cancer, with one of the cancers diagnosed <50 years;
- CRC diagnosed in a patient with two or more first-degree relatives with LS-related cancers, regardless of age.

  *includes CRC, endometrial, gastric, ovarian, pancreas, ureter and renal pelvis, biliary tract, brain (glioblastoma), small bowel, sebaceous adenoma/carcinoma

  **presence of tumor-infiltrating lymphocytes, Crohn's-like lymphocytic reaction, mucinous/signet-ring cell differentiation, medullary growth pattern

Initial tumor analysis can be performed by either IHC staining for the mismatch repair proteins, a PCR-based MSI assay, or both. MSI and IHC are best validated in colorectal cancer tissue for the detection of LS; however, these tests can also be performed in endometrial tumors and other LS-associated tumors. MSI and IHC testing performed in combination is the most specific for LS, detecting approximately 95–99% of cases [10].

Approximately 15% of sporadic (non-hereditary) colorectal cancers have high levels of MSI. These are most often associated with loss of MLH1 and/or *PMS2* proteins in the tumor on IHC analysis. Sporadic mechanisms can account for the majority of these MSI high tumors, including hypermethylation of the *MLH1* promoter and *BRAF* V600E mutations. Sporadic hypermethylation of the *MLH1* promoter occurs most often in older patients with predominantly proximal colon tumors. Hypermethylation of the *MLH1* promoter accounts for approximately 80% of MSI-high tumors, meaning that most MSI-high tumors can be attributed to sporadic methylation [10;11]. However, hypermethylation of the *MLH1* promoter can also be seen rarely in patients with Lynch syndrome, in which a germline *MLH1* mutation exists on one allele and sporadic methylation provides the 'second hit'. In other sporadic MSI-high tumors, the *BRAF* gene acquires a somatic mutation, typically V600E. This somatic mutation drives mismatch repair gene methylation, which also results in a tumor that is MSI-high, with loss of MLH1 protein expression [12]. The presence of a *BRAF* V600E mutation reduces the likelihood that a young patient has Lynch syndrome, but does not exclude the possibility. Therefore, young patients with a strong family history warrant close evaluation for Lynch syndrome, even if a *BRAF* mutation or *MLH1* hypermethylation is present in the tumor.

Ideally, MSI and IHC for the mismatch repair enzymes are performed first on the tumor tissue to guide further genetic analysis. Figure 16.1 displays a recommended testing strategy for patients who undergo MSI and IHC analysis [11]. In rare cases, tumor tissue may not be available or access to pathology-based screening tests may be limited. For patients with a personal history of cancer, it may be reasonable to proceed with comprehensive germline genetic testing of the four mismatch repair genes. Currently, genetic testing detects mutations in only 50–70% of individuals with diagnostic tumor studies [11]. Therefore, approximately 30–50% of patients with a presumptive diagnosis of Lynch syndrome based on abnormal tumor studies (Figure 16.1) have negative germline genetic test results. A negative result is considered non-diagnostic, or inconclusive, and does not rule out the possibility of Lynch syndrome in individuals whose tumors have not been analyzed.

If a mutation is identified in a family with LS, at-risk relatives are recommended to undergo predictive genetic testing at adulthood (18 years or older). Genetic testing is not recommended in minors for several ethical reasons, including that Lynch syndrome is not characterized by childhood onset cancers; thus there are no surveillance or management recommendations for individuals under 18 years of age who test positive for LS. For individuals with tumor studies suggestive of LS but no detectable mutation, all at-risk relatives are recommended to undergo LS surveillance, as predictive genetic testing is not available (Figure 16.1).

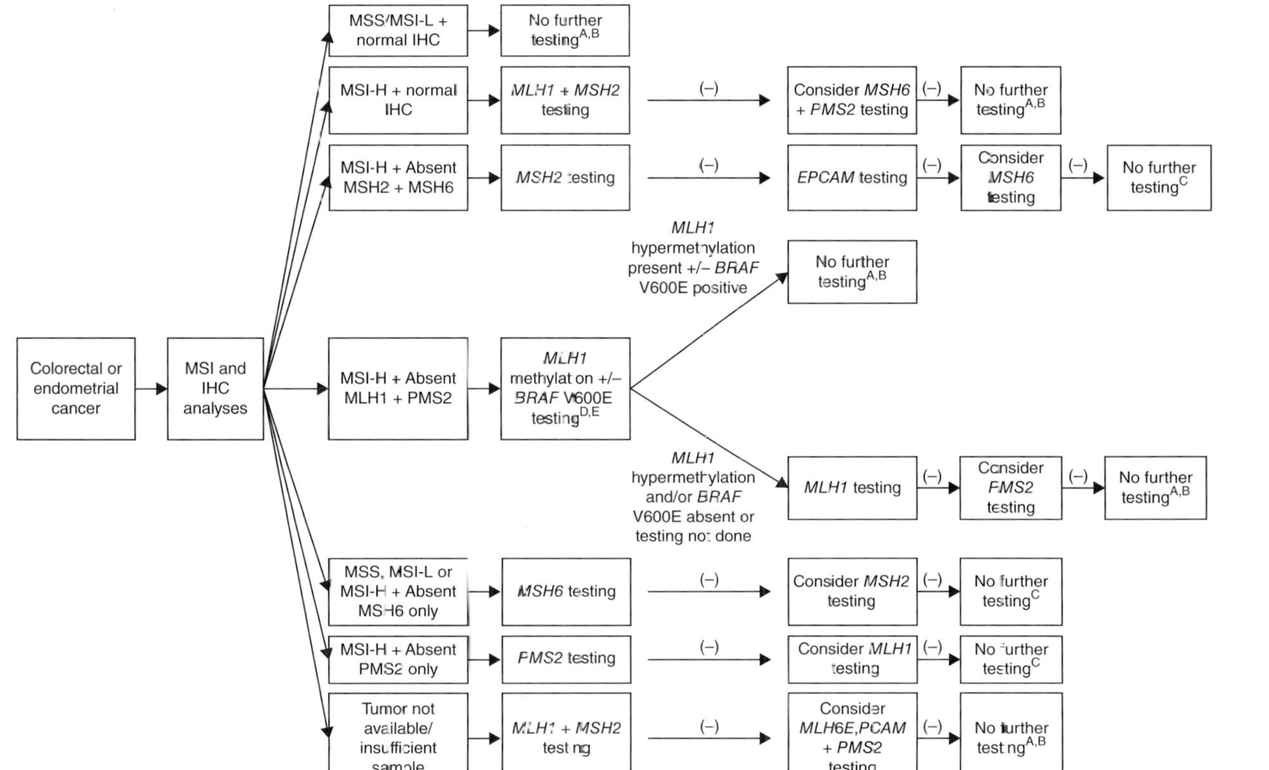

Figure 16.1 (a) If strong family history (e.g. Amsterdam criteria) is present, additional testing may be warranted in the proband or consider tumor testing in another affected family member due to the possibility of a phenocopy. (b) Management should be based on individual and family risk assessment. (c) Affected individual and at-risk family members should follow Lynch syndrome management recommendations. (d) *BRAF* testing is not appropriate in endometrial cancers. (e) If strong family history is present, direct germline testing may be indicated instead of additional tumor studies [8]. With kind permission from Springer Science+Business Media.

Clinical Vignette #2

A 32-year-old female presents for genetic consultation. She was recently diagnosed with a rectal adenocarcinoma on colonoscopy, which was performed to evaluate a change in bowel habits. The colonoscopy report is also significant for multiple polyps, confirmed to be tubular adenomas, numbering approximately 20 throughout the left colon. Her family history is significant for her mother with colorectal cancer diagnosed at age 45 and thyroid cancer at age 50.

Discussion

The presence of multiple adenomatous polyps (10–15+) in the young patient with CRC is typically more suggestive of attenuated familial adenomatous polyposis (AFAP) or MutYH-associated polyposis (MAP), particularly if the tumor is left-sided and a family history of multiple polyps is present. The number, location, and type of polyps are important to note. Adenomatous polyps are most highly concerning for AFAP and/or MAP. Hyperplastic, sessile serrated, or inflammatory polyps do not typically occur in patients with AFAP; however, one or two may be noted amongst a majority of adenomas. Hyperplastic polyposis, or a combination of adenomas with a preponderance of hyperplastic polyps, is most often seen as its own clinically distinct polyposis syndrome, for which no gene has been identified.

Familial Adenomatous Polyposis (FAP)

FAP, an autosomal dominant condition caused by mutations in the *APC* gene, is characterized by hundreds to thousands of adenomatous colon polyps, beginning on average at age 16 years [13]. Over 90% of individuals who have FAP will develop adenomatous (pre-cancerous) polyps in the colon. By age 35, 95% of patients have multiple adenomas. Without endoscopic intervention or colectomy, the risk of CRC approaches 100% in patients with FAP, with a preponderance of left-sided cancers. Approximately two-thirds of cases of FAP are inherited from an affected parent; one-third, however, are due to *de novo* germline mutations in the *APC* gene [14].

Extracolonic characteristics are also seen in FAP. Gastric fundic gland polyps occur in approximately 50% of patients with FAP [15]. Approximately 50–90% of patients with FAP develop duodenal adenomas, typically periampullary, which are associated with an increased risk of small bowel adenocarcinoma (4–12%). Duodenal adenocarcinomas in patients with FAP develop at a mean age of 45–52 years; however, the range reported is

17–81 years [16]. Additional extracolonic cancers in patients with FAP include pancreas (~1%), thyroid (typically papillary type; however, cribiform variant is also seen, 1–2%), CNS (typically medulloblastoma, <1%), and liver (hepatoblastoma, 1.6%) [17;18;19].

A subset of FAP, attenuated FAP (AFAP), is characterized by patients with a fewer number and more proximally located colonic polyps, a lower but significant risk of CRC, and a later age of diagnosis than classic FAP. Individuals with AFAP typically have an average of 25 adenomas. The lifetime risk for CRC in patients with attenuated FAP has not been established; the cumulative risk of CRC by 80 years is estimated to be approximately 70% [20]. Patients with AFAP typically have fewer of the extracolonic manifestations associated with classic FAP.

Approximately 30% of patients with attenuated FAP have a deleterious mutation in the *APC* gene. Of the remaining 60% of individuals with AFAP who do not have an *APC* mutation identified, some have *MUTYH*-associated polyposis (MAP) and others have non-diagnostic genetic testing [21].

MUTYH-Associated Polyposis (MAP)

MAP is caused by biallelic mutations in the mut-Y homolog gene (*MUTYH* or *MYH*), involved in DNA base-excision repair. Patients with MAP develop multiple colorectal adenomas, typically 20–100, usually beginning after age 40. MAP is often clinically indistinguishable from AFAP based on the number of colon adenomas. MAP is distinguished from other CRC cancer predisposition syndromes because it is inherited in an autosomal recessive pattern. Individuals with MAP must inherit a *MYH* mutation from both parents, meaning that patients with MAP often have no family history of CRC or polyposis, or only affected siblings. The risk for extracolonic cancers is not clearly defined, although cancers of the small bowel, thyroid, stomach, and breast have been reported [22]. One study has found that approximately 2% of all patients with CRC diagnosed under age 50 carry biallelic *MYH* mutations [23]. This is an important consideration for the young patient who has a MSI tumor, particularly if he or she presents with synchronous colorectal adenomas. The risk of CRC for monoallelic *MYH* carriers is also unclear, although estimated to be two times the general population risk (10–15%) [24].

Evaluation

In the young patient with multiple polyps and a family history of polyps and/or CRC consistent with autosomal dominant inheritance, genetic testing for FAP is appropriate. Genetic testing of the *APC* gene should include sequencing and deletion/duplication analysis. If an *APC* mutation is detected, at-risk children are recommended to undergo genetic testing at age 10 for classic FAP and in the late teens for AFAP [13;25]. In families with no detectable mutation, endoscopic surveillance is recommended for all at-risk relatives.

In some cases, there is no clear autosomal dominant inheritance, or the status of polyps in other family members in unknown. If such a patient has no identifiable mutations in the *APC* gene, it is appropriate to consider proceeding to *MYH* genetic testing. The testing strategy for MAP differs from other hereditary CRC syndromes, as MAP is autosomal recessive. Testing is available for the two common mutations in the Caucasian population (Y179C and G396D previously reported as Y165C and G382D) [22]. Testing can be initiated with the common mutations with reflex to full gene sequencing, or may begin with full gene sequencing. Once an individual is identified as having biallelic *MYH* mutations, his parents are presumed to be monoallelic carriers and his siblings are at 25% risk of having MAP and at 50% risk of being carriers. The children of the affected individual are obligate carriers of at least a single *MYH* mutation. The partner of the affected individual may undergo carrier testing to determine risk to offspring, as there is a 1–2% population carrier frequency of *MYH* mutations [27].

In some patients with oligopolyposis (<20 polyps), no mutations are identified in the *APC* or *MYH* genes. Endoscopic surveillance following attenuated FAP surveillance guidelines is recommended for all at-risk relatives in these families [3].

Genetic counseling and testing

Professional organization consensus statements, including American Society of Clinical Oncology, American College of Medical Genetics, American Society of Human Genetics, and Evaluation of Genomic Applications in Practice and Prevention (EGAPP) Working Group, recommend criteria for offering genetic testing/counseling including:

1 CRC in three individuals, one of whom is a first-degree relative of the other two, with two generations affected and one case diagnosed at under 50 (ASCO) [27]; and
2 personal or family history of a cancer or cancers known to be associated with specific genes or mutations, such as sebaceous skin lesions, endometrial cancer at a young age, small bowel, upper urinary tract, and/or colorectal in the context of a compelling family history, young age at onset, and familial clustering of related tumors (ACMG) [28].

The EGAPP Working Group in 2009 found sufficient evidence to recommend that individuals with newly diagnosed CRC be offered genetic testing for LS for the purpose of reducing morbidity and mortality in their relatives [29].

Genetic counseling is a process that addresses the risk of occurrence of a genetic disorder in a family. Genetic counselors are trained to help families understand the probability of an inherited condition, the risks and benefits of genetic testing, the natural history of the genetic condition, the recommended management strategies, and the risk to relatives. Genetic counselors also assist in the decision-making process and facilitate coping with the diagnosis of a hereditary condition. Genetic counseling can also be performed by another health care provider with specialized training in cancer genetics and risk assessment.

Psychosocial implications

The genetic counseling process addresses psychosocial issues raised through the diagnosis of a hereditary cancer syndrome. The majority of patients who undergo genetic counseling and testing are also dealing with a diagnosis of cancer. Psychosocial issues that can frequently arise include cancer worry, anxiety, depression, anger, fear, guilt, perception of cancer as influenced by family experiences with cancer, risk perception for cancer for self and others, whether the patient is competent to provide informed consent, presence or absence of support network, and family communication. These elements have been thoroughly explored in the literature [30;31]. Sivell et al. suggests that cancer genetic risk assessment services, such as genetic counseling, help to reduce distress in patients, and improve the accuracy the perceived risk of cancer, as well as knowledge of cancer and genetics [32].

References

1 Surveillance, Epidemiology, and End Results (SEER) Program (*www.seer.cancer.gov*) SEER*Stat Database: Incidence – SEER 9 Regs Research Data, Nov 2011 Sub (1973–2009) <Katrina/Rita Population Adjustment> – Linked To County Attributes – Total US, 1969–2010 Counties, National Cancer Institute, DCCPS, Surveillance Research Program, Surveillance Systems Branch, released April 2012, based on the November 2011 submission.

2 Jasperson et al. Hereditary and familial colon cancer. *Gastroenterology* 2010 June; 138(6): 2044–58.

3 Reproduced/adapted with permission from the NCCN Clinical Practice Guidelines in Oncology (NCCN Guidelines®) for Guideline Name 2.2012.© 2012 National Comprehensive Cancer Network, Inc. All rights reserved. The NCCN Guidelines® and illustrations herein may not be reproduced in any form for any purpose without the express written permission of the NCCN. To view the most recent and complete version of the NCCN Guidelines, go online to *NCCN.org*. NATIONAL COMPREHENSIVE CANCER

NETWORK®, NCCN®, NCCN GUIDELINES™, and all other NCCN Content are trademarks owned by the National Comprehensive Cancer Network, Inc.

4 Win et al. Determining the frequency of de novo germline mutations in DNA mismatch repair genes. *J Med Genet.* 2011 Aug; 48(8): 530–4.

5 Umar et al. Revised Bethesda Guidelines for hereditary nonpolyposis colorectal cancer (Lynch syndrome) and microsatellite instability. *J Natl Cancer Inst* 2004 Feb; 96(4): 261–8.

6 Stoffel et al. Calculation of risk of colorectal and endometrial cancer among patients with Lynch syndrome. *Gastroenterology* 2009 Nov; 137(5): 1621–7.

7 Capelle et al. Risk and epidemiological time trends of gastric cancer in Lynch syndrome carriers in the Netherlands. *Gastroenterology* 2010 Feb; 138(2): 487–92.

8 Weissman et al. Genetic Counseling Considerations in the Evaluation of Families for Lynch syndrome – A Review. *J Gen Counsel* 2011; 20(1): 5–19.

9 Rumilla et al. Frequency of deletions of EPCAM (TACSTD1) in MSH2-associated Lynch syndrome cases. *J Mol Diagn* 2011 Jan; 13(1): 93–9.

10 Boland et al. The biochemical basis of microsatellite instability and abnormal immunohistochemistry and clinical behavior in Lynch Syndrome: from bench to bedside. *Fam Cancer* 2008; 7(1): 41–52.

11 Weissman et al. Identification of individuals at risk for lynch syndrome using targeted evaluations and genetic testing: National Society of Genetic Counselors and the Collaborative Group of the Americas on Inherited Colorectal Cancer Joint Practice Guideline. *J Genet Counsel.* 2011 Nov.

12 Maestro et al. Role of the BRAF mutations in the microsatellite instability genetic pathway in sporadic colorectal cancer. *Ann Surgl Oncol* 2006 May; 14(3): 1229–36.

13 Petersen et al. Screening guidelines and premorbid diagnosis of familial adenomatous polyposis using linkage. *Gastroenterology* 1991; 100: 1658–64.

14 Bisgaard et al. Familial adenomatous polyposis (FAP): frequency, penetrance, and mutation rate. *Hum Mutat* 1994; 3: 121–5.

15 Offerhaus et al. Upper gastrointestinal polyps in familial adenomatous polyposis. *Hepatogastroenterology* 1999; 46: 667–9.

16 Kadmon et al. Duodenal adenomatosis in familial adenomatous polyposis coli. A review of the literature and results from the Heidelberg Polyposis Register. *Int J Colorectal Dis* 2001; 16: 63–75.

17 Giardello et al. Increased risk of thyroid and pancreatic carcinoma in familial adenomatous polyposis. *Gut* 1993; 34: 1394–6.

18 Hamilton et al. The molecular basis of Turcot's syndrome. *N Engl J Med* 1995; 332: 839–47.

19 Aretz et al. Somatic APC mosaicism: a frequent cause of familial adenomatous polyposis (FAP). *Hum Mutat* 2007; 28: 985–92.

20 Neklason et al. American founder mutation for attenuated familial adenomatous polyposis. *Clin Gastroenterol Hepatol* 2008; 6: 46–52.

21 Lefevre et al. Implication of MYH in colorectal polyposis. *Ann Surg* 2006; 244: 87–9.

22 Sieber et al. Multiple colorectal adenomas, classic adenomatous polyposis, and germ-line mutation in MYH. *N Engl J Med* 2003; 348: 791–9.

23 Balaguer et al. Identification of MYH mutation carriers in colorectal cancer: a multicenter, case-control, population-based study. *Clin Gastroenterol Hepatol* 2007 Mar; 5(3): 379–87.

24 Jenkins et al. Risk of colorectal cancer in monoallelic and biallelic carriers of MYH mutations: a population-based case-family study. *Cancer Epidemiol Biomarkers Prev* 2006 Feb; 15(2): 312–4.
25 Burt et al. Genetic testing and phenotype in a large kindred with attenuated familial adenomatous polyposis. *Gastroenterology*.2004; 127: 444–51.
26 Aretz et al. *MUTYH*-associated polyposis: 70 of 71 patients with biallelic mutations present with an attenuated or atypical phenotype. *Int. J Cancer* 2006; 119: 807–14.
27 ASCO Subcommittee on Genetic Testing for Cancer Susceptibility. Statement of the American Society of Clinical Oncology. *J Clin Oncolo* 1996; 14: 1730–6.
28 Joint Test and Technology Transfer Committee Working Group (ACMG/ASHG). *Gen Med* 2010 Dec; 2(6): 362–6.
29 Evaluation of Genomic Applications in Practice and Prevention (EGAPP) Working Group. Recommendations from the EGAPP Working Group: genetic testing strategies in newly diagnosed individuals with colorectal cancer aimed at reducing morbidity and mortality from Lynch syndrome in relatives. *Gen Med* 2009 Jan; 11(1): 35–41.
30 Chivers Seymore et al. What facilitates or impedes family communication following genetic testing for cancer risk? A systematic review and meta-synthesis of primary qualitative research. *J Genet Couns* 2010 Aug; 19(4): 330–42.
31 Trepanier et al. Genetic cancer risk assessment and counseling: recommendations of the National Society of Genetic Counselors. *J Genet Couns* 2004 Apr; 13(2): 83–114.
32 Sivell et al. How risk is perceived, constructed and interpreted by clients in clinical genetics, and the effects on decision making: systematic review. *J Genet Couns* 2008; Feb 17(1): 30–63.

CHAPTER 17

Best practices of supportive care while receiving chemotherapy

Maura Polansky
The University of Texas MD Anderson Cancer Center, Houston, TX, USA

Clinical Vignette #1

Chemotherapy-induced diarrhea

A 57-year-old woman with advanced colorectal cancer presents for management of her disease. You and the patient have elected to initiate systemic chemotherapy.

Which patients are at increased risk of severe diarrhea including chemotherapy agents prescribed and patient characteristics?

Discussion

Colorectal cancer patients with baseline bowel dysfunction, including diarrhea due to surgery (particularly low anterior resection, colostomy, ileostomy, subtotal colectomy), may be at increased risk of diarrhea from chemotherapy. Patients with diarrhea due to malabsorption, including those who have had a small bowel resection or cholecystectomy, may also be at increased risk. If this patient has any of these characteristics, the clinician should take a through history regarding pre-existing diarrhea and attempt to provide adequate management of this before initiating chemotherapy.

Patients who will be receiving irinotecan, 5 fluorouracil and combination therapies including these agents, for treatment of colorectal cancer, are at significant risk of diarrhea. Also those receiving capecitabine or cetuximab are also at considerable risk [1].

Colorectal Cancer: Diagnosis and Clinical Management, First Edition. Edited by John H. Scholefield and Cathy Eng.

What initial recommendations, including patient education and medications, for management of diarrhea should be provided?

Discussion

Patient education should include ensuring patients understand what constitutes diarrhea (change in frequency, consistency or volume of stools) and the importance of adequate treatment to minimize the risk of complications, including hospitalization or even death.

Loperamide should be used as a first line for treatment of diarrhea. Patients should be instructed to take 4 mg with initial incidence of diarrhea and 2 mg after each additional loose stool or every 4 hours for a maximum of 16 mg daily [1]. Patient should also attempt to ensure adequate hydration by drinking 8–10 glasses of liquids per day. They should also be instructed on initial management of diarrhea and what they should do if they develop diarrhea refractory to initial management strategies.

If the patient calls to report persistent diarrhea with use of loperamide, what additional interventions should be considered?

Discussion

First, a patient history should be obtained to determine the grade of diarrhea (Table 17.1) and if any complicating signs or symptoms are present, including cramping, grade 2 or higher nausea or vomiting (Table 17.2), fever, sepsis, bleeding or symptoms of dehydration such as dizziness. A review of

Table 17.1 NCI criteria for diarrhea [6].

Grade	1	2	3	4	5
Without Ostomy	Increase <4 stools/day over baseline	Increase of 4–6 stools/day	Increase ≥7 stools per day; incontinence; hospitalization indicated	Life-threatening consequences; urgent intervention indicated	Death
With Ostomy	Mild increase in output	Moderate increase in output	Severe increase in ostomy; hospitalization indicated output; limited self care ADL	Life-threatening consequences; urgent intervention indicated	Death

Table 17.2 NCI criteria for nausea and vomiting [6].

Grade	1	2	3	4	5
Nausea	Loss of appetite without alteration in eating habits	Oral intake decreased without significant weight loss, dehydration or malnutrition	Inadequate oral caloric or fluid intake; tube feeding, TPN or hospitalization indicated	-	-
Vomiting	1–2 episodes* in 24 hrs	3–5 episodes* in 24 hrs	≥6 episodes* in 24 hrs; tube feeding, TPN or hospitalization indicated	Life-threatening consequences; urgent intervention indicated	Death

*episodes separated by 5 minutes

loperamide use should be performed to ensure adequate dosing. Patients who have persistent diarrhea in spite of loperamide at 16 mg daily should be evaluated for dehydration and/or electrolyte disturbances. Patients who also experience nausea or vomiting are at particular high risk of complications and may require a face-to-face visit in the clinic or emergency center. IV fluids and/or electrolyte replacement may be indicated. Patients with severe diarrhea, sepsis, fever or neutropenia may require hospitalization. For patients on capecitabine, the drug may need to be withheld until the diarrhea has resolved.

A patient history should be taken to ensure there are no additional causes of diarrhea, which may include medication such as laxatives, infectious causes including *c. difficile*, other medications or malabsorption.

If the patient provides a history consistent with maximum dosing of loperamide and no other causes of diarrhea has been identified, an additional agent should be added. Diphenoxylate atropine may also be used early in the management of chemotherapy induced diarrhea [2]. It is dosed at diphenoxylate atropine 2.5/0.25 mg 2 tablet initial dose and 1–2 tablets every 6 hrs for a maximum of 8 tablets per day. An oral fluoroquinolone is recommended for 7 days for patients with diarrhea uncontrolled for more than 24 hrs or with complicating symptoms [1].

Patients and clinicians should ensure adequate hydration is maintained. Small frequent meals, avoidance of dairy (due to an increased rate of hypolactasia from chemotherapy) and avoidance of high-fiber foods is typically advised [3]. Although lactose intolerance may result for chemotherapy administration, it may not be the cause of diarrhea associated with pelvic radiation [4].

What other medications could be considered if diarrhea continues with adequate administration of loperamide and diphenoxylate atropine?

Discussion

Initiation of opioids can be considered for these patients, including paregoric and tincture of opium. Paragoic is dosed at 5–10 mL 1–4 times daily and tincture of opium 0.6 mL daily. Both agents have the potential for abuse and are classified as schedule III and II, respectively.

Octeotide has been used for refractory diarrhea. This is a non-FDA approved indication and optimal dosing and administration has not been established. Some studies have utilized short-acting subcutaneous injections with doses ranging from 50–2500 micrograms 2–3 times daily. Continuous infusion of high-dose octreotide has also been found to be effective for patients with diarrhea refractory to loperamide, diphenoxylate atropine and opiates. Escalating dosing has been reported at 50 micrograms/hrs for 12 hrs, then 1000 microgram/hr × 12 hrs, then 150 microgram/hr for 72 hrs. Additional 72 hrs of therapy was used if diarrhea recurred [1;2].

Clinical Vignette #2

Nausea and vomiting

A 72-year-old man with a history of resected stage III colorectal cancer presents to your clinic for adjuvant therapy. You have decided to initiate treatment with FOLFOX (oxapliatin, 5 fluorouracil, and leucovorin) for 6 months.

What risk factors should you consider in determining the risk of nausea and vomiting for this patient?

Discussion

Oxaliplatin is considered a moderate emetic risk drug, while 5 fluorouracil carries low emetic risk. Patients receiving a regimen with moderate emetic risk have a 30–90% risk of vomiting without anti-emetic prophylaxis. While the risk of vomiting is diminished with the use of effective antiemetic prophylaxis, they often still experience nausea. Patients at increased risk of chemotherapy-induced nausea and vomiting include women, the young, non-alcohol drinkers, and those with a history of motion sickness [5].

What initial anti-emetics should be used for administration as part of his pre-treatment therapy to prevent chemotherapy induced nausea and vomiting?

Discussion

Since this regimen is expected to result in nausea or vomiting in 30–90% of patient, premedication is essential. The NCCN guidelines (version 1.2012) recommend the use of a serotonin antagonist and dexamethasone [5]. In addition, lorazepam and/or an H2 blocker or a proton pump inhibitor may also be included.

What patient education (including instructions for PRN medications) should be provided to patients to manage nausea or vomiting?

Discussion

Patients should understand that the goal is to prevent and minimize nausea and vomiting. Patients may have a preconceived idea that nausea and vomiting are always experienced by patients undergoing therapy. Patients may not understand the risk of severe nausea (without vomiting), which may result in dehydration and malnutrition.

Patients should be counseled on the risks of uncontrolled nausea and vomiting and they should be encouraged to following recommendations for treatment of breakthrough side effects. They should also be instructed to continue using these medications on schedule until side effects have resolved. They should also be instructed to call or seek medical attention for uncontrolled nausea or vomiting or symptoms of dehydration. Patients with both diarrhea and nausea and vomiting may be at high risk of complications from dehydration and electrolyte imbalances.

Breakthrough medications may include benzodiazepines (lorazepam), cannabinoid, phenothiazine, serotonin 5-HTE3 antagonists, steroids (dexamethasone) or other agents including haloperidol, metoclopramide and others [5]. Other non-pharmacologic strategies include eating cold foods, eating small, frequent meals, avoiding alcohol and encouraging fluid intake to avoid dehydration.

The patient calls on day 10 complaining of persistent n/v, what other potential causes should be considered in patients with poorly controlled nausea and vomiting?

Discussion

Patients with nausea/vomiting that is more severe than predicted, persists beyond the anticipated duration of delayed chemotherapy-induced nauseas/vomiting or does not respond to anti-emetics should be evaluated for other potential causes. Bowel obstruction, constipation, gastroparesis, brain metastases, hypercalcemia, side effects of other medications (including opiates), dyspepsia and anticipatory nausea/vomiting are all potential causes of nausea/vomiting in this patient population.

What strategies may be used for management of anticipatory nausea/vomiting?

Discussion

Patients with anticipatory nausea and vomiting may complain of symptoms prior to arriving for chemotherapy or before infusion of chemotherapeutic agents. It is important to optimize anti-emetic regimens in these patients. Benzodiazepines may be initiated the evening before chemotherapy. Behavioral therapy and acupressure may also be helpful [5].

References

1 Benson AB, Ajani JA, Catalano RB, Engelking C, Kornblau SM, Martenson MA, et al. Recommended guidelines for the treatment of cancer treatment-induced diarrhea. *J Clin Oncol* 2004; 22: 2918–26.

2 Petrelli NJ, Rodrigeuz-Bigas M, Rustum Y, Herrera L, Creaven P. Bowel rest, intravenous hydration, and continuous high-dose infusion of octreotide acetate for the treatment of chemotherapy-induced diarrhea in patient with colorectal cancer. *Cancer* 1993; 72(5): 1543–6.

3 Osterlund P, Ruotsalainen T, Peuhkuri K, Korpela R, Ollus A, Ikonen M, et al. Lactose intolerance associate with adjuvant 5-fluorouracil-based chemotherapy for colorectal cancer. *Clin Gatroenterol and Hepatol* 2004; 2: 696–703.

4 Stryker JA, Bartholomen M. Failure of lactose-restricted diets to prevent radiation-induced diarrhea in patients undergoing whole pelvis irradiation. *Int J Rad Oncol Biol Phys* 1985; 12: 789–92.

5 NCCN Clinical Practice Guidelines in Oncology Antiemesis Version 1.2012.

6 Common Terminology Criteria for Adverse Events version 4.03. Published: June 14, 2010.

CHAPTER 18

Palliative care vignettes

Jenny Wei[1] & Egidio Del Fabbro[2]
[1] *University of Texas, MD Anderson Cancer Center, Houston, TX, USA*
[2] *Virginia Commonwealth University, Richmond, VA, USA*

Clinical Vignette #1

AB, a 53-year-old male diagnosed 10 months ago with metastatic colorectal cancer to his liver and retroperitoneum, underwent colectomy, chemoradiation, and is currently being treated with a Phase I investigational therapy. His course has been complicated by abdominal pain, which is controlled by morphine sulfate extended release 30 mg twice daily and morphine sulfate immediate release 7.5 mg every 2 hours as required for breakthrough pain. His symptoms were well controlled until two days ago, when he was admitted for abdominal pain and emesis. An abdominal CT scan showed evidence of peritoneal carcinomatosis, ascites and partial small bowel obstruction. He was started on morphine Patient Controlled Analgesia (PCA) with settings equivalent to the morphine equivalent daily dose of his home regimen, 1 mg per hour continuous infusion and 2 mg RN bolus every 2 hours as needed. The dose of morphine escalated as he continued to complain of worsening abdominal pain. On day 2 he developed confusion, myoclonus, and agitation. On hospital day 4, laboratory data revealed an elevated creatinine value of 2.1 mg/dL (185 μmol/L). His renal function prior to this hospitalization was normal.

Discussion

Morphine is metabolized in the liver to normorphine, morphine-3-glucuronide (M3G), and morphine-6-glucuronide (M6G). M6G accounts for the major component of clinical analgesia and although M6G has fewer side effects than its parent drug, accumulation can cause respiratory depression. M3G has no analgesic effect and is thought to be responsible for neuroexcitatory effects such as delirium, myoclonus, and even seizures. Delirium, myoclonus, allodynia, and hyperalgesia are all manifestations of

Colorectal Cancer: Diagnosis and Clinical Management, First Edition. Edited by John H. Scholefield and Cathy Eng.

opioid-induced neurotoxicity (OIN). Since the kidneys excrete all morphine metabolites, doses should be titrated with caution in patients with renal impairment. Intravenous opioids such as Fentanyl and Methadone are safer to use in patients with decreased creatinine clearance, because they utilize both the renal and the hepatic system for elimination. Although limited data have demonstrated the safety of Fentanyl in renal failure, Methadone is preferable, since gradual accumulation of Fentanyl is possible with long-term use. Of note, although Fentanyl and Methadone are the 'safest' in renal failure and have the advantage of not requiring any major dose adjustments, they are not dialyzable, so caution is required [1].

Opioid rotation is often used to achieve a balance of effective pain control with minimal or acceptable side effects, in response to delirium, uncontrolled pain, and OIN [2]. This switch from one opioid to another is based on the principle of incomplete cross-tolerance between opioids, such that a lower equi-analgesic dose of the 'new' opioid can be used to treat pain. In practice this results in a 30–50% reduction of the MEDD after rotation, which enables effective pain control with less sedation, while the toxic opioid metabolites of the old opioid are being excreted. It is important that clinicians are well-versed in the equi-analgesic doses of opioids before electing an opioid switch. If in doubt, the palliative care team should be consulted for guidance.

Management

The patient was rotated from morphine to a Fentanyl PCA with 50 mcg per hour basal, 75 mcg per hour as needed nurse-administered bolus, and no demand dose. Demand doses, controlled by patients, should be avoided in delirium. After intravenous hydration, his renal function returned to baseline and Dexamethasone 4 mg was given twice daily, as corticosteroids may allow for maintenance of bowel patency and temporary resolution of malignant bowel obstruction [3]. Nausea and emesis were controlled with metoclopramide, bowel movements increased, and he was continued on transdermal fentanyl at home, because of concerns that disease progression would again precipitate nausea and emesis. Because of peritoneal carcinomatosis, ascites and declining performance status, he was not considered to be a candidate for surgery.

In the case of complete obstruction, haloperidol and octreotide would have been preferable to control nausea and secretions, instead of a pro-kinetic agent such as metoclopramide [4]. Haloperidol can be given i.v. or subcutaneously along with octreotide at a starting dose of 100 mcg q8h. Octreotide has demonstrated superiority compared to anticholinergics in small randomized trials and is the medical management of choice for bowel obstruction due to malignancy.

Although medical management alone is often effective, venting gastrostomy tubes have the advantage of allowing patients to derive some pleasure from the taste of liquids. Placement of a venting tube is feasible, even in patients with ascites and peritoneal carcinomatosis [5].

Clinical Vignette #2

A 49-year-old male recently diagnosed with stage IIIb colon cancer after presenting with intermittent rectal bleeding, is treated with surgical resection and chemotherapy, and then referred to the palliative care clinic for management of fatigue and cachexia. He reports minimal abdominal pain and some sedation on twice daily extended release morphine. In the past, attempts at lowering the dose of morphine have resulted in unbearable pain escalation. He has daily bowel movements with the aid of laxatives. His most distressing symptoms are poor appetite and profound fatigue. He has noticed loss of muscle mass and complains that he is rarely able to fully participate in activities with his family and although he occasionally still has desire for food, this is limited by early satiety and dysgeusia.

Discussion

Cancer-related fatigue is a multidimensional symptom with multiple contributing factors including depressed mood, pain, insomnia, dyspnea, cachexia, anemia, and medication side effects (Figure 18.1). Treatment of fatigue should focus on correcting reversible causes (i.e. anemia, dehydration, drug side effects, hypothyroidism, hypercalcemia and depression), because there are limited pharmacological interventions specifically for fatigue. The psycho stimulant methylphenidate demonstrated promise in open label trials [6]; however, subsequent randomized controlled trials showed no benefit over placebo. Nevertheless, Methylphenidate has been shown to be an effective therapy for opioid induced sedation in selected patients and may be helpful for fatigue and depressed mood. Because of the narrow balance between desirable and undesirable effects, caution should be exercised when using methylphenidate for opioid induced sedation [7].

Corticosteroids may be useful in short-term therapy of patients with very advanced cancer but are prone to cause side effects such as proximal myopathy and glucose intolerance when used long term. Non-pharmacologic interventions such as exercise, psychosocial interventions (e.g. counseling on coping strategies), and hormone replacement are also important to consider. Exercise can improve physical performance in patients with advanced cancer

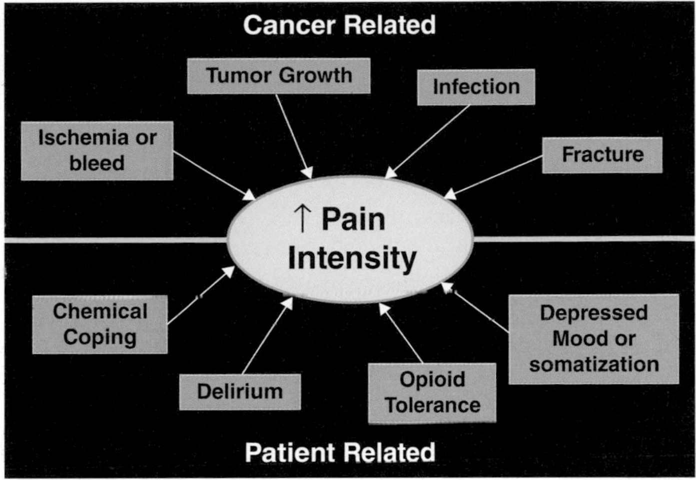

Figure 18.1 Contributors to increased pain in patients with cancer.

[8]; however, most studies for cancer-related fatigue have been conducted in patients with breast cancer and good performance status. Hypogonadism is common in male patients with cancer, and is associated with increased symptom burden [9] and decreased quality of life (QOL). Testosterone replacement therapy (TRT) is effective for fatigue and muscle loss in non-cancer patients, but as yet, no randomized controlled trials (RCTs) have been completed in cancer patients.

The symptoms of fatigue and poor appetite often occur together as a 'symptom cluster' [10], along with other symptoms such as early satiety and dysgeusia that are characteristic of the cachexia syndrome. Cancer cachexia is defined as a multifactorial syndrome characterized by an ongoing loss of skeletal muscle mass (with or without loss of fat mass) that cannot be fully reversed by conventional nutritional support, and leads to progressive functional impairment [11]. Multimodality therapy using pharmacological and non-pharmacological interventions is the optimal approach to treat the cachexia syndrome [12]. A randomized controlled trial showed that nutritional counseling may provide sustained benefits to colorectal patients receiving radiation [13]. Other symptoms such as depression, nausea, and constipation could also exacerbate cachexia by further decreasing appetite and caloric intake (Nutritional Impact Symptoms). These symptoms often improve with relatively inexpensive medications [14].

As regards specific drug therapies for cachexia, no single agent has been found to be consistently effective. Systematic reviews suggest megestrol acetate improves appetite and weight but not QOL, or other clinical outcomes such as lean body mass or function. Unfortunately progestational agents also increase the risk of thromboembolic disease, hypogonadism, and hypoadrenalism. Small trials of non-steroidal anti-inflammatory drugs (NSAIDs) (ibuprofen [15], indomethacin, celecoxib) and thalidomide have improved clinical outcomes in cachectic patients with solid tumors. Other novel agents under investigation include Selective Androgen Receptor Modulators (SARMs) and ghrelin agonists. Ghrelin and Ghrelin agonist have the potential for improving multiple mechanisms contributing to cachexia including appetite, gastric motility and immune modulation and have been well tolerated in preliminary clinical trials.

Management

Laboratory tests included serum levels of TSH, vitamin B_{12}, bioavailable testosterone and vitamin D. Besides a low testosterone level, a depression screen was positive for depressed mood. Testosterone was replaced with a topical gel after discussion of the risks and potential benefits of TRT. In addition to exercise and sunlight exposure, a trial of Methylphenidate 2.5 mg twice daily was prescribed to counter opioid induced sedation, and nutritional impact symptoms of early satiety (metoclopramide) and depression (mirtazapine) were treated. Antihistamines were discontinued and benzodiazepines tapered. After 6 weeks, his fatigue had improved, and caloric intake was better after treatment. He also reported an improved appetite, compliance with a daily exercise regimen, and more active participation in family activities.

References

1 King S, Forbes K, Hanks GW et al. A systematic review of the use of opioid medication for those with moderate to severe cancer pain and renal impairment: a European Palliative Care Research Collaborative opioid guidelines project. *J Palliat Med* 2011; 25: 525–52.

2 de Stoutz N et al. Opioid rotation for toxicity reduction in terminal cancer patients, *J Pain Symptom Manage* 1995; 10: 378–84.

3 Feuer DDJ, Broadley KE. Corticosteroids for the resolution of malignant bowel obstruction in advanced gynecological and gastrointestinal cancer. *Cochrane Database Syst Rev* 2000; 1:D001219.

4 O'Connor B, Creedon B et al. Pharmacological treatment of bowel obstruction in cancer patients. *Expert Opin Pharmacoth*. 2011; 12: 2205–14.

5 Ripamonti CI, Easson AM, Gerdes H. Management of malignant bowel obstruction. *Eur J Cancer* 2008; 44: 1105–15.

6 Bruera E, Driver L, Barnes E et al. Patient-controlled methylphenidate for the management of fatigue in patients with advanced cancer: a preliminary report. *J Clin Oncol* 2003; 21: 4439–43.

7 Stone P, Minton O. European Palliative Care Research collaborative pain guidelines. Central side effects management: what is the evidence to support best practice in the management of sedation, cognitive impairment and myoclonus? *Palliat Med* 2011; 25: 431–41.

8 Oldervoll LM, Loge JH, Lydersen S et al. Physical exercise for cancer patients with advanced disease: a randomized controlled trial. *Oncologist* 2011; 16: 1649–57.

9 Del Fabbro E, Hui D, Nooruddin ZI, et al. Associations among hypogonadism, C-reactive protein, symptom burden, and survival in male cancer patients with cachexia: a preliminary report. *J Pain Symp Man* 2010; 39: 1016–24.

10 Walsh D, Rybicki L. Symptom clustering in advanced cancer. *Support Care Cancer* 2006; 14: 831–6.

11 Fearon K, Strasser F, Anker SD et al. Definition and classification of cancer cachexia: an international consensus. *Lancet Oncol* 2011; 12: 489–95.

12 Del Fabbro E More is better: a multimodality approach to cancer cachexia. *Oncologist* 2010; 15: 119–21.

13 Ravasco P, Monteiro-Grillo I, Vidal PM et al. Dietary counseling improves patient outcomes: a prospective, randomized, controlled trial in colorectal cancer patients undergoing radiotherapy. *J Clin Oncol* 2005; 23: 1431–8.

14 Del Fabbro E, Hui D, Dalal S et al. Clinical outcomes and contributors to weight loss in a cancer cachexia clinic. *J Palliat Med* 2011; 14: 1004–8.

15 McMillan DC, O'Gorman P, Fearon KC et al. A pilot study of megestrol acetate and ibuprofen in the treatment of cachexia in gastrointestinal cancer patients. *Br J Cancer* 1997; 76: 788–90.

Index

Colorectal Cancer: Diagnosis and Clinical Management, First Edition. Edited by John H. Scholefield and Cathy Eng.